SYMBOLS AND NOTATIONS USED II
A Quick Review

T0249695

α–Alpha level, or probability of a type I error

A–Baseline phase in the single-case experimental method

B–Treatment phase in the single-case experimental method

C, D, etc.–Alternative treatment phases in the single-case experimental method (i.e., alternatives to treatment phase B)

CG–Control group

CI–Confidence interval

CV–Criterion variable

$\overset{X}{\textbf{Case}}$–Currently existing group of participants with outcome of interest present in a retrospective case-control design

$\overset{\bullet}{\textbf{Control}}$–Currently existing group of participants with outcome of interest absent in a retrospective case-control design

CompG–Single group of participants in a longitudinal design

CompG1–Comparative group 1 in a cross-sectional design

CompG2–Comparative group 2 in a cross-sectional design

$\overset{X_1}{\textbf{CompG1}}$–Comparative group 1 in a prospective cohort design

X₁ CompG1–Comparative group 1 in a retrospective cohort design

$\overset{X_2}{\textbf{CompG2}}$–Comparative group 2 in a prospective cohort design

X₂ CompG2–Comparative group 2 in a retrospective cohort design

DV–Dependent variable

EG–Experimental group

EG₁, EG₂, etc.–Experimental group 1, experimental group 2, and so forth

ES–Effect size

H_A or H₁–Alternative hypothesis

H₀–Null hypothesis

H_R–Research hypothesis

IRB–Institutional review board

IV–Independent variable

MRAW–Massage research agenda workgroup

MT–Massage therapy

MTRC–Massage therapy research competencies

MTRD–Massage therapy research database

μ–Population mean (lowercase Greek letter mu)

N–Population size

n–Sample size

NHST–Null hypothesis significance test(ing)

O_Post–Postobservation/measurement/test

O_Pre–Preobservation/measurement/test

p–P value, probability level, or level of significance

P1, P2, etc–Participant #1, participant #2, and so forth

PV–Predictor variable

r–Pearson correlation coefficient

r²–Coefficient of determination

r₁₂.₃–Partial correlation coefficient; correlation between dependent variable 1 and dependent variable 2, with the influence of dependent variable 3 "partialed" out

R–Multiple correlation coefficient

R²–Multiple coefficient of determination

RA or R–Random assignment

RC–Research category

RCT–Randomized controlled trial

RD–Research design

RM–Research method

RP–Research procedure

RS–Research strategy (in the context of a subdivision under research category)

RS–Random selection (in the context of a feature of randomization)

X–Experimental level of the independent variable

●–Nonexperimental level of the independent variable

X₁, X₂, etc.–Experimental level 1 of the independent variable, experimental level 2 of the independent variable, and so forth

X̄–Sample mean (read as X bar)

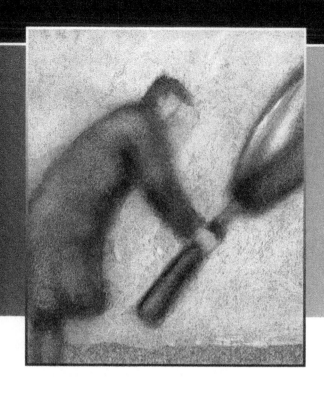

RESEARCH METHODS FOR MASSAGE AND HOLISTIC THERAPIES

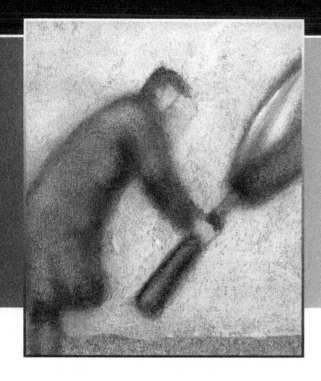

RESEARCH METHODS FOR MASSAGE AND HOLISTIC THERAPIES

Glenn M. Hymel, EdD, LMT
Professor and Former Chair
Department of Psychology
Loyola University
New Orleans, Louisiana

with **83** *illustrations*

ELSEVIER
MOSBY

ELSEVIER
MOSBY

11830 Westline Industrial Drive
St. Louis, Missouri 63146

RESEARCH METHODS FOR MASSAGE AND HOLISTIC THERAPIES   ISBN-13: 978-0-323-03292-6
Copyright © 2006, Mosby Inc.   ISBN-10: 0-323-03292-3

All rights reserved. No part of this publication may be reproduced or transmitted in any form
or by any means, electronic or mechanical, including photocopying, recording, or any information
storage and retrieval system, without permission in writing from the publisher.
Permissions may be sought directly from Elsevier's Health Sciences Rights Department in
Philadelphia, PA, USA: phone: (+1) 215 239 3804, fax: (+1) 215 239 3805,
e-mail: healthpermissions@elsevier.com. You may also complete your request on-line via
the Elsevier homepage (http://www.elsevier.com), by selecting 'Customer Support' and then
'Obtaining Permissions'.

Notice

Neither the Publisher nor the Author assumes any responsibility for any loss or injury and/or damage to
persons or property arising out of or related to any use of the material contained in this book. It is the
responsibility of the treating practitioner, relying on independent expertise and knowledge of the patient,
to determine the best treatment and method of application for the patient.

The Publisher

International Standard Book Number 0-323-03292-3

Publishing Director: Linda Duncan
Acquisitions Editor: Kellie Fitzpatrick
Developmental Editor: Jennifer Watrous
Editorial Assistant: Elizabeth Clark
Publishing Services Manager: Melissa Lastarria
Project Manager: Gail Michaels
Designer: Amy Buxton

Working together to grow
libraries in developing countries

www.elsevier.com | www.bookaid.org | www.sabre.org

ELSEVIER   BOOK AID
            International   Sabre Foundation

Transferred to Digital Printing 2011

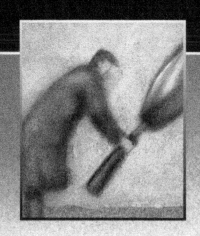

DEDICATION

This book is lovingly dedicated to
my parents,
ROSE MAE TRICHE HYMEL AND
CLEMENT ETIENNE HYMEL,
in gratitude for the gift of life,
the wisdom of their guidance,
the saintly examples of their own lives, and
the unconditional love I've always received;

and

my daughters, sons, and three grandsons,
JUDY, DONNA, STEVEN, MICHAEL,
SEAN, JASON, AND ANDREW,
truly my greatest blessings in life and
the source of inspiration for everything I do.

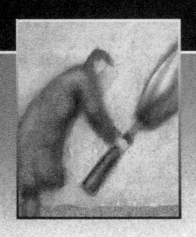

REVIEWERS

CLINT CHANDLER, LMP, CNMT
Associate Faculty
Cortiva Institute of Colorado
Greenwood Village, Colorado

TRISH DRYDEN, M. ED, RMT
Coordinator
Centre for Applied Research in Health,
Technology, and Education
School of Applied Arts and Health Sciences
Centennial College
Toronto, Ontario
Canada

NADINE FORBES, MS
National Director of Education
Steiner Education Group
Baltimore, Maryland

SANDY FRITZ, MS, NCTMB
Founder, Owner, Director, and Head Instructor
Health Enrichment Center
School of Therapeutic Massage and Bodywork
Lapeer, Michigan

JEFFREY A. SIMANCEK, BS, CMT
Massage Therapy Department Chair
Olympia Career Training Institute
Grand Rapids, Michigan

MAUREEN STOTT, LMT
Instructor
Department of Education/Financial Aid
Connecticut Center for Massage Therapy
Newington, Connecticut
CT Licensed Therapist
Therapeutic Massage Center of Vernon
Vernon, Connecticut

KRISTOPHER VAN DER VEER, DC, BSc. HK
Professor
Kine Concept Institute Ottawa
Ottawa, Canada

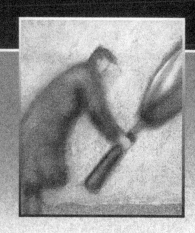

FOREWORD
by Leon Chaitow

Two different imperatives are the driving forces behind this important book: the need for ever-improving competencies in the application of massage and bodywork and the need for evidence that validates and supports the methods and techniques used in therapeutic massage in particular and manual therapies in general. The question is how these imperatives are to be satisfied?

Without competence and an optimal skill base, the safety and efficacy of the methods used in therapeutic massage would be compromised, and results would be poor. Competence derives from skills that are substantiated by an evidence base that emerges from a combination of research and clinical experience. Research data and clinical audit can be used to inform educators, therapists, regulating authorities, insurance reimbursement sources, and media outlets, as well as other health care professionals with whom collaboration and integration may be possible and desirable. Ultimately research should be available to inform the public.

Evidence derived from a variety of sources, including clinical results as well as basic research, needs to demonstrate that what is being done when massage is applied is safe, efficacious, and cost effective.

If training standards are low, there will be lack of confidence in the methods of any profession. Similarly, if professional or ethical behavior is poor, the methodologies used are of an unproven nature, or potentially useful methods are applied inappropriately, there will be a loss of confidence in the profession. It is therefore vital for any emerging health care profession that national and local licensing authorities be supportive and insurance reimbursement be available. Additionally, and most importantly, other health care professions need to feel confident and comfortable in any move toward collaboration and integration. These objectives can result only when those applying treatment methods are well trained and their techniques are appropriate to the needs of their clients. In an era of "evidence-based medicine" this cannot simply be assumed; it has to be shown to be so by research and clinical audit.

Massage is now conceived by the public to be one of the safest, most effective, most trusted (and widely used) forms of complementary health care. However, a degree of resistance to its wider use in medical settings remains (Field 2000, Eisenberg 1998). The evolution to this position of public and media acceptance over the past 50 years has seen massage and bodywork change from being a part of fringe medicine to the slightly more respectable "alternative medicine" before it emerged as complementary to mainstream medicine–becoming in a more recent evolution a part of integrated health care.

The impetus for these shifts has derived largely from a combination of improved quality of training and enhanced professional and ethical standards, supported and encouraged by a trickle of research evidence demonstrating the range and potential of hands-on touch therapy. Much of this evidence has come from people such as Tiffany Field, PhD, and her team at the Touch Research Institute, University of Miami. With limited financial support despite ongoing funding from sources such as Johnson & Johnson, this team has demonstrated the value of touch therapies such as massage in a wide range of conditions (Field 2000, Rich 2002).

To paraphrase Kahn's rhetorical question (in Rich 2002), if massage is effective, safe and benign, why research it? Kahn's answer is that the widespread use of massage makes it essential that more research be performed.

Kahn also explains the relative dearth of research papers on the topic, and lack of funding is not the only cause. Most importantly, she maintains that there is less research into massage than there should be because there are not enough researchers involved in the field, not enough research proposals, and not enough pressure on funding agencies. To put it simply, there is not enough enthusiasm. This book should go a long way toward remedying that deficit, as it is written with a patent enthusiasm, which will hopefully be infectious.

Other questions needing more answers include the following:

- What are the benefits of massage?
- If there are benefits, what are the mechanisms?
- How do benefits differ from those obtained by other (often infinitely more expensive) methods?
- Are there potential dangers, and if so what?

Researching a topic such as massage is far from easy because of variables inherent in the interaction between client and therapist. In real life each treatment should reflect the current individual needs of the client as perceived by the therapist, whose clinical approach is likely to vary to some extent from that of any other therapist.

A potential criticism of the methods used in Touch Research Institute's trials is that they almost always entail the use of a standard protocol, involving a fixed and, frequently, fairly limited amount of time per treatment session, with specified strokes applied in a predetermined sequence. Such protocols make sense in research settings, but do not reflect what happens in a real-life massage treatment. Yet despite the limitations imposed by use of such standardized methodologies (to overcome the accusation that apples are not being compared with other apples but with oranges instead) the results of most of Field's studies have been extremely supportive of the value of massage therapy. How is this impasse to be overcome?

A different choice might be to focus attention on outcomes rather than on the fine detail of methodology. Renowned osteopathic researcher Irvin Korr (1991) suggested that measurement of objective findings, relative to the client's condition, as well as assessment of the client's subjective feelings relative to the symptoms, before and after an individualized treatment, could help to avoid the problem of a "standardized" therapeutic input.

More recently Ernst (2002) has expressed similar thoughts, saying that the gold standard of researchers, the randomized control trial, could be modified to compare outcomes, in which some clients receive a standard protocol of care while others receive individualized attention based on the therapists' perception of needs. These examples suggest that more meaningful research into systems such as massage can be achieved if sufficient attention is given to posing well-structured and appropriate questions.

What Glenn Hymel has done in this remarkable text is to cover the entire spectrum of research and audit needs, associated with all levels of documenting and investigating the profession he so clearly loves. He has defined a very real need for the massage therapy profession to become research literate–better able to understand the methods and outcomes– as well as for its members to participate actively in the process, ideally under the auspices of suitably qualified professionals. He has explained the complex processes involved in quantitative, qualitative, and integrative research approaches and has also offered detailed analysis and direction for those researchers drawn to work in this as yet relatively unexplored field. Researching massage therapy and manual methods requires an understanding of the categories, strategies, methods, designs, and procedures. It also demands recognition of the problems of resources.

At present research funding is difficult to obtain, and fundamental research without funding is almost impossible. The lack of funding excludes all but the most dedicated of researchers from involvement and precludes large studies. Much has to be achieved on a shoestring, often involving small-scale projects. Organizations such as the Massage Therapy Foundation have a variety of initiatives that aim to overcome these limitations and obstacles.

The detailed advice contained in this book will, if adopted, help in overcoming current limitations. This book should help to change the climate by encouraging an enthusiasm for research. It may well lead therapists who are trained in the disciplines of massage but not research literate to undertake advanced study to enable participation in or actually conducting of research.

At the very least it should lead to an appreciation of the methods involved, as well as help consumers of research information discern "good" from "bad" research when faced with articles and papers in peer-reviewed journals. This is extremely important, since a clear understanding of new evidence can help the therapist to modify what is done clinically, as well as allow a deeper understanding of the nature of the conditions being treated and the methods used, leading to more meaningful communication with clients, as well as with other health care professionals.

Among the practical aids that this book contains are many pages that can assist in the complicated task of describing research outcomes in ways that are clear and logical to others. If the language used and the format adopted, particularly in relation to presentation of statistical information, is not readily comprehensible, then the very best of research methodology will be wasted. Ultimately research has to be well conducted and well described and easily accessible to those who need to see it. The book certainly offers educators the tools with which to instruct the next generation of therapists and potential researchers to meet those needs.

It also, and most importantly, provides existing researchers with guidelines pertaining to the special needs and methods required for the investigation of complex holistic systems such as massage.

Ultimately research competence requires an understanding of the body of knowledge that Glenn Hymel has laid before us. It also calls for an enthusiasm and passion that he has demonstrated in compiling this very important text.

LEON CHAITOW, ND, DO
Editor, Journal of Bodywork &
Movement Therapies
University of Westminster, London

References

Eisenberg, D., David, R., Ettner, S. (1998). Trends in Alternative Medicine in use in USA 1990–1997. *Journal of American Medical Association*, 280, 1569–1575.

Ernst, E. (2003). Obstacles to research in complementary and alternative medicine. *Medical Journal of Australia*, 179, 279.

Field, T. (2000). *Touch therapy*. Edinburgh: Churchill Livingstone.

Korr, I. (1991). Osteopathic research: The needed paradigm shift. *Journal American Osteopathic Association*, 91, 156–171

Rich, J. (Ed.). (2002). Massage Therapy: *The evidence for practice*. St. Louis: Mosby.

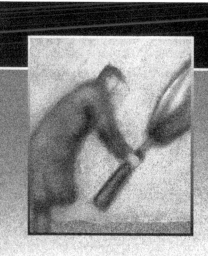

FOREWORD

by Sandy Fritz

I am so glad that Glenn agreed to write this book. I remember being introduced to Glenn by my Elsevier editor, Kellie, at an AMTA conference. When I learned that he was interested in doing a textbook on research, one that would be suitable for use in therapeutic massage instruction, I wondered how this "educational angel" appeared.

When I write textbooks, I have to sift and sort through volumes of research to be able to justify and make relevant the information that is presented. Since I write both entry-level and advanced level texts, I appreciate the almost impossible task of describing the nature of research in such a way that it is easily understood and relevant, regardless of where the reader is in the learning journey.

When Glenn was writing the text, he would send chapters for me to review. As I read, I would note when my brain could no longer follow the terminology and sequence of the content. I have had research design and statistics classes, and if I was getting lost so would students. I sent comments back to Glenn, who received them well and made changes in the manuscript. Discussions with the editorial staff were ongoing, especially concerning whether the content was too complex. I remember saying that of all of the Elsevier authors currently writing textbooks for the therapeutic massage education, Glenn had the hardest job. This content is complex, and he was doing a great job in making it understandable. With the completion of this textbook, Glenn has accomplished a task I thought was nearly impossible—a textbook that I could both understand and teach from and that students could realistically understand as well.

This is not a book you will read on a relaxing day when the goal is for your mind to wander into the vastness of the story. This book will take reading over and over to really understand, but that is the nature of the topic. Glenn has organized the information into "bite-size" pieces, inserted a sense of humor, created diagrams and illustrations, and provided analogies and metaphors. He has used relevant research as an example and carried those themes throughout the text. I doubt that the presentation can get any more effective.

The text serves two purposes. The most important is to allow the massage professional to understand enough about the research process to critically read research and be able to translate the theoretical information into concrete practical use. Most massage professionals will not conduct research although a few may participate in various research studies. However, all massage professionals need to assess, analyze, develop treatment strategies, and effectively chart the progress and outcomes of the therapeutic interaction with the client. This process is really individual research based on the case study method, which each of us should be doing in the context of client care. Even when readers do not expect to conduct research, understanding the process will enhance their professional skills.

The second purpose of this text is to prepare those who are interested in participating in research. The advancement of understanding the mechanism of the benefits of therapeutic massage and various other forms of manual therapy is necessary for the ongoing evolution of the profession. This text provides an avenue for massage and manual therapy professionals to begin the educational process to be part of a research team.

I do not feel that I could be a good researcher. The meticulous attention to detail, the vastness of knowledge, and the ability to persist in finding concreteness in abstraction is beyond me. However, without the researchers, I could not write practical application textbooks. I am forever grateful for professional research contributions to the growth of therapeutic massage acceptance and credibility.

This text lays the groundwork for the next evolution of professional growth for the massage and bodywork profession. Readers, please appreciate how hard a task it has been to create this book to assist you in undertaking the important task of learning about the research process. Thank you Glenn, for being capable and willing to write this wonderful text.

SANDY FRITZ, MS, NCTMB
Founder, Owner, Director,
and Head Instructor
Health Enrichment Center
School of Therapeutic Massage and Bodywork
Lapeer, Michigan

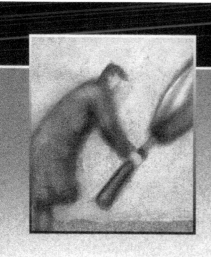

PREFACE

The "incubation" phase for the development of this research methods textbook has been rather extensive. Thirty-one years of teaching at the university level have provided me with ample opportunity to cultivate a sense of what might resonate well with students where research issues are concerned. And then there were the delights of teaching mathematics at the secondary school level in an even earlier "lifetime."

I have always had a particularly keen interest over the years in teaching research and statistics. A large part of the attraction has been the almost aesthetic nature of the order and regularity that defines these two areas of study. Equally exciting is the opportunity to work with students who for a variety of reasons frequently enter such courses somewhat frightened and terribly worried about "what's in store for them." Furthermore, the somewhat recent emphasis in the massage therapy profession and related fields regarding scientific inquiry simply adds to the urgency for resource materials that are comprehensive yet clear, well organized, and relevant to the practitioner's concerns. I've tried to accomplish precisely that in the development of this book.

On another personal note, my entrance into the massage therapy profession was rather delayed when compared with my other professional efforts over the years. I completed my studies at the Blue Cliff School of Therapeutic Massage in the New Orleans area in the late 1990s and have been playing "catch up" ever since, trying earnestly to acquire the knowledge and skills I recognize as so extensive among my more experienced colleagues in the profession. Another source of motivation in this most rewarding world of touch has been my own lived experiences where the realities of injury, pain, and disability are concerned. And in that regard let me hasten to acknowledge and honor the fact that indeed every one of us "has a story" leading us to the choices and decisions we make.

I consider myself extremely blessed, then, to have the opportunity to combine the experiences of so many years in an academic setting with a newly-acquired health science profession that quite literally touches the lives of others in so many meaningful ways. It is for my current and future colleagues that this book tries to provide a degree of clarity about how we might all go about the task of advancing the scientific basis for our chosen profession.

As our title indicates, my intended audience in writing this book includes not only massage therapists but also other related health science professionals. These include but are certainly not limited to such colleagues as physical therapists, chiropractors, osteopaths, physiatrists, naturopaths, occupational therapists, holistic nurses, and acupuncturists. They also include those colleagues in the basic and behavioral sciences whose work is so critical to informing effective health care delivery. The intent, then, is to include in the scope of those served by this book professionals from the alternative, integrative, and allopathic health care communities.

As you will soon notice, the first chapter speaks to several questions having to do with the what, how, why, why now, where, and a few other concerns about which most prospective readers of this book probably wonder. I will refrain from elaborating on what is covered in detail later; however, I believe there may be some value to acknowledging briefly in this preface at least an overview of what lies ahead.

This book spans a total of 10 chapters and four appendixes. The chapters are grouped and sequenced with a view toward covering the three generally recognized major research categories. These include the quantitative (or numerical data–based) approach to research, the qualitative (or verbal data–based) approach, and the integrative (or synthesis-based) approach. The four appendixes represent "tools" that are critical to the research process. They are intentionally segregated from the flow of the 10 chapters so as to not interrupt the logical and consistent progression from one research approach to the next. The inclusion of such topics as electronic literature searching, ethics, research report format, and measurement and statistics in the appendixes certainly does not minimize their critical importance to the research process.

For the record, a number of ancillaries in print, electronic, and manipulative form are available as support materials for both instructors and students.

The ancillary in manipulative form, the *Tactile Card*, tries to accommodate those individuals whose preferred sensory learning modality is tactile. This ancillary engages the student, for example, in learning various research designs by manipulating cut-out pieces that are positioned on a card stock insert to the book. Further details regarding the book's expansive collection of ancillaries are available elsewhere.

I would like to conclude this preface by referring to a quote by George Bernard Shaw that I hope will set the tone for everything that follows in this volume. It reads as follows: "Some people see things as they are and ask 'Why?'; others dream things that never were and ask 'Why not?'"

Bringing the incredible healing power of touch to others most in need, both physically and emotionally, is a privilege, an honor, and indeed a sacred trust. In that regard, let us always endeavor to count ourselves among those who "dream things that never were and ask 'Why not?'"

GLENN M. HYMEL

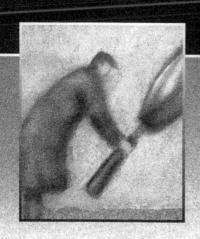

PREFACE FOR THE INSTRUCTOR

AIDS FOR "MANAGING" THIS BOOK

INSTRUCTIONAL DESIGN FEATURES

Partly because you have read to this point in the book, you are deserving of a "confession," or disclosure of sorts, regarding the dire state of courses and books on research methods as typically taught and written. For a variety of reasons, historically these courses and books are among the most poorly presented. Without going into the many reasons this dreadful reality is the case, let it suffice to say that one of the major reasons for this unfortunate situation is that the type of structure that should naturally organize a research course or book frequently is not there. An advantage to your current text (as presumably you will soon realize) is the almost obsessive attention that has been given to sequencing the material in a way that reflects the logical and natural unfolding of the research process in its several forms.

To help bring about this logical and natural unfolding of the research process, your book relies on several learning aids as you move from chapter to chapter.

You should find the following tools in virtually all of the remaining chapters and appendixes to be quite helpful as you work your way through the material: a concept map and detailed outline of the topics and subtopics covered; a list of performance objectives that indicates the behaviors students should be able to demonstrate; an introductory section at the outset of the chapter or appendix that quickly reviews the material just completed in the previous chapter and its relation to the new material you are just starting; a deductive approach (from the general to the specific) to covering the material

within each chapter and across chapters of the book; frequent graphic flowcharts and diagrams to help you see the "big picture" of what is being discussed; review/summary tables that give an overview of the narrative development of topics; bare bones boxes that provide the essential features of a given topic; a reliance on multiple examples of possible research scenarios and illustrative excerpts from the published research literature; occasional humor break boxes to provide some jocularity; a concluding section at the end of the chapter that projects where we go from there; bibliographic listings of references cited as well as additional recommended resources, including both print and electronic forms; and recommended Web sites and software application packages for further information.

BASIC AND STRETCHING (INTERMEDIATE) LEVELS OF COVERAGE

Another aid of sorts in each of the book's 10 chapters and 4 appendixes is the distinction made between (a) those topics that are basic or foundational to the research process and (b) those that represent somewhat of a "stretching" beyond the basics. The vast majority of any given chapter's topical coverage should be considered basic. The stretching topics represent an intermediate level and are flagged in any given chapter and appendix by way of this icon: This is certainly not intended to discourage delving into these topics but simply to acknowledge their positioning beyond what might be reasonably considered foundational.

An important point needs to be made here regarding the sequencing of topics covered in Chapters 2–10 as well as Appendixes A–D. Chapters 2–4 constitute the book's Part Two, titled "A Conceptual Framework for Understanding the Research Process." These are foundational chapters, and although they are quantitatively based, they still serve the purpose of laying the groundwork for the remainder of the book. Chapters 5–7 comprise Part Three, titled "The Quantitative Research Category." Chapters 8–9 comprise Part Four, titled "Qualitative and Integrative Research Categories: Options Beyond the Quantitative." Finally, Chapter 10 is a stand-alone chapter comprising Part Five, "Advancing the Massage Therapy Research Agenda." Appendixes A–D are clustered together because they represent the essential tools for the research process: electronic literature searching, ethical principles governing research, research report format and styles, and measurement and statistics.

Although an integral part of the book, the four appendixes are separated by design from the sequence of the 10 chapters so as not to interrupt the logical progression across the several research categories, strategies, and methods. The intent here is for the reader to access any one or more of the appendixes at any point in the book as the need arises. In this sense, then, each of the four appendixes may be considered a tool in the service of virtually any chapter topic. If the tools constituting the 4 appendixes had been interspersed among the 10 chapters, the desired flow across the research categories, strategies, and methods might have been disrupted.

CLOCK-HOUR LEVELS OF COVERAGE: 45, 30, AND 15

The complete coverage of the book's 10 chapters and four appendixes (A–D) should be possible within the context of an approximately 45–clock-hour course. This is intended to parallel a standard academic course offering the equivalent of 3 semester hours of credit, with a ratio of 1 semester hour of credit per 15 clock hours of instruction. Of course, the awarding of clock hours of credit or semester hours of credit is really quite variable and should reflect whatever is accepted practice in a given school setting.

Other options available are those of 30– and 15–clock-hour courses. The existing demands of a school's curriculum may allow only a course offering less than the full 45 hours recommended for complete coverage of the book's contents. A 30–clock-hour course would be tantamount to a

---

BOX 1   RECOMMENDED BASIC COVERAGE OF TOPICS REFLECTING 30 & 15 CLOCK-HOUR COURSES/SEMINARS/ WORKSHOPS

30–Clock-Hour Course (Basic Topical Coverage Only)
   Only basic topical coverage in Chapters 1–10 and Appendixes A–D
15–Clock-Hour Mini-Course or Continuing Education Seminar/ Workshop
   Only basic topical coverage in the following chapters and appendixes:
   Chapter 1: Why Research and Why Now?
   Chapter 2: The Research Continuum: A Deductive Approach to Viewing the Research Process
   Chapter 3: An Overview of the True Experimental/Randomized Controlled Trial Research Method
   Chapter 4: A More Focused View of the True Experimental/ Randomized Controlled Trial Research Method
   Chapter 7: The Descriptive-Oriented Research Strategy
   Chapter 8: The Qualitative Research Category and Its Contextual/ Interpretive-Oriented Research Strategy
   Chapter 10: Advancing Massage Therapy Research Competencies: Recent Contexts and Projected Directions
   Appendix A: Electronic Literature Searching: Sources and Strategies
   Appendix B: Ethical Principles Governing Research in the Biomedical and Behavioral Sciences
   Appendix C: Research Report Format and Stylistic Requirements

---

somewhat abbreviated yet potentially rigorous treatment of the topics. The 15–clock-hour use of only select topics in the book would accommodate, for example, a very brief introduction to research in a school's curriculum or a continuing education seminar or workshop for professional development purposes. Box 1 identifies the recommended basic coverage of topics appropriate to both the 30- and 15–clock-hour course or workshop possibilities.

CURRICULUM KIT–SPECIFIC LEVELS OF COVERAGE

The *Massage Therapy Research Curriculum Kit* (Achilles & Dryden, 2003) is organized in terms of three possible options for use that reflect 6-, 15-, and 24-hour commitments. Although the rationale and intent of this book are somewhat different from those of the kit, sections of this book may support and inform the coverage provided in the curriculum kit. Box 2 suggests certain topics in this book that may prove useful to users of this curriculum resource.

Box 2 RECOMMENDED BASIC COVERAGE OF TOPICS IN THIS BOOK CORRESPONDING TO THE 6-, 15-, AND 24-HOUR OPTIONS AVAILABLE TO USERS OF THE MASSAGE THERAPY RESEARCH CURRICULUM KIT (ACHILLES & DRYDEN, 2003)

Curriculum Kit's 6-Hour Option (Modules 1 and 2)

Only basic topical coverage in the following chapters and appendixes:

Chapter 1: Why Research and Why Now?

Chapter 2: The Research Continuum: A Deductive Approach to Viewing the Research Process

Chapter 3: An Overview of the True Experimental/Randomized Controlled Trial Research Method

Chapter 10: Advancing Massage Therapy Research Competencies: Recent Contexts and Projected Directions

Appendix A: Electronic Literature Searching: Sources and Strategies

Curriculum Kit's 15-Hour Option (Modules 1, 2, 3.1, 4.1, and 5.1)

Only basic topical coverage in the following chapters and appendixes:

Chapter 1: Why Research and Why Now?

Chapter 2: The Research Continuum: A Deductive Approach to Viewing the Research Process

Chapter 3: An Overview of the True Experimental/Randomized Controlled Trial Research Method

Chapter 4: A More Focused View of the True Experimental/Randomized Controlled Trial Research Method

Chapter 7: The Descriptive-Oriented Research Strategy

Chapter 8: The Qualitative Research Category and Its Contextual/Interpretive-Oriented Research Strategy

Chapter 10: Advancing Massage Therapy Research Competencies: Recent Contexts and Projected Directions

Appendix A: Electronic Literature Searching: Sources and Strategies

Appendix B: Ethical Principles Governing Research in the Biomedical and Behavioral Sciences

Appendix C: Research Report Format and Stylistic Requirements

Curriculum Kit's 24-Hour Option (Modules 1, 2, 3.1, 3.2, 4.1, 4.2, 5.1, and 5.2)

Only basic topical coverage in the following chapters and appendixes:

Chapter 1: Why Research and Why Now?

Chapter 2: The Research Continuum: A Deductive Approach to Viewing the Research Process

Chapter 3: An Overview of the True Experimental/Randomized Controlled Trial Research Method

Chapter 4: A More Focused View of the True Experimental/Randomized Controlled Trial Research Method

Chapter 7: The Descriptive-Oriented Research Strategy

Chapter 8: The Qualitative Research Category and its Contextual/Interpretive-Oriented Research Strategy

Chapter 9: The Integrative Research Category and its Synthesis-Oriented Research Strategy

Chapter 10: Advancing Massage Therapy Research Competencies: Recent Contexts and Projected Directions

Appendix A: Electronic Literature Searching: Sources and Strategies

Appendix B: Ethical Principles Governing Research in the Biomedical and Behavioral Sciences

Appendix C: Research Report Format and Stylistic Requirements

Appendix D: Measurement and Statistics as Research Tools

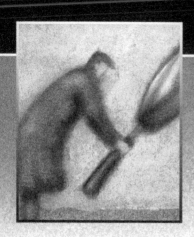

ACKNOWLEDGMENTS

One always runs the risk of "sins of omission" when attempting to recall and acknowledge those individuals who have played a major part in the authoring of a book. It is with a certain degree of concern, then, that I now try to recognize those persons who—knowingly or unknowingly—have assumed a significant role in the completion of this project.

Undoubtedly, my immediate family members have been at the forefront of the support, encouragement, understanding, and patience I needed in order to complete this book. I would think, also, that my seemingly nonstop unavailability while buried in my "office cave" for such a long period was at times considerably more demanding on them than it was on me. The dedication page for this book is just a small gesture of the heartfelt gratitude I extend to my parents, daughters, sons, and grandsons for their unconditional love.

On the professional front, certain colleagues—both present and past—have played a strategic role in a variety of ways. Mary M. Brazier, PhD, has been a faculty colleague of mine for the past 20 years and Chair of Loyola's Psychology Department from 1994-2004. In both capacities her support and encouragement have been consistent and invaluable, yet always in the context of her not hesitating to remind me of my considerable limitations. Frank E. Scully, PhD, as Dean of Loyola's College of Arts and Sciences, is in my judgment the model academic dean. Over the past several years he has not hesitated in the least to critique my professional performance in very demanding ways; however, it has always been done in a constructive manner with an optimal and genuine degree of support and confidence that has made all the difference. Stephen M. Scariano, PhD, Loyola's "statistics guru"

and my fellow gadfly at this fine institution, has consistently and vociferously supported my ambitions and efforts over many years. And such unflinching support has always seemed to come at times when I needed it the most. Finally, I must recognize W. George Gaines, EdD, my mentor and dissertation advisor from many, many, many years ago. Dr. Gaines—George—has always been in my mind the consummate university professor, and has remained for over three decades a most valued colleague, cherished friend, and trusted confidant.

Fellow health care professionals in the New Orleans area who must likewise be acknowledged for their role in support of my efforts on this book include John Muggivan, LCSW, whose exceptional intuitive and clinical skills are matched only by his personal sensitivity and integrity; Robert J. Jeanfreau, MD, the exemplar par excellence to which all internal medicine and primary care physicians should aspire; and Chad W. Millet, MD, whose skills as a gifted surgeon have given so very many people a new lease on life.

I must also recognize my son, Michael, whose computer science expertise and easy-going disposition quite literally came to my rescue at several strategic points during the preparation of the book's manuscript. Ms. Andrea Lee, the Administrative Assistant for Loyola's Psychology Department, has been consistently encouraging and always a sensitive listener when I felt the need to express my frustrations over the slow progress of the book's preparation. Also, the conscientious assistance of two of our current psychology majors—Ms. Amanda Rodrigue and Mr. Paul Bileci—has come at a critical stage as the book's manuscript preparation came to a close.

The entire editorial team at Mosby/Elsevier has been most encouraging, patient, and helpful in their support of my work on this book. In particular, I am most indebted to Ms. Kellie F. Fitzpatrick as Health Professions Editor, Ms. Jennifer Watrous as Developmental Editor, and Ms. Gail Michaels as Project Manager for the personally sensitive and professionally insightful way in which they have directed this book project. I look forward to the privilege of continuing to work with them on future projects. Additionally, I am grateful to the several reviewers listed elsewhere in the book for their conscientious critiques of the manuscript and helpful suggestions.

Finally, I extend my gratitude to my many other relatives, friends, and colleagues who were–in different ways and to varying degrees–supportive of what may have seemed at times to be a fanatical effort on my part in crafting this book. In that regard, perhaps all I can do now is borrow from the title and spirit of Lance Armstrong's book, *It's Not About the Bike*, and say quite honestly that on my end "it was never only about the book."

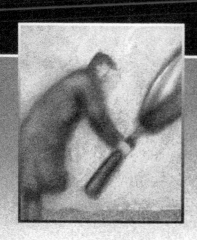

ABOUT THE AUTHOR

Glenn M. Hymel, EdD, LMT, is Professor and former Chairman of the Department of Psychology at Loyola University New Orleans. Glenn earned his baccalaureate and master's degrees from Loyola University New Orleans and his doctorate degree from the University of New Orleans. His principal areas of specialization include educational psychology, research design and statistics, school counseling, personal adjustment psychology, and philosophical psychology. Dr. Hymel's work at the elementary, secondary, tertiary, and professional school levels has focused primarily on mastery learning, competency-based education, instructional design, and test-preparation skills. Glenn has published extensively in major psychology and education journals, and his research has been presented at numerous international and national conferences over considerably more years than he is comfortable with acknowledging. Glenn is a graduate of the Blue Cliff School of Therapeutic Massage in Metairie, La., and has a particular practice and research interest in stress management as well as fibromyalgia, chronic fatigue, and chronic pain populations. He currently serves on the Massage Therapy Foundation's Board of Trustees and chairs the Foundation's Massage Therapy Research Database Committee as well as the Research Grant Proposal Review Committee.

When not succumbing to his workaholic tendencies, Glenn enjoys weight training, swimming, cycling, and reading. He also takes delight in "primitive gardening," science fiction movies, and stand-up comedy routines—as an observer, that is, not as a performer (except for his occasional, and usually futile, attempts at interjecting humor into his teaching efforts).

To contact the author . . .

I would sincerely appreciate receiving comments and suggestions regarding this book from students, instructors, practitioners, researchers, or whoever may feel so moved by the Spirit. Whether your reactions represent "bouquets" or "brickbats," your input regarding what has worked and what hasn't is invaluable for future improvements to this book. If your reactions are indeed favorable to the life-draining effort required to write this book, then please know that I will remain humble and vigilant. If your reactions, however, are less than favorable—in fact, even critical—then rest assured that my feelings and self-concept will not be irreparably damaged and I will try my best to keep it all in proper perspective. In either case, you may contact me electronically at hymel@loyno.edu or via snail mail at the following address: Department of Psychology, Loyola University, 6363 St. Charles Ave., New Orleans, LA 70118. For those of you who really eschew the depersonalization of e-mail and traditional postal delivery and prefer to opt instead for direct conversation, feel free to call me at 504-865-3257. If you choose the latter option, though, please be forewarned that you may encounter an electronically voice-simulated rendition of yours truly if indeed I am unavailable to take the call.

GLENN M. HYMEL

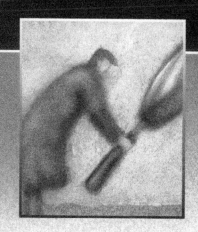

CONTENTS

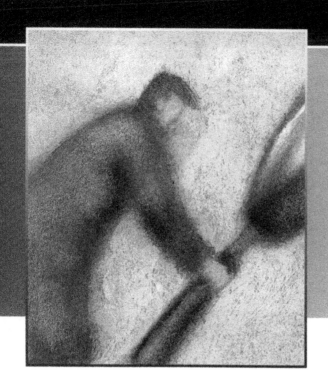

PART ONE

INTRODUCTION: THE GUIDING QUESTIONS FOR THIS BOOK

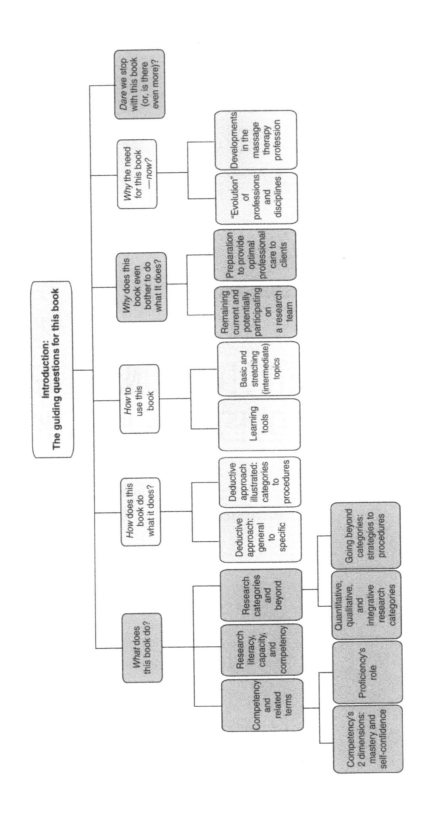

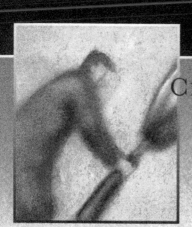

1

WHY RESEARCH AND WHY NOW?

OBJECTIVES

Upon completion of this chapter, the reader will have the information necessary to perform the following tasks:

1 Characterize (a) the basics of the research process;
   (b) the nature of competency; (c) the relationship among
   research literacy, research capacity, and research competency;
   and (d) the progressive sequence of research strategies,
   methods, designs, and procedures for each research category.

2 Define quantitative research, qualitative research,
   and integrative research.

3 Diagram, discuss, and illustrate the deductive approach as an
   explanation of the progression from research categories to
   research strategies, methods, designs, and procedures.

4 Explain why this book creates the potential for you to participate
   on a research team, as well as prepares you to provide optimal
   professional care to clients.

5 Identify and discuss at least three recent and ongoing
   professional developments that give insight as to why the
   massage profession is focusing on the advancement of research
   competencies.

6 Identify and discuss at least five learning tools provided
   in this book.

KEY TERMS

Basic topics
Competency
Deductive approach
Integrative research
Mastery
Proficiency
Qualitative research

Quantitative research
Research capacity
Research category
Research competencies
Research design
Research literacy
Research method

Research procedure
Research strategy
Research universe
Self-confidence
Stretching topics

WHAT DOES THIS BOOK DO?

This book provides an introduction to various concepts, principles, and procedures that are critical to understanding the research process. The principal focus will be on the approaches to research that are most fundamental to massage and other holistic and integrative therapies. We will also look at professionals working in basic and behavioral science disciplines that are the most relevant to the current work done in therapeutic massage and bodywork, regardless of the context within which the manual therapy intervention occurs.

COMPETENCY AND RELATED TERMS

The various topics covered in the text provide you with basic competencies for two very specific professional roles: (a) the role of a critical reader or consumer of the research literature that is already available or currently being proposed and (b) the role of active participant and valued member of a research team engaged in advancing the scientific basis of your profession. Because we have just referred to the notion of competencies as a basis for two possible professional roles, let's clarify what we mean by the construct *competency* as well as certain related terms, namely *mastery, self-confidence,* and *proficiency.*

Reflecting the works of Morrison (1931) and White (1959), Anderson and Block (1977) characterize **competency** as follows:

> Competency ... *is a two-dimensional construct (cf. White, 1959). The first dimension is ... mastery. In other words,* mastery *can be thought of as the intellectual component of competency. A competent learner has acquired a variety of learning products. However, competency also consists of the attainment of* self-confidence *or the sense of being able to cope. This attainment of self-confidence is the emotional or affective component of competency (emphases added). (p. 165)*

This reference to **mastery** reflects Morrison's original characterization of competency as implying not only that a *desired learning outcome* has been achieved but also that an *acceptable level of performance* has been reached.

Anderson and Block (1977) continue their discussion of competency with the following explanation of **proficiency** and its relationship to mastery:

> Proficiency *refers to the* efficiency *with which the individual makes use of the acquired learning products. While* mastery *refers to the* effectiveness *of the learning process in producing the desired learning product, proficiency refers to the efficiency of the learning product once it has been acquired (emphasis added)....*
>
> *In essence, then we see the relationship among mastery, competency, and proficiency as follows: Mastery is a precondition for both competency and proficiency. The positive affective consequences that usually accompany mastery help to produce a competent individual. Finally, through practice and continued use of a particular learning, competent individuals become proficient. (p. 165)*

To summarize what we have just covered, the term competency implies the following: (a) some new learning has been acquired at an acceptable level of performance and (b) the learner consequently now has a heightened **self-confidence** or sense of being able to deal with the newly acquired learning. With continued practice and refinement, the competent learner becomes even more efficient and spontaneous—or proficient—in using the newly acquired learning.

Consider, for example, competency regarding what constitutes a dependent variable in a published research study. In this instance competency implies that the reader can accurately and consistently recognize the one or more dependent variables in a research article. Additionally, the reader has a sense of confidence about being able to continue recognizing a study's dependent variable as distinct from the other variables. With further practice, the reader should be able to use this particular research competency even more efficiently and spontaneously—or more proficiently—in reading research articles.

We have digressed somewhat into the issues of mastery and self-confidence as components of competence as well as the relationship to proficiency. This is critical, however, due to the need to clarify certain terminology at the outset. It is also particularly important given the existing distinctions in the massage therapy literature between such terms as *research literacy* and *research capacity* (cf. Dryden & Achilles, 2003).

RESEARCH LITERACY, RESEARCH CAPACITY, AND RESEARCH COMPETENCY: THE RELATIONSHIP

As mentioned earlier in the "Preface to the Instructor," the Massage Therapy Research Curriculum Kit is a resource developed by Dryden and Achilles (2003) under the sponsorship of the Massage Therapy Foundation. It provides recommended topical coverage, learning activities, and related materials for advancing research competencies in the profession. In so doing, this resource distinguishes between **research literacy** and **research capacity** as follows: "Research literacy is the ability to find, understand, and critically evaluate research evidence for application in professional practice. Research capacity is the ability to conduct research" (Dryden & Achilles, 2003, p. 1; cf., also, Achilles & Dryden, 2002). This distinction is helpful and appropriate to the mission of the curriculum kit, which provides a very general overview of certain research issues. The kit's primary focus is on literacy issues aimed at developing critical consumers of the research literature already available.

Our current text is related to, yet expands considerably beyond, the kit's focus. Accordingly, our coverage in this book speaks to **research competencies** involving (a) the mastery of important learning outcomes at acceptable levels of performance and (b) the self-confidence usually associated with such mastery. With additional practice, you can eventually use these research competencies more efficiently and spontaneously, i.e., more proficiently. The result, then, should be that of massage and holistic therapists possessing an array of competencies corresponding to those procedures defining the research process. This, in turn, should allow the two professional roles discussed earlier to become a possibility: the critical consumer of the already available research literature and the valued member of an actively-engaged research team.

For the most part, then, your completion of this text should allow you to have at least a fundamental preparation regarding the research process. This type of basic preparation is prerequisite not only to your being able to read and understand most of the research literature available but also to your being positioned to contribute actively to the scientific advancement of your profession.

RESEARCH CATEGORIES AND BEYOND

The **research universe** involves, at the most general level, three subsets of research categories: quantitative, qualitative, and integrative (Figure 1-1). The primary emphasis of this book is **quantitative research**, which is well established in massage, health professions, and the sciences. Quantitative research emphasizes an objective and unbiased approach to scientific investigation. This approach depends primarily on the statistical analysis of numerical data once the measurements have been demonstrated to be valid and reliable. We will also address **qualitative research**, which has recently started to attract recognition and is certainly a viable genre of research. Qualitative research is philosophically driven by subjective, contextual, and highly individualistic perceptions of all that is observed and experienced. This research is based primarily on verbal data that by their nature lend themselves to alternative interpretations on

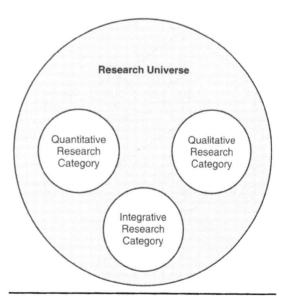

FIGURE I-I ■ Three categorical subsets of the research universe: quantitative research category, qualitative research category, and integrative research category.

the part of both the observed and the observer. Finally, we will focus on **integrative research**, which synthesizes, in various ways, earlier research that has already been completed. The essential distinctions among these three research categories will be introduced in Chapter 2. We will also cover related research strategies, methods, designs, and procedures, looking at each area in detail.

HOW DOES THIS BOOK DO WHAT IT DOES?

DEDUCTIVE APPROACH: MOVING FROM GENERAL TO SPECIFIC

We will take a **deductive approach** to covering the many topics that are critical to understanding the research process, moving from a general focus to progressively more specific topics.

Figure 1-2 shows the type of progression that occurs when a deductive approach is used to explore any complex issue. The starting point is the "panoramic view," or general level, followed by increasingly detailed levels of specificity. For our purposes, four specificity levels are shown beyond the general level.

DEDUCTIVE APPROACH ILLUSTRATED: CATEGORIES TO PROCEDURES

As mentioned earlier, the most general way of thinking about research considered in this text is the **research category**. We then consider—in increasing detail—various research strategies, methods, designs, and procedures. There are five levels in total, then, at which we think about the research process as we work our way through this book. Figures 1-3 and 1-4 provide a look at these five levels and the terminology we will use as we progress from the general to the most specific.

To elaborate, in the general level of *quantitative research category*, one possible **research strategy** is the *difference-oriented research strategy*, or specific level 1 (SL1). An example of difference-oriented research

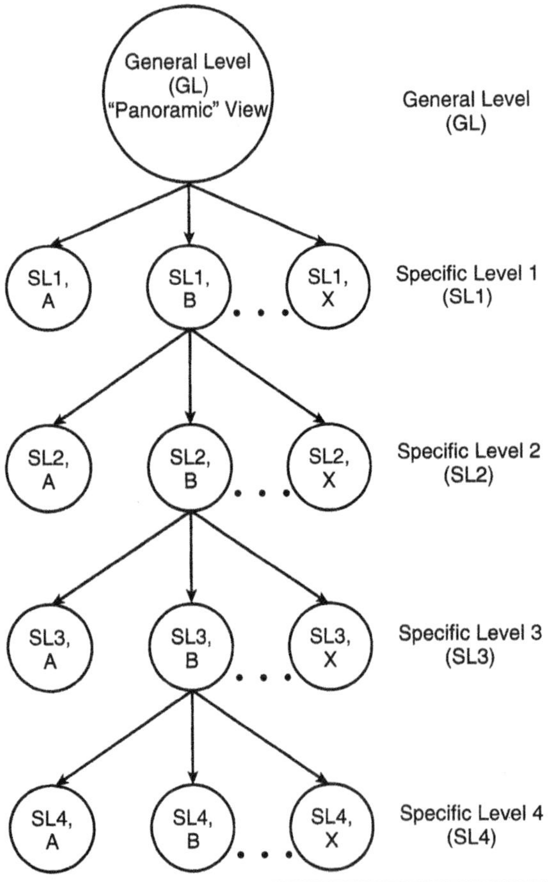

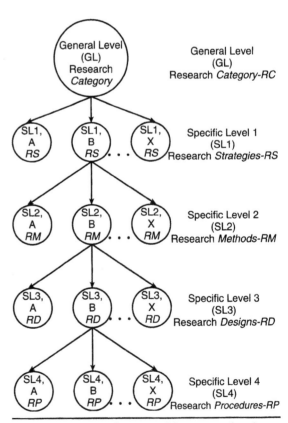

FIGURE 1-2 ■ Generic display of the progression from general to specific in the deductive approach.

FIGURE 1-3 ■ Deductive view of the progression from the general level of research category to the specific levels of research strategies, methods, designs, and procedures.

FIGURE 1-4 ■ Another view of the progression from research category to research procedures.

is a study investigating whether the presence and absence of chair massage is related to a difference in stress levels among clerical workers in a corporate setting. One viable **research method** affiliated with this strategy is the *true experimental or randomized controlled trial (RCT) research method,* a specific level 2 (SL2). A prevalent **research design** associated with this method is the *randomized, control group, pretest-posttest design,* designated in Figure 1-3 as specific level 3 (SL3). Finally, **research procedures**, the specific level 4 (SL4), ideally include such procedures as *random selection, random assignment, pretesting* on relevant variables, a *manipulated independent variable* (in this case the presence or absence of chair massage intervention), and *posttesting* of the dependent or outcome variable(s).

Please keep in mind that this is simply an introductory or preliminary explanation of the deductive approach. The specific strategies, methods, designs, and procedures in this example will be discussed later in this book.

HOW TO USE THIS BOOK

LEARNING TOOLS

This text sequences material in a way that reflects the logical and natural unfolding of the research process in its several forms. To do this, we rely on several learning tools a few of which are presented in this chapter. We will continue to use these tools in the remaining chapters as well as incorporating other tools. As you work your way through this book, you will find the following in each chapter: a concept map and detailed outline of the topics and subtopics covered; a listing of learning objectives indicating the concepts and skills in which you should be able to demonstrate competency; an introductory section that presents a review of the material completed in the previous chapter and relates it to the new material in the current chapter; a deductive approach (from the general to the specific) to covering the material within each chapter and across chapters of the book; frequent graphic flow charts and diagrams to help you understand the "big picture" that is being discussed;

review/summary tables that give an overview of the narrative development of topics; Bare Bones boxes that provide the essentials of a given topic; multiple examples of possible research scenarios and illustrative excerpts from the published research literature; occasional Humor Break boxes to provide comic relief; a concluding section at the end of the chapter that projects where we go from there; listings of references cited as well as additional recommended resources, including both print and electronic forms; and recommended Web sites and software application packages for further information.

BASIC AND STRETCHING (INTERMEDIATE) TOPICS

Another feature you will find in each chapter involves the distinction made between those topics that are **basic**, or *foundational,* to the research process and those that *stretch* beyond the basics. The vast majority of the material in this book is basic. **Stretching topics**, however, represent an intermediate level and are marked with a stretching icon. This icon is certainly not intended to discourage delving into these topics, but instead is meant to acknowledge that the material goes beyond what might be reasonably considered foundational.

An important point needs to be made regarding the sequencing of topics covered in Chapters 2-10, as well as Appendixes A-D. Part Two, A Conceptual Framework for Understanding the Research Process, comprises Chapters 2-4, three foundational chapters that are quantitatively based but still serve the purpose of laying the groundwork for the remainder of the book. Part Three, The Quantitative Research Category, comprises Chapters 5-7. Part Four, Qualitative and Integrative Research Categories: Options Beyond the Quantitative, comprises Chapters 8 and 9. Finally, Part Five, Advancing the Massage Therapy Research Agenda, is Chapter 10, a stand-alone chapter. Appendixes A-D include the essential tools for the research process, namely, electronic literature searching, ethical principles governing research, research report format and styles, and measurement and statistics. Although the appendixes are separate

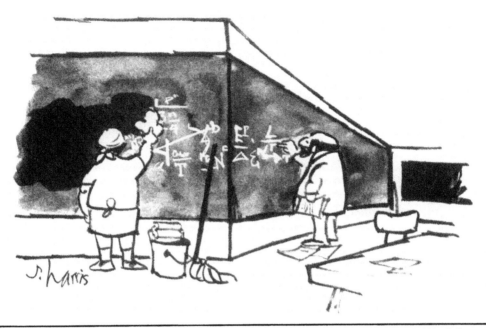

HUMOR BREAK ■ Such are the perils of not protecting the sequence of our work. (From Harris, S. [1992]. *Chalk up another one: The best of Sidney Harris*. New Brunswick, NJ: Rutgers University Press.)

from the main chapters, they nonetheless provide information that is critical to your understanding of chapter material and the research process. You should access one or more of the appendixes at any point in the book as the need arises.

WHY DOES THIS BOOK EVEN BOTHER TO DO WHAT IT DOES?

REMAINING CURRENT AND POTENTIALLY PARTICIPATING ON A RESEARCH TEAM

In all likelihood you have invested the time, energy, and resources to pursue a career in therapeutic massage with the intention of cultivating as high a degree of competence and professionalism as possible. Assuming that is the case, then a critical part of your education and training involves acquiring the knowledge and skills that will allow you over the span of your career to remain current regarding developments in your profession. This, in turn, may perhaps lead you to contribute actively to your profession's advancement as a member of a research team. The research process is a major part of the knowledge base and skills acquisition that will allow you to develop professionally to the fullest.

PREPARATION TO PROVIDE OPTIMAL PROFESSIONAL CARE TO CLIENTS

Of course, the ultimate aim of all of your professional educational experiences is to position yourself to provide optimal professional care to your clients in as well-informed a manner as possible. To do otherwise would be a grave injustice not only to yourself but, more critically, to those clients entrusted to your care. The major goal of this book is to foster your professional growth in such a way that the very best scientific evidence that pertains to your work as a health science professional is readily accessible and understandable to you.

WHY THE NEED FOR THIS BOOK — NOW?

As important as the *what, how,* and *why* questions are, this introductory chapter would certainly be lacking if the *why now* question were not acknowledged and answered, especially because of the increased recent attention, particularly in the massage therapy profession, to the importance of the research process.

EVOLUTION OF PROFESSIONS AND DISCIPLINES

The current attention to the research process in the massage therapy profession is actually very much overdue. As frequently occurs during the initial growth spurts experienced in any given health care profession or supporting discipline, practitioners begin to recognize that continued development of that profession or discipline depends on a solid research foundation. Individual therapists in their practice must have the competence to stay informed of relevant research findings. Likewise, a profession as a whole must also be vigilant to ensure that the education and training of its members include the knowledge and skills to allow them, at the very least, to function as intelligent and informed consumers of what the research literature has to say.

DEVELOPMENTS IN THE MASSAGE THERAPY PROFESSION

The massage therapy profession is at a juncture in its development. Partial evidence of this is the decision by the Commission on Massage Therapy Accreditation (COMTA) mandating that its accredited schools give evidence effective March 2003 of curricular provisions for ensuring research literacy among their graduates (Ostendorf & Schwartz, 2001). This mandate was partly in response to the recommendations of the multidisciplinary Massage Research Agenda Workgroup (MRAW), convened in 1999 by the then American Massage Therapy Association Foundation (recently renamed the Massage Therapy Foundation). These recommendations are reported in the Foundation's publication titled the *Massage Therapy Research Agenda* (see AMTA Foundation & Kahn, 2002, in Chapter 10). And as a follow-up to these two initiatives by COMTA and the AMTA Foundation, a relatively recent article in the *Journal of Bodywork & Movement Therapies* comprehensively surveys eight professional areas of focus that are critical to advancing massage therapy research competencies (Hymel, 2003).

Additional current evidence of the heightened recognition of the importance of acquiring research competency is the *Massage Therapy Research Curriculum Kit* (Dryden & Achilles, 2003) that was commissioned by the AMTA Foundation partially in response to COMTA's research mandate. Furthermore, topics addressed at professional conferences and meetings over the past several years have increasingly included a research focus. This increased attention to the research process within the massage therapy profession has not been restricted only to the regional and national levels, but has progressively encompassed international efforts to bring colleagues together for the expressed purpose of advancing scientific inquiry.

DARE WE STOP WITH THIS BOOK? (OR IS THERE EVEN MORE?)

Yes, Virginia, there is indeed considerably more to the intricacies of research in the health science professions. As mentioned earlier, this book surveys at an introductory level those concepts, principles, and procedures that are basic to research categories spanning the quantitative, qualitative, and integrative realms. Each of these three research categories could easily justify a complete book unto itself if the subject were pursued in greater depth. However, this would not be consistent with the book's central goal. Our goal, once again, is to provide an introduction to those essential competencies needed for consuming the research already available and, perhaps, eventually allowing you to engage in scientific inquiry as a member of a research team.

Throughout the majority of this book an effort is made to guide you to additional recommended resources that provide opportunities for more in-depth study. The successful mastery of the full scope of what has been laid out in this book will provide you with the foundation for confidently pursuing in greater detail any of the research strategies covered.

So, our journey together has just begun. Enjoy!

REFERENCES

Achilles, R., & Dryden, T. (2002). Research literacy for complementary and alternative practitioners: Results of the national needs assessment. *Hand in Hand: The Newsletter of the Canadian Massage Therapist Alliance,* Summer, 4–6, 9, & 13.

AMTA Foundation, & Kahn, J. (2002). *Massage therapy research agenda.* Evanston, IL: AMTA Foundation.

Anderson, L. W., & Block, J. H. (1977). Mastery learning. In D. J. Treffinger, J. K. Dent, & R. E. Ripple (Eds.), *Handbook on teaching educational psychology* (pp. 163–185). New York: Academic Press.

Dryden, T., & Achilles, R. (2003). *Massage therapy research curriculum kit.* Evanston, IL: AMTA Foundation.

Hymel, G. M. (2003). Advancing massage therapy research competencies: Dimensions for thought and action. *Journal of Bodywork & Movement Therapies, 7*(3), 194–199.

Morrison, H. C. (1931). *The practices of teaching in the secondary school* (2nd ed.). Chicago: University of Chicago Press.

Ostendorf, C., & Schwartz, J. (2001). COMTA begins move toward competencies. *Massage Therapy Journal, 40,* 116–120.

White, R. W. (1959). Motivation reconsidered: The concept of competence. *Psychological Review, 66,* 297–333.

ADDITIONAL RECOMMENDED RESOURCES

Block, J. H. (1978). Learning for competence. *Victorian Institute of Educational Research Bulletin, 40,* 27–43.

Cassidy, C. M., & Hart, J. A. (2003a). Methodological issues in the scientific investigation of massage and bodywork therapy: Part I. *Journal of Bodywork & Movement Therapies, 7*(1), 2–10.

Cassidy, C. M., & Hart, J. A. (2003b). Methodological issues in investigations of massage/bodywork therapy: Part II–Making research designs and data credible: Model fit validity, combining scientific soundness with the explanatory model of massage and bodywork therapies. *Journal of Bodywork & Movement Therapies, 7*(2), 71–79.

Cassidy, C. M., & Hart, J. A. (2003c). Methodological issues in investigations of massage/bodywork therapy: Part III–Qualitative and quantitative designs for MBT and the bias of interpretation. *Journal of Bodywork & Movement Therapies, 7*(3), 136–141.

Cassidy, C. M., & Hart, J. A. (2003d). Methodological issues in investigations of massage/bodywork therapy: Part IV–Experimental research designs. *Journal of Bodywork & Movement Therapies, 7*(4), 240–250.

White, R. T. (1979). Achievement, mastery, proficiency, competence. *Studies in Science Education, 6,* 1–22.

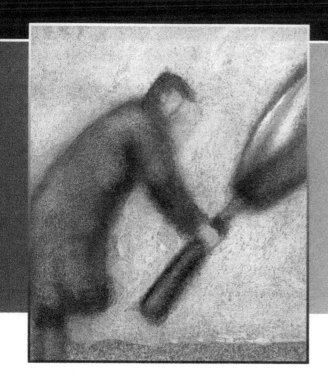

PART TWO

A CONCEPTUAL FRAMEWORK FOR UNDERSTANDING THE RESEARCH PROCESS

2 *The Research Continuum: A Deductive Approach to Viewing the Research Process,* 12

3 *An Overview of the True Experimental/Randomized Controlled Trial Research Method,* 20

4 *A More Focused View of the True Experimental/ Randomized Controlled Trial Research Method,* 36

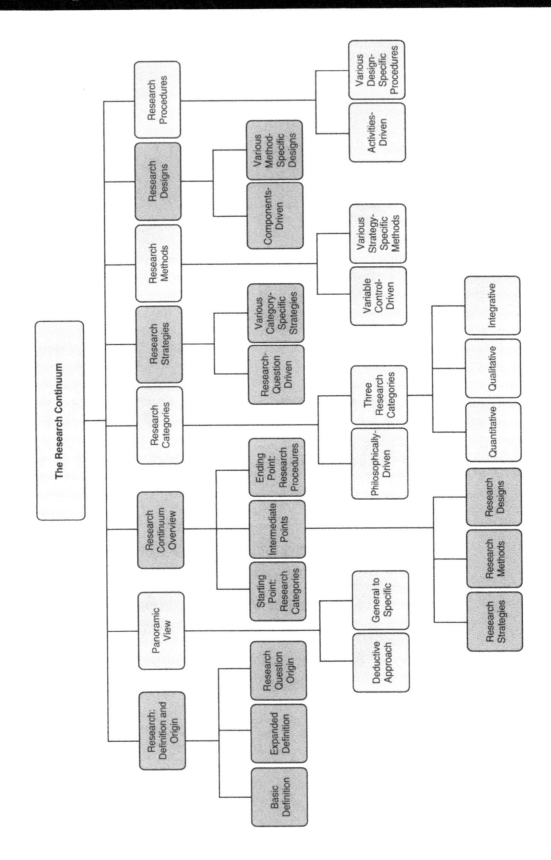

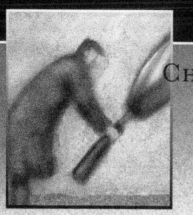

2

THE RESEARCH CONTINUUM: A DEDUCTIVE APPROACH TO VIEWING THE RESEARCH PROCESS

OUTLINE

OBJECTIVES

Upon completion of this chapter, the reader will have the information necessary to perform the following tasks:

1 Define research.

2 Identify and explain the point of origin of any research endeavor.

3 Discuss the research process as a deductive approach.

4 Flowchart the research continuum, displaying the progression from research category to research procedures, with an emphasis on labeling its starting and ending points as well as its three intermediate points.

5 Identify and explain each of the three research *categories* and discuss the one or more research *strategies* that define it.

6 Identify and explain the distinguishing features of any given research *strategy* and discuss the two or more research *methods* that define it.

7 Identify and explain the distinguishing features of any given research *method* and discuss — if applicable — the two or more research *designs* that define it.

8 Identify and explain the distinguishing features of any given research *design* and discuss — if applicable — the two or more research *procedures* that define it.

9 Identify and explain the distinguishing features of any given research *procedure*.

10 Discuss and provide one example of the distinction in research terminology across various basic science, behavioral science, and health science professions.

11 Explain why analysis of the research procedures used in a study is an essential skill for understanding the research process and, thereby, mastering the research language.

RESEARCH: DEFINITION AND ORIGIN

Our journey through the research process starts with defining exactly what we mean by the term **research**. Because there are three research categories and various subdivisions under each, as we have already seen, a single definition is challenging but certainly not out of the question. At its most basic level, then, research is a process that explores one or more areas of interest (called *factors* or *variables*) by analyzing numerical or verbal data to advance our understanding.

More specifically, we might define research as an activity that allows us to accomplish one or more of the following tasks: (a) to characterize a variable of interest through numerical or verbal data, (b) to investigate a possible relationship between two or more variables, and (c) to integrate or synthesize data from already published sources concerning one or more variables of interest.

As illustrations of these three tasks, please consider the following. In the first instance, we might find the percentage of adults surveyed nationwide who have used therapeutic massage as a form of complementary and alternative health care. Or we might use a detailed interview to document a client's individual experience and perception of therapeutic massage over a designated period of time as an intervention for chronic low-back pain. In the second instance, a research team might explore the nature of the relationship—if any—between aquatic therapy and increased range of motion for clients recovering from bilateral hip replacement surgery. Finally, the third task might involve a massage therapist completing an exhaustive state-of-the-art review and synthesis of what the professional literature has to say about therapeutic massage as a viable intervention for clients suffering from fibromyalgia.

Across all three possible tasks that define the research process is a **point of origin** that gives direction and meaning to the entire research effort.

That point is the **research question** being posed. For example, if one were to ask about the relationship between trigger point therapy and the alleviation of migraine headaches, then one possible research effort might be to investigate whether or not a meaningful difference exists between trigger point therapy and a conventional drug-specific intervention relative to the alleviation of migraines. The origin, then, is always the research question on which all of the research activities are based.

THE DEDUCTIVE APPROACH

As we observed in Figures 1-2 and 1-3 in the previous chapter, a helpful way to begin understanding

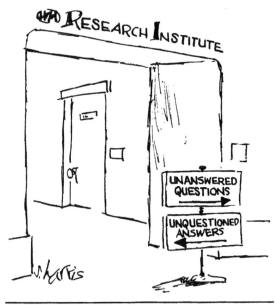

HUMOR BREAK ■ Our most important research questions may be "hiding" in our unchallenged solutions. (From Harris, S. [1991]. *"You want proof? I'll give you proof!": More cartoons from Sidney Harris.* New York: W.H. Freeman.)

the research process is to visualize a movement from an initial general level to several more detailed and specific levels that must be considered. Figure 1-4 and the outline for this chapter, likewise, convey the same "panoramic view" of the desired sequence as we work our way through the various research options.

THE RESEARCH CONTINUUM

The starting point in our discussion of the research process is the **research category** from which everything else flows. The ending point in terms of detail is the specific **research procedures** one would have to carry out to complete the research effort. Sandwiched in between are the intermediate points that progress from **research strategies** to **methods** to **designs**. Figure 2-1 displays these various points in the **research continuum** and sets the stage for us to be able to specify precisely where we are in the research process.

RESEARCH CATEGORIES, STRATEGIES, METHODS, DESIGNS, AND PROCEDURES: WHAT DRIVES THEM AND HOW ARE THEY RELATED?

RESEARCH CATEGORIES: THE MOST GENERAL LEVEL

At the most general level, we encounter three possible research categories: (a) the *quantitative* research category, (b) the *qualitative* research category, and (c) the *integrative* research category. The distinguishing feature that drives each of these three categories is its *philosophical orientation*.

More specifically, the *quantitative* category of research is **philosophically driven** by a view of reality and truth that emphasizes the objective and unbiased approach to scientific investigation. This orientation is rooted primarily in numerical data that are statistically analyzed once the measurements have been demonstrated to be valid and reliable. The vast majority of research that has historically dominated the basic, behavioral and health sciences is of this type (Peat, Mellis, Williams, & Xuan, 2002).

Somewhat in contrast is the *qualitative* category of research, which is philosophically driven by a perspective on reality and truth that relies on subjective, contextual, and highly individualistic perceptions of all that is observed and experienced. This perspective is based primarily on verbal data that by their nature lead to alternative interpretations on the part of both the observed and the observer. Historically, this qualitative approach has been emphasized in disciplines such as anthropology and sociology, but with a somewhat recent emergence in psychology and various health science professions (Creswell, 1998).

The integrative category of research is a hybrid perspective on reality and truth. This view recognizes the equally valuable possibilities that exist in both the objective analysis and the subjective interpretations of whatever experiences are being investigated. The focal point in this orientation may encompass both numerical and verbal data, but with a concerted effort to synthesize research that has already been generated in the quantitative and/or qualitative realms. In a sense, then, this category of research highlights the two themes that (a) the whole may be greater than the sum of its parts and (b) patterns of meaning may unfold in an area of research if a synthesizing approach is taken. Publications by authors such as Marks and Sykes (2004), Mulrow and Cook (1998), and Paterson, Thorne, Canam, and Jillings (2001) give us guidelines for this integrative category of research.

Figure 2-2 displays the philosophically driven nature of each of these three research categories, which we address with more detail in Chapters 5 through 9.

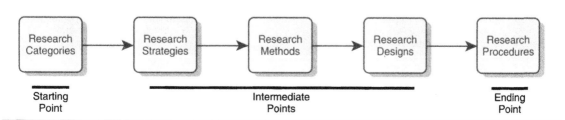

FIGURE 2-I ■ The research continuum from research categories to research procedures.

- Research Categories:Philosophically Driven
  - • Quantitative:Objective Analysis,Primarily Numerical Data
  - • Qualitative:Subjective and Contextual Interpretation,Primarily Verbal Data
  - • Integrative:Synthesizing Effort Valued,Objective and/or
    Subjective Orientation,Numerical and/or Verbal Data

FIGURE 2-2 ■ Research categories and their philosophical orientations.

RESEARCH STRATEGIES

Any one of the three research categories is made operational—or brought to life—by one or more of its defining **research strategies**. A *research strategy* is the first level of specificity or detail beyond the general research category to which it belongs, and it is driven by the *research question* that the strategy is investigating.

The *quantitative* category involves three possible research strategies, each reflecting the type of research question that gives it direction and meaning. These three strategies are (a) the *difference-oriented* research strategy, (b) the *association-oriented* research strategy, and (c) the *descriptive-oriented* research strategy. The *qualitative* category includes only one research strategy: the *contextual/interpretive-oriented* strategy. Likewise, the *integrative* category of research has only one research strategy, which is called *synthesis-oriented* strategy. Figure 2-3 identifies these research question-driven strategies and their affiliated research categories. These categories are covered in detail in Parts Three and Four of this book.

RESEARCH METHODS

Research methods represent the next level of specificity in our research continuum. Any given research strategy is implemented by one or more **research methods**. Any particular research method is **variable control driven**. This simply means that the investigator's degree of control over the several variables (aspects or features subject to change) of the study is precisely what defines the research method.

Methods Used in the Quantitative Research Category

The three strategies included in the *quantitative* category each have two or more related methods. Specifically, the *difference-oriented* strategy encompasses four possible research methods: (a) the *true experimental—or randomized controlled trial*—method, (b) the *quasi-experimental* method, (c) the *single-case experimental* method, and (d) the *nonexperimental comparative groups* method. The *association-oriented* strategy includes two research methods: (a) the *correlational* method and (b) the *predictive* method. The *descriptive-oriented* strategy employs four possible methods: (a) the *single-case quantitative analysis* method, (b) the *survey* method, (c) the *naturalistic/structured observational* method, and (d) the *case report* method. Figure 2-4 displays the research strategies and their variable control-driven methods within the quantitative research category.

- Quantitative Research Category
  - • Difference-Oriented Research Strategy
  - • Association-Oriented Research Strategy
  - • Descriptive-Oriented Research Strategy
- Qualitative Research Category
  - • Contextual/Interpretive Research Strategy
- Integrative Research Category
  - • Synthesis-Oriented Research Strategy

FIGURE 2-3 ■ Research categories and their research question-driven strategies.

- Quantitative Research Category
  - • Difference-Oriented Research Strategy
    - • • True Experimental
      (or Randomized Controlled Trial)
      Method
    - • • Quasi-Experimental Method
    - • • Single-Case Experimental Method
    - • • Nonexperimental Comparative
      Groups Method
  - • Association-Oriented Research Strategy
    - • • Correlational Method
    - • • Predictive Method
  - • Descriptive-Oriented Research Strategy
    - • • Single-Case Quantitative
      Analysis Method
    - • • Survey Method
    - • • Naturalistic/Structured
      Observational Method
    - • • Case Report Method

FIGURE 2-4 ■ The quantitative research category: its affiliated research strategies and variable control-driven methods.

- Qualitative Research Category
  - • Contextual/Interpretive-Oriented Research Strategy
    - • • Case Study Method
    - • • Phenomenological Method
    - • • Grounded Theory Method
    - • • Ethnographic Method

FIGURE 2-5 ■ The qualitative research category: its affiliated research strategy and variable control-driven methods.

Methods Used in the Qualitative Research Category

As indicated earlier, the *qualitative* category involves only one strategy, the *contextual/interpretive-oriented* strategy. This strategy includes four methods: (a) the *case study* method, (b) the *phenomenological* method, (c) the *grounded theory* method, and (d) the *ethnographic* method. Figure 2-5 shows the qualitative research category as well as its affiliated research strategy and variable control-driven methods.

Methods Used in the Integrative Research Category

In a somewhat similar fashion, the *integrative* category involves one strategy, the *synthesis-oriented* strategy. The five research methods included within this category are (a) the *traditional narrative review* method, (b) the *critical systematic review* method, (c) the *meta-analytic systematic review* method, (d) the *best-evidence synthesis* method, and (e) the *qualitative systematic review* methods including *meta-syntheses* and *meta-summaries*. Figure 2-6 identifies the research strategy and its variable control-driven methods affiliated with the integrative category.

At this point you may be wondering how to make sense of the many names and labels of research terms just thrown at you. It is very important for you to keep in mind that our primary interest now is simply to overview a framework, or a way of thinking about and organizing all that remains in this book as we discuss the research process. The next few chapters will give you more than

enough opportunity to revisit this information in detail.

RESEARCH DESIGNS

Continuing with our deductive approach, which moves from the general to the specific, many—though not all—research methods can be further subdivided into *research designs*. Any given *research design* can be called **components driven**. This simply means that to implement a certain research method, various options—or research designs—are sometimes available that involve including or excluding certain components or parts of a study. It is precisely those components that the investigator chooses and that define the research design. One design, for example, may involve as a component a measure of shoulder pain before massage therapy is introduced, whereas in another design the premeasure might be omitted. That single component, involving either the presence or absence of a premeasure, can distinguish one design from another.

At this point in our progression from research categories to research procedures, it would not be helpful to list the particular research design subdivisions that are possible under each of the research methods already identified. Such specific discussion will be considerably more understandable once you reach Parts Three and Four of the book.

RESEARCH PROCEDURES

As with research designs, the discussion of *research procedures* is best delayed until later chapters due to the high degree of specificity involved. At this stage it is sufficient to simply acknowledge that any given research design involves implementing several research procedures, which in turn involve certain activities. Any given *research procedure* is **activities driven**. For example, one design that we will address later in the book involves the research procedure of randomization, which can, in turn, include both random selection and the random assignment

- Integrative Research Category
  - • Synthesis-Oriented Research Strategy
    - • • Traditional Narrative Review Method
    - • • Critical Systematic Review Method
    - • • Meta-Analytic Systematic Review Method
    - • • Best-Evidence Synthesis Method
    - • • Qualitative Systematic Review Methods
      - • • • Qualitative Meta-Synthesis Method
      - • • • Qualitative Meta-Summary Method

FIGURE 2-6 ■ The integrative research category: its affiliated research strategy and variable control-driven methods.

of participants in the study, or simply random assignment.

MASTERING THE RESEARCH LANGUAGE: DISTINCTIONS IN TERMINOLOGY ACROSS VARIOUS DISCIPLINES AND PROFESSIONS

At this point in our journey, it is understandable if the terms being used seem rather intimidating. That is to be expected because every discipline and profession has its own language, which has been developed to facilitate communication among those professionals. The same is true for the language spoken and written by researchers of various disciplines and professions.

One feature of this research language issue is that professionals in, for example, the behavioral sciences may use one name to refer to a given research method, whereas professionals in the health sciences may apply a different expression to basically the same research method. Perhaps the best example is the use of the expression "true experimental" in the behavioral sciences and the expression "randomized controlled trials" in the health sciences. Both expressions refer to essentially the same research method, which is highly valued in both realms. As we move through the remaining chapters, particularly Chapters 5 to 9, we will give a great deal of attention to acknowledging the differences in terminology used in the research process as we cross disciplines and professions.

FUNCTIONAL ANALYSIS OF THE RESEARCH PROCEDURES USED: THE ESSENTIAL SKILL FOR UNDERSTANDING THE RESEARCH PROCESS

The terminology challenge mentioned in the preceding section is best addressed by recognizing that one needs to focus on the precise procedures used in any given research study in order to understand the research process. Regardless of the expression used—be it true experimental or randomized controlled trial as an illustration—the critical task is to recognize what functions or activities are being accomplished in a given study as the study's procedures are being carried out. With that in mind, the following chapters emphasize not only the procedures that define various research methods and their designs, but the rationale or justification for such procedures. Your most important learning task in this regard is being able to analyze in a

functional way those procedures that are intended to serve the research study at hand.

WHERE DO WE GO FROM HERE?

AN OVERVIEW OF THE TRUE EXPERIMENTAL/ RANDOMIZED CONTROLLED TRIAL METHOD

The next chapter provides an overview of the true experimental/randomized controlled trial method that is one of four research methods included under the difference-oriented research strategy. As you may recall, the difference-oriented research strategy is only one of three research strategies that constitute the quantitative research category.

In exploring this particular research method, we will focus on a specific type of research design known as the randomized, control group, posttest-only design. We will highlight such research procedures as the random assignment of participants to treatment and control groups as well as the use of a treatment intervention that is manipulated (or governed) by the researcher.

REASONS WHY THIS METHOD IS SO HIGHLY VALUED IN SCIENTIFIC INQUIRY

The basic, behavioral, and health sciences have historically held in highest respect the quantitative research category and its difference-oriented research strategy. Within that strategy, the true experimental/randomized controlled trial research method has occupied a highly regarded position. This is because it alone has the extensive degree of control over features of the study that is essential for the researcher—potentially—to arrive at cause-and-effect conclusions. This early overview is important for establishing the concepts, principles, and procedures that are the most inclusive and necessary for ensuring a study that is objective, unbiased, and potentially most valuable.

At this point a quick disclaimer of sorts is needed. We make the preceding assertions in the context of the philosophical orientation of the quantitative research category. Admittedly, there are competing philosophical orientations that would—in their own contexts—justifiably disagree with the designation of the true experimental/randomized controlled trial method as a highly regarded standard for researchers. This fact is certainly recognized and represents one reason why this book addresses not only the quantitative but the qualitative and integrative research categories as well. We must, however, start the scrutiny of the research process somewhere, and for the reasons cited, we'll begin the next chapter with an overview of the true experimental/randomized controlled trial method.

REFERENCES

Creswell, J. W. (1998). *Qualitative inquiry and research design: Choosing among five traditions.* Thousands Oaks, CA: Sage.

Harris, S. (1991). *"You want proof? I'll give you proof!": More cartoons from Sidney Harris.* New York: W. H. Freeman.

Marks, D. F., & Sykes, C. M. (2004). Synthesizing evidence: Systematic reviews, meta-analysis and preference analysis. In D. F. Marks & L. Yardley (Eds.), *Research methods for clinical and health psychology* (Chap. 11, pp. 185–209). Thousand Oaks, CA: Sage.

Mulrow, C., & Cook, D. (Eds.). (1998). *Systematic reviews: Synthesis of best evidence for health care decisions.* Philadelphia: American College of Physicians.

Patterson, B. L, Thorne, S. E., Canam, C., & Jillings, C. (2001). *Meta-study of qualitative health research: A practical guide to meta-analysis and meta-synthesis.* Thousand Oaks, CA: Sage.

Peat, J. K., Mellis, C., Williams, K., & Xuan, W. (2002). *Health science research: A handbook of quantitative methods.* Thousand Oaks, CA: Sage.

ADDITIONAL RECOMMENDED RESOURCES

Cooper, H., & Hedges, L. V. (Eds.). (1994). *The handbook of research synthesis.* New York: Russell Sage Foundation.

Creswell, J. W. (2003). *Research design: Qualitative, quantitative, and mixed methods approaches* (2nd ed.). Thousand Oaks, CA: Sage.

Glasziou, P., Irwig, L., Bain, C., & Colditz, G. (2001). *Systematic reviews in health care: A practical guide.* New York: Cambridge University Press.

Thomas, R. M. (2003). *Blending qualitative & quantitative research methods in theses and dissertations.* Thousand Oaks, CA: Corwin Press.

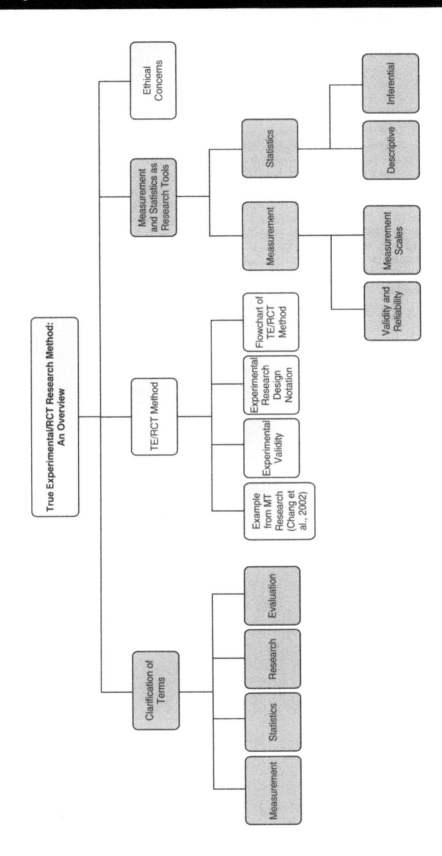

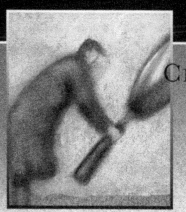

CHAPTER

3

AN OVERVIEW OF THE TRUE EXPERIMENTAL/RANDOMIZED CONTROLLED TRIAL RESEARCH METHOD

OUTLINE

OBJECTIVES

Upon completion of this chapter, the reader will have the information
necessary to perform the following tasks:

1 Define the following terms: *measurement, statistics, research,*
  and *evaluation.*

2 Working from the model provided by the example research
  study (Chang, Wang, and Chen, 2002), discuss the following
  features of that study in the context of its representing a true
  experimental/randomized controlled trial research method:
  a. research question and professional literature review
  b. population and sample
  c. random selection and random assignment as manifestations
    of randomization
  d. variables, from a research design perspective, including
    independent, dependent, extraneous, control, confounding,
    and intervening variables
  e. research hypothesis, null (or statistical) hypothesis,
    and alternative hypothesis
  f. parameter and statistic
  g. statistical analyses to include such concepts as the following:
    statistical testing and inference, alpha (α) level or probability
    of a Type I error, P value or level of significance, statistical
    power or power analysis, confidence interval, and effect size
  h. internal validity and external validity
  i. experimental research design notation

3 Working from the example, interpret and discuss a schematic
  illustration in the form of an annotated flowchart that reflects only
  select features of, and a slight modification in, this particular study.

Accessible population
Alpha (α) level (or probability of Type I error)
Alternative hypothesis
Confidence interval
Confounding variable
Control variable
Dependent variable
Descriptive statistics
Determinants of statistical usage
Effect size
Evaluation
Experimental research design notation
Experimental validity

External validity
Extraneous variable
Hypothesis
Independent variable
Inferential statistics
Institutional review board
Internal validity
Intervening variable
Measurement
Null (or statistical) hypothesis
p value (or level of significance)
Parameter
Professional literature review

Random assignment
Random selection
Randomization
Reliability (of measurement)
Research
Research hypothesis
Research question
Sample
Statistic
Statistical power (or power analysis)
Statistics
Validity (of measurement)

4 Define and discuss the two technical characteristics of a measuring instrument known as validity and reliability.

5 Explain how measurement scales as well as research strategy through research design considerations serve as critical determinants of the statistical technique(s) used in a study.

6 Distinguish between the two families of statistical techniques: descriptive statistics and inferential statistics.

7 Discuss at least three of the major ethical considerations that are prevalent in contemporary behavioral science and health science research.

8 Explain how the issues discussed in this chapter provide a foundation for moving on to the next chapter's more focused view of the concepts, principles, and procedures involved in the true experimental/randomized controlled trial research method.

WHERE HAVE WE BEEN AND WHERE ARE WE NOW? THE CONNECTION

The previous chapter used a deductive (general-to-specific) approach to viewing the research process. In so doing, we used a research continuum that proceeded from the most general level of research categories to the most specific level of research procedures. We briefly considered the research categories as being philosophically diverse and labeled as quantitative, qualitative, and integrative—with the quantitative research category acknowledged as the one that has historically dominated basic, behavioral, and health science research.

This chapter provides an overview of the quantitative research category by considering the abstract of a published research study that illustrates both the difference-oriented research strategy and, within that particular strategy, the true experimental/randomized controlled trial research method. Again, please keep in mind that the intent here is simply to provide an initial view of this highly valued type of research method. A more detailed and elaborate discussion of this method of scientific inquiry follows in the next chapter.

MEASUREMENT, STATISTICS, RESEARCH, AND EVALUATION: A CLARIFICATION OF TERMS

Measurement and statistics are tools that are critical to both the processes of research and evaluation. The term **measurement** refers to the procedure whereby numerical and/or verbal data are collected so as to show, in as valid and reliable a manner as possible, a factor or variable of interest to an investigator. As an illustration, any testing effort of an outcome of interest (for example, range of motion) is considered an instance of measurement. Once the measurement data are collected, the applied area of mathematics known as **statistics** is used to analyze and better understand what the data set is demonstrating. This is accomplished by using one or more mathematical techniques that can be selected from the areas of descriptive statistics and/or inferential statistics. For example, in the instance of descriptive statistics, calculating the arithmetic average or mean of a numerical data set would serve to describe for us the central tendency of the scores in the data set. In the instance of inferential statistics, a technique could be used that tells us if the outcome measures of participants in a study's two comparison groups are indeed different in a mathematically meaningful way. (Appendix D provides considerably more detail on both measurement and statistics as critical research tools.)

Chapter 2 provided a definition of research that spans the quantitative, qualitative, and integrative categories. As discussed, **research** is a process that attempts to advance our understanding of one or more factors of interest (called variables) by analyzing numerical and/or verbal data. This is done for the purpose of (a) characterizing one or more variables of interest, (b) investigating a possible relationship between or among two or more variables, or (c) integrating or synthesizing data from already published sources concerning one or more variables. An illustration of the second purpose just cited is that of a massage therapist serving as a member of a research team that investigates whether or not a significant relationship exists between therapeutic massage intervention and the reduction in episodes of migraine headaches (cf. Hernandez-Reif, Dieter, Field, Swerdlow, & Diego, 1998).

Any evaluative effort may follow immediately on the heels of measurement and statistical analysis or as a sequel to a research effort. In either case, **evaluation** is that process of making a value judgment or an assessment of merit concerning one or more variables of interest that have been measured and analyzed. An example might be a corporate policy decision to include in a company's health coverage package reimbursement provisions for employees who use therapeutic massage for chronic pain management. Such a decision might stem at least partially from the corporation's human resource

office being aware of research demonstrating massage therapy as a viable intervention for managing chronic pain (e.g., Cherkin et al., 2001).

THE TRUE EXPERIMENTAL/RANDOMIZED CONTROLLED TRIAL RESEARCH METHOD: A HOLISTIC VIEW

AN EXAMPLE FROM THE MASSAGE THERAPY RESEARCH LITERATURE

As an illustration of a true experimental/randomized controlled trial, Box 3-1 provides the abstract from a study by Chang, Wang, and Chen (2002). Once you have examined this excerpted abstract, we will discuss those aspects and procedures that define this study as representing a difference-oriented research strategy from the quantitative research category.

Research Question and Professional Literature Review

The starting point in any research study is the **research question** that the investigator poses at the outset. Closely affiliated with the research question is the **professional literature review**, a comprehensive examination of the professional literature that is relevant to the research question at hand. Actually, the formulation of the research question and the review of the relevant professional literature occur concurrently, in a sense, for the following reasons. Stating the research question in a specific and operational way calls for the researcher to already be somewhat familiar with studies that earlier researchers have conducted in a particular research problem area. Likewise, one would need at least the beginnings of a research question in mind to know exactly where in the vast professional literature to search for studies relevant to one's problem area.

Appendix A provides a detailed explanation of what is involved in accessing or "mining" the vast store of professional knowledge that relates to massage therapy and related health science fields. Specifically, the appendix provides guidelines for identifying those resources available in the form of bibliographic databases and making optimal use of them by way of focused search strategies that can lead to the acquisition of relevant research documents.

In the study by Chang et al. (2002), the implied research question is as follows: What are the effects of massage on the degree of pain and anxiety experienced during childbirth? More specifically, is there a statistically significant difference between participants in an experimental group receiving massage

Box 3-1   EXCERPT FROM ABSTRACT FOR A STUDY ILLUSTRATING A RANDOMIZED CONTROLLED TRIAL CONDUCTED BY CHANG, WANG, AND CHEN (2002) THAT INVESTIGATED THE EFFECTS OF MASSAGE ON PAIN AND ANXIETY DURING CHILDBIRTH

Aims. To investigate the effects of massage on pain reaction and anxiety during labour.

Background. Labour pain is a challenging issue for nurses designing intervention protocols. Massage is an ancient technique that has been widely employed during labour, however, relatively little study has been undertaken examining the effects of massage on women in labour.

Methods. A randomized controlled study was conducted between September 1999 and January 2000. Sixty primiparous women expected to have a normal childbirth at a regional hospital in southern Taiwan were randomly assigned to either the experimental ($n = 30$) or the control ($n = 30$) group. The experimental group received massage intervention whereas the control group did not. The nurse-rated present behavioural intensity (PBI) was used as a measure of labour pain. Anxiety was measured with the visual analogue scale for anxiety (VASA). The intensity of pain and anxiety between the two groups was compared in the latent phase (cervix dilated 3-4 cm), active phase (5-7 cm) and transitional phase (8-10 cm).

Results. In both groups, there was a relatively steady increase in pain intensity and anxiety level as labour progressed. An *t-test* demonstrated that the experimental group had significantly lower pain reactions in the latent, active and transitional phases. Anxiety levels were only significantly different between the two groups in the latent phase. Twenty-six of the 30 (87%) experimental group subjects reported that massage was helpful, providing pain relief and psychological support during labour.

Conclusions. Findings suggest that massage is a cost-effective nursing intervention that can decrease pain and anxiety during labour, and partners' participation in massage can positively influence the quality of women's birth experiences.

Keywords: massage, labour pain, anxiety, partner participation, childbirth

From Chang, M. Y., Wang, S. Y., & Chen, C. H. (2002). Effects of massage on pain and anxiety during labor: A randomized controlled trial. *Journal of Advanced Nursing, 38*(1), 68–73.

and those in a control group not receiving massage relative to the degree of pain and anxiety experienced during childbirth? Regarding the literature review, the 24 citations in the body of the research report itself and listed in the references section at the end of the article identify the efforts of other researchers who have addressed a similar research interest.

Another important aspect of the research question in this study is that it is a difference-oriented research question. This terminology is used because the research question is basically asking if there is a *difference* between the two comparison groups (i.e., the experimental group receiving the massage intervention and the control group not receiving massage), relative to the outcome measures of degrees of pain and anxiety. Because this research question is difference oriented, it is necessary that the researchers use a *difference-oriented research strategy*. Included under the difference-oriented research strategy is the true experimental, or randomized controlled trial, research method. Details as to why the research method in this study is considered a true experimental or randomized controlled trial method are addressed later in this chapter.

Population and Sample

Although this study's report identifies a total of 60 women who participated in the research, the abstract and body of the report are silent on the size of the original group from which the participants were recruited. That information would have allowed us to identify the number of potential study participants in the **accessible population** (also known as the set or universe or macrocosm of potential participants). As reported, though, we can easily recognize that the **sample** (also known as the subset or microcosm of actual participants) included 60 women who would, in turn, be members of the two comparison groups having 30 participants each.

Randomization: Random Selection and Random Assignment

This study recruited the 60 participants from a regional hospital in a sequential manner (in other words, as they became available by virtue of their admission to the hospital to give birth). As hinted earlier, one alternative to the sampling method used would have been for the researchers to identify a set number of maternity patient admissions anticipated over the span of a designated time period, thus allowing the identification of a set number of potential study participants that would have constituted the study's accessible population. With that feature of the study in place, the researchers would then have had the option to *randomly select* the 60 participants from the larger set/universe/macrocosm of patients defining the accessible population. The ramifications of using **random selection** will become apparent later in this chapter when we turn our attention to a study's external validity.

As the study was conducted, though, the available participants totaled 60 and represented the study's sample. **Random assignment** was then used to allocate 30 of the participants to the experimental group that received the massage intervention and 30 to the control group that did not receive massage. The terminology of random assignment of participants to comparison groups means that each of the 60 subjects had an equal and nonzero chance of being assigned to either comparison group. The ramifications of using random assignment, likewise, will be addressed later in this chapter when we consider the study's internal validity.

Variables From a Research Design Perspective

Those aspects or features of interest in this study that have the potential to vary or change are the study's *variables*. The subsections that follow focus on several types of variables that can be identified from a research design perspective. This clarification is important because variables may also be considered from other perspectives, namely, a measurement perspective and a conceptual/theoretical perspective. These other two perspectives are addressed later in this book.

Independent Variable.

The **independent variable** (IV) in this study is the extent to which massage therapy is provided to each of the 60 participants. Because we are dealing with two comparison groups, one that is receiving massage and the other that is not, we can say that the IV has two levels—or, is being manifested in two ways—namely, the presence and the absence of the massage therapy intervention. Level 1, then, of our IV is the presence of the massage intervention that serves to define our experimental group (EG); level 2 of our IV is the absence of the massage intervention that in turn defines our control group (CG). Accordingly, we have only one IV, yet two levels of the IV that represent our two comparison groups. In this particular study, we can also say that the researchers are manipulating our one IV in that they actually govern (or determine) the two ways in which the IV is being manifested. The existence of a *manipulated IV* is precisely what one encounters when any type of treatment or intervention is used in a research study, be that treatment a massage modality, instructional method, drug dosage, medical procedure, or psychotherapeutic intervention. Possible synonyms for independent variable include *stimulus variable, input variable, treatment variable,* or *causal variable.*

Dependent Variable.

In a true experimental/randomized controlled trial, the manipulated IV is considered to be a potential cause of some outcome or effect being measured among the participants. The study's outcome is viewed as a potential effect of the impact of the manipulated IV. This particular variable, then, is identified as the study's **dependent variable** (DV) because it represents an outcome or effect that presumably is dependent on, or caused by, the manipulated IV. Possible synonyms for dependent variable include such expressions as *response variable, output variable, outcome variable, consequent variable,* or *effect variable.* In the Chang et al. (2002) study, the researchers investigated two DVs: pain and anxiety intensity during labor.

Extraneous Variable.

In studies comparable to the one we are considering, the researchers are principally—though not exclusively—interested in whether or not there is a meaningful relationship between the IV and the DV. However, many other variables are present in the study beyond the manipulated IV and the DV. These other variables may relate to characteristics of the study's participants as well as to characteristics of the setting or circumstance in which the study is being conducted. They are present in the study, though not the principal or primary focus of the researchers' interest, and, hence, are considered to be extraneous to the study's major emphasis. Accordingly, any one of these variables is referred to as an **extraneous variable** simply because it is extraneous to the study's main interest.

Extraneous variables that pertain to characteristics of the study's participants, sometimes also referred to as personological or organismic variables, include individual differences in traits and features that distinguish one person from another. These person-specific features include, to name only a few in a vast array of perhaps hundreds, such variables as health status, lifestyles and work habits, intelligence, socioeconomic status, race, gender, ethnicity, motivational and compliance tendencies, behavioral habits affecting one's health, genetic inclinations, aptitudes, avocational interests, occupation, family of origin, self-esteem, and academic background.

Likewise, characteristics of the setting or circumstance in which a study is conducted may indeed be extraneous to the study's primary concern. Examples in this realm of extraneous variables may include such situation-specific features as time of day, climatic conditions, unanticipated noise or lighting fluctuations, personal interaction dynamics of participants and others, unintentional influences of the study's personnel on the participants, and ergonomic features of furniture and surroundings.

In the results section of the Chang et al. (2002) study, the researchers acknowledged among the 60 participants several demographic and obstetric characteristics such as age of mother, maternal weight, gestation age, newborn weight, and duration of labor. Each of these factors represents an extraneous variable in this particular study.

Control Variable. If ignored, any extraneous variable in a study has the potential to confuse the manner in which the completed study is eventually interpreted. Researchers therefore must address these extraneous variables in such a way as to ensure that the comparison groups are equivalent at the outset of a study on as many of the extraneous variables as possible. Although there are several procedures for bringing about this so-called equivalence of comparison groups, one approach that is essential to any true experimental or randomized controlled trial is that of randomly assigning participants to the comparison groups. Such a procedure was used in this abstracted study, with the resulting assignment of 30 participants to the experimental group and 30 to the control group. This feature of **randomization** allows the researcher a certain degree of latitude in assuming—though not guaranteeing—that the two comparison groups are essentially equal on extraneous variables that are particularly relevant to the study. In other words, this procedure of random assignment allows one to view the potentially problematic extraneous variables as having been "controlled" in that the assumption—again, not a guarantee—is that the comparison groups are basically similar on any given extraneous variable. Accordingly, those variables that are so controlled are referred to as **control variables**.

Confounding Variable. If an extraneous variable is not appropriately controlled, then the potential exists for that variable to be *un*equally present in the comparison groups. This occurrence would result in the original extraneous variable becoming what is known as a **confounding variable**. If this scenario develops, then any differences between the two groups on a dependent variable might well be the result of the uncontrolled extraneous variable, now labeled the confounding variable, because that variable is having the impact of confusing or confounding our proper interpretation of the study. The result here is that the true relationship between the IV and DV would be somewhat disguised due to the possibility

that another variable (i.e., the confounding variable) has influenced the outcome of the study in an unanticipated way. In our abstracted study, any one or more of the several demographic and obstetric features (e.g., age of mother, maternal weight, gestation age, newborn weight, and duration of labor) could potentially function as a confounding variable if not adequately controlled.

Intervening Variable. An **intervening variable** in a study is the factor that is proposed or theorized as a plausible explanation for why the researchers obtained the results that were indeed uncovered. In more common parlance, the intervening variable is the variable that explains "why we got what we got" in a study. A synonym for the intervening variable, then, is the *explanatory variable*. It is that variable that *intervened* at some point between the onset of the IV and the eventual measurement of the DV and now represents a viable explanation of why the IV had the impact it had on the DV. In massage therapy research in general, the appeal to so-called underlying mechanisms typically captures the idea of intervening variables in that a proposed underlying mechanism represents a potential explanation of what factor came into play to explain why the results of the study were what they were (see, e.g., Field, 2000).

In the abstracted study we are now using, several intervening variables were acknowledged as possible explanations for the study's findings. Among the possible explanations considered in the discussion section of the report itself were psychosocial factors impacting the participating nurses/midwives, the participants themselves, and their spouses. Also considered were physiological factors related to the gate control theory of pain management as well as increased levels of endorphins and increased vagal activity.

Hypotheses

The research procedure of formulating hypotheses is critical to any scientific investigation. Just as a study's research question is informed by the researchers' familiarity with the relevant professional literature, a study's hypotheses likewise reflect the pertinent literature and are specific to the research question being investigated.

In its most basic form, a **hypothesis** is a statement that (a) is founded or justified by way of some conceptual, theoretical, experiential, or research basis and (b) predicts a research outcome regarding the study's sample or population. Although not always stated directly or explicitly, the hypotheses for a study typically assume three forms that are critical to the research process. The following three subsections identify these hypotheses, and where appropriate they make reference to the excerpted abstract's study presented in Box 3-1.

Research Hypothesis. At the outset of a study, specifically when the research question is being formulated in the context of what the relevant professional literature has to say about the problem area, the researchers formulate the study's research hypothesis. The **research hypothesis** is simply a well-justified prediction of the study's anticipated outcome in the context of the study's sample. In a sense it is the researchers' predicted answer to the study's research question in the context of the sample. In a difference-oriented research strategy, for example, the research question being addressed is difference oriented in the manner described earlier in this chapter. Accordingly, the research hypothesis likewise is difference oriented.

As an illustration, the excerpted abstract implies a research hypothesis that could be stated as follows: There will be a statistically significant difference between participants in an experimental group receiving massage and those in a control group not receiving massage relative to the degrees of pain and anxiety intensity experienced during childbirth. More specifically, the participants in the experimental group receiving massage will demonstrate significantly lesser degrees of pain and anxiety intensity during childbirth than will those participants in the control group not receiving massage.

This research hypothesis (a) provides a predicted answer to the study's research question, (b) is founded on or justified by some conceptual, theoretical, experiential, or research basis reflected in the professional literature, and (c) speaks to one or more characteristics or properties of the sample used in the study. Contrary to an unfounded fear that some students of the research process have regarding a research hypothesis, such a prediction at the outset of a study neither compromises the objectivity of the study nor suggests any bias on the part of the researchers. Typical studies are not conducted in some sort of intellectual vacuum. A study is planned and implemented against the backdrop of an intellectual history and in the context of a current intellectual milieu. Consequently, some attempt at predicting a well-founded outcome to a study is to be expected and must be reported by the researchers at the study's conclusion, even if the actual results of the study are contrary to what was predicted from the outset. Intellectual honesty and professional ethics demand no less of researchers with respect to acknowledging objectively the actual results of a study, regardless of how contrary they might be to the researchers' initial predictions.

A decision to confirm or disconfirm a study's research hypothesis is not made as a result of testing the research hypothesis directly. Instead, it is the null hypothesis that we test statistically, as we will discuss in the following section.

Null (or Statistical) Hypothesis. The **null (or statistical) hypothesis** is that prediction of a study's outcome that (a) asserts the absence of a statistically significant relationship between or among the study's variables, (b) speaks to one or more characteristics or properties of the study's population, (c) is the focal point in a study's statistical analysis, and (d) provides the basis for inferring a decision back to the study's research hypothesis and alternative hypothesis (with the latter hypothesis still awaiting our discussion in the next subsection).

For example, the Chang et al. (2002) study implies a null hypothesis that could be stated as follows: There will be no statistically significant difference between participants in that segment of the population represented by the experimental group receiving massage and participants in that segment of the population represented by the control group not receiving massage relative to the degrees of pain and anxiety intensity experienced during childbirth.

This formal statement of the null hypothesis is saying that, in the population represented by the sample, there is no statistically significant relationship between the IV of extent of massage therapy intervention and the DVs of degrees of pain and anxiety intensity experienced during childbirth. This prediction takes the operational form of stating that in the population represented by the sample, there is no statistically significant difference between the two levels of the IV relative to the two DVs under investigation. Again, it is this null statement that is subjected to a study's statistical analysis. The decision thus made regarding the null hypothesis becomes the basis for inferring a decision back to both the research hypothesis and the alternative hypothesis. If the statistical test of a study's null hypothesis results in its being rejected, then the researchers may infer a confirmation of the research and alternative hypotheses.

Having already mentioned the alternative hypothesis in this section, the time is perhaps overdue for us to clarify precisely what this hypothesis entails.

Alternative Hypothesis. The alternative hypothesis might be viewed as somewhat of an intermediary between the research hypothesis and the null hypothesis. More to the point, the **alternative hypothesis** is a prediction of a study's anticipated outcome in the context of the population. In a sense, then, it is the researchers' predicted answer to the study's research question in the context of the population (as opposed to the study's sample).

For example, the implied alternative hypothesis in our abstracted study could be stated as follows: There will be a statistically significant difference between participants in that segment of the population represented by the experimental group receiving massage and participants in that segment of the population represented by the control group not receiving massage relative to the degrees of pain and anxiety intensity experienced during childbirth. More specifically, participants in that segment of the population represented by the experimental group receiving massage will demonstrate significantly lesser degrees of pain and anxiety intensity during childbirth than will those participants in that segment of the population represented by the control group not receiving massage.

The research hypothesis and the alternative hypothesis have in common the fact that each is making an identical prediction of a statistically significant difference between the levels of the IV relative to the study's two DVs in favor of the experimental group. It is precisely in this sense that the alternative hypothesis is considered, quite literally, an alternative to the prediction of the null hypothesis.

The research hypothesis and the alternative hypothesis, however, certainly do differ in that the research hypothesis is predicting an outcome in terms of the study's sample, whereas the alternative hypothesis is predicting an outcome in the context of the study's population. The alternative and null hypotheses have in common the fact that each is predicting an outcome regarding the study's population.

Parameter and Statistic

The terms *parameter* and *statistic* have specific meanings in any discussion of the research process. **Parameter** refers to any characteristic, property, or feature of a population, whereas **statistic** pertains to any characteristic, property, or feature of a sample.

For example, part of our illustrative study focuses on the average or mean degree of pain intensity experienced by the participants during childbirth. The mean degree of pain during childbirth can be

considered a feature or property of the population from which our sample was derived. In the context of the study's population, the mean degree of pain is considered to be a parameter. In a somewhat comparable way, the mean degree of pain during childbirth can be viewed as a feature or property of the sample that has been derived from the study's population. In the context of the study's sample, the mean degree of pain is considered to be a *statistic*.

A verbal analogy here may be helpful for remembering the distinction between parameter and statistic. We could say, "parameter is to population as statistic is to sample." Expressed in another form, the analogy might look like this:

parameter : population :: statistic : sample

In the context of hypotheses, our earlier discussion should now allow us to recognize that the research hypothesis is always a prediction that is specific to a sample statistic, whereas the null and alternative hypotheses are always predictions that are specific to a population parameter.

Statistical Analysis

Statistical Testing and Inference. The research process involves both measurement procedures and statistical analyses as vital tools for collecting data on variables of interest and for analyzing the data so as to make our understanding of the variables clearer. For example, the massage and childbirth study involved the measurement of pain and anxiety intensity levels as the two DVs, and then proceeded to statistically analyze the data sets in order to test the study's null hypothesis.

The appropriate use of measurement and statistical testing are critical research procedures that allow investigators to make two important inferences: (a) The statistical analysis of data collected on a given DV enables the researchers to test the null hypothesis. The decision made regarding the null hypothesis—namely, to reject or fail to reject the null—then permits an inferential decision back to both the alternative and research hypotheses. (b) If indeed a study has employed random selection of participants from an accessible population for the purpose of forming the sample, then the statistical analysis of the study's hypotheses allows an inference of what is learned about the sample back to the accessible population.

Alpha (α) Level or Probability of a Type I Error. An important feature of scientific inquiry involves the statistical analysis of data for hypothesis-testing purposes.

It is the realization that the statistical conclusion arrived at is never absolute and is always couched in probability terms. When testing a null hypothesis, for example, a decision to reject the null is always accompanied by an admission that there is a certain probability that we may be making an error in doing so. That probability level, also known as the **alpha (α) level (or probability of Type I error)**, is established before the actual analysis is completed. If the decision is to reject the null, alpha indicates the probability or likelihood that we are committing a *Type I error* (i.e., rejecting the null when in reality it should not be rejected). In the behavioral sciences, an alpha level of .05 is customary; in many of the basic and health science areas of research, though, a lower and more demanding alpha is set (e.g., at .01).

p Value or Level of Significance.

In addition to establishing an alpha level when testing a null hypothesis, there is another type of probability context in which any decision regarding the null is made. The *p* **value (or level of significance)** signifies the likelihood or probability of obtaining by chance the results of our statistical analysis if indeed our null hypothesis is actually valid. In a sense, researchers are searching for statistical results in a study that have such a low likelihood or probability of having occurred by chance that it becomes more tenable to conclude that the results were driven by some nonchance reality, namely, the reality of an authentic relationship between or among the variables being studied.

In our childbirth study, for example, the statistical analysis indicated that the experimental group receiving massage had significantly lower pain reactions across all three labor phases than did the control group. Translated, this means that the statistical analysis of the data collected on the pain intensity DV had such a low likelihood or probability of occurring by chance (if indeed the null hypothesis is true) that it was more reasonable or tenable to conclude that some *non*chance reality is responsible for our findings. That *non*chance reality in this instance is the strong and convincing likelihood that a significant relationship exists between our IV and DV, thereby allowing a conclusion that the massage intervention—as contrasted with its absence—is responsible for lowering the participants' pain level in the experimental group.

Statistical Power (or Power Analysis).

Still another type of probability context in which a null hypothesis is

tested is the statistical power present when the analysis occurs. The **statistical power (or power analysis)** that exists when the data on a given DV are being statistically analyzed refers to the probability or mathematical odds that the analysis will result in a rejection of the null hypothesis when in reality the null is false and, hence, should be rejected. Unfortunately, not all research reports provide for this type of calculation. It is critical, though, for a power analysis to be performed by researchers because it relates in part to the number of participants needed in a study for an appropriate probability (usually at least .80) to exist for rejecting the null if indeed it should be rejected.

Confidence Interval.

Researchers in the basic, behavioral, and health sciences typically supplement or augment their hypothesis testing with the calculation of a **confidence interval**. Although various types of confidence intervals may be reported in the results section of a research report, in its most basic form we can consider a confidence interval as referring to a range of numerical values that has a certain probability of *capturing* the true population parameter under investigation in a study. For example, a 95% confidence interval (CI) would identify both the lower and upper limits of that range of numerical values that we are 95% confident actually contain or capture the true population parameter under investigation in a study (e.g., the population mean of pain intensity level).

Effect Size.

In a manner similar to reporting confidence intervals as a supplement to hypothesis testing, researchers across various science areas should also report in their analysis what is known as an **effect size**. Here, too, there are several variations of this particular statistical concept, but in its basic form an effect size refers to the degree or extent of influence or *effect* of the IV on the DV in a study. An effect size may be quantified as (a) the proportion of variation on the DV measures that can be explained or accounted for by the IV and/or (b) the size of the difference between the means of two comparison groups as indicated in standard deviation units.

EXPERIMENTAL VALIDITY

The **experimental validity** of a difference-oriented study refers to the degree of control that researchers are positioned to exercise over the several variables present in an investigation. In the context of a true experimental or randomized controlled trial, two types of experimental validity designated as internal validity and external validity are of paramount importance. The internal validity issue in these studies is typically a more important concern than the external validity issue, although the integrity of each type of validity should be ensured if at all possible.

Internal Validity

The issue of **internal validity** in a difference-oriented study involves the extent to which the dependent variable measures can be traced exclusively back to the influence of the independent variable. The greater the degree of internal validity in a study, the better positioned a researcher is to relate the IV to the DV in a cause-and-effect fashion. The heightened level of internal validity is precisely what defines the true experimental or randomized controlled trial as such a highly valued approach to research. More specifically, the two critical research procedures that serve to increase a study's internal validity are the use of random assignment and a manipulated IV.

The *random assignment* of participants to the comparison groups in a study helps to control the extraneous variables that otherwise run the risk of functioning as confounding variables. As mentioned earlier in this chapter, the random assignment of participants to the comparison groups or levels of the IV allows one to assume—though not guarantee—that the comparison groups are essentially equivalent on the major extraneous variables pertinent to the study. Once the *manipulated IV* is then introduced, the comparison groups can now be thought of as differing, by intent and design, on only that one single variable, namely, the manipulated IV. The experimental group is now defined as receiving the experimental or treatment level of the manipulated IV being studied, whereas the control group is not. If a difference eventually occurs between the two comparison groups relative to the DV, then we can reasonably infer that this effect in all likelihood is traceable back to the manipulated IV (i.e., the only earlier variable on which the participants differed). This sequence and line of reasoning, then, becomes the basis for possibly inferring a causal relationship between the manipulated IV and the DV.

The childbirth study abstracted earlier does indeed contain these two essential research procedures for elevating the study's internal validity. The 60 participants in the sample were randomly assigned to the experimental and control groups,

and the IV was manipulated to establish—by intent and design—a planned distinction or difference between the two groups on that one single variable. The stage was then set for any difference between the two groups on either the pain intensity DV or the anxiety level DV to be traced back to the manipulated IV that involved the presence versus the absence of massage intervention.

External Validity

The issue of **external validity** in a study considers the extent to which the conclusions reached can be generalized from the sample back to the accessible population from which the sample was derived. A study is implemented in the context of both (a) those participants who actually constitute the sample and (b) the setting or circumstances that operationally define the research procedures used. Understandably, one would be interested in generalizing as extensively as possible from the comparatively limited sample back to the original accessible population.

The random selection of participants from the accessible population is the research procedure most critical to elevating the external validity of a study. This is the case largely because random selection allows the researchers to assume that the resulting sample so derived is an unbiased and representative subset or microcosm of the larger population (set or macrocosm). This assumption is based on the role of random selection in ensuring that each member of the accessible population has an equal and nonzero chance of being included in the sample. Properly performed, random selection allows chance factors alone to operate in determining which participants in the accessible population become members of the sample, thereby protecting against any systematically biased influence on the selection process.

The childbirth study that we have been considering did not use the procedure of random selection, but instead recruited participants sequentially as they entered the maternity ward in a regional hospital. Consequently, the ability of the researchers to generalize with confidence the study's findings back to an accessible population is seriously compromised to a large extent. This is the case because (a) the accessible population was not thoroughly defined as a known set of potential participants in terms of size and characteristics of the group and, consequently, (b) there was no way of mathematically ensuring that each member of the sample had the same probability as other members of being selected.

Having seen the relationship between random assignment and internal validity as well as the connection between random selection and external validity, a verbal analogy would be useful to study. We could say, "random assignment is to internal validity as random selection is to external validity." Expressed in another form, the analogy would look like this:

random assignment : internal validity :: random
selection : external validity

EXPERIMENTAL RESEARCH DESIGN NOTATION

The holistic view that we are taking in this chapter of the true experimental or randomized controlled trial type of study has involved quite an accumulation of concepts, principles, procedures, and terminology that might come across as somewhat intimidating. A strong recommendation at this point is for you to keep foremost in mind the overarching context within which our discussion is occurring.

If we were to rely only on narrative descriptive labels, we could say that the Chang et al. (2002) study is (a) a randomized, control-group, posttest-only research design that is (b) one of several possible designs affiliated with the true experimental/randomized controlled trial research method that is included in (c) the difference-oriented research strategy that is recognized as (d) belonging to the quantitative research category.

Experimental research design notation that takes the following form can economically display the specifics of the preceding paragraph:

$$RA \quad EG \quad X \quad O_{Post}$$
$$RA \quad CG \quad \bullet \quad O_{Post}$$

This display is interpreted as follows: The *RA* indicates the random assignment of participants to both the experimental group (*EG*) and the control group (*CG*) as in the childbirth study. The *X* designates the experimental level of the manipulated IV that in the childbirth study is the presence of massage for those 30 participants in the experimental group. The $\bullet$ represents the nonexperimental level of the manipulated IV that in the study is the absence of massage for those 30 participants in the control group. The O_{Post} at the end of each horizontal row indicates that both the experimental group and the control group were postobserved, or posttested, on each of the DVs.

This research design notation display allows us to *read* the design of the study as being a *randomized, control-group, posttest-only research design*. That realization, in turn, becomes the prompt for us to

recognize that such a research design logically belongs to the *true experimental/randomized controlled trial research method* because of the use of random assignment and a manipulated IV. Furthermore, this recognition then leads us to recall that any research method examining the relationship between an IV and a DV must, of necessity, belong to the *difference-oriented research strategy* family. This is because the relationship between an IV and a DV is explored by investigating whether or not there is a difference between or among the two or more levels of the IV relative to the DV. Now we recognize that this particular research strategy is one of three possible research strategies constituting the *quantitative research category*.

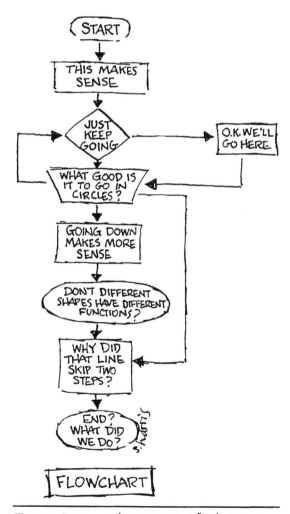

HUMOR BREAK ■ A warm-up exercise in flowcharting to prepare for the very next section! (From Harris, S. [1991]. *"You want proof? I'll give you proof!": More cartoons from Sidney Harris.* New York: W. H. Freeman.)

SCHEMATIC ILLUSTRATION OF THE TRUE EXPERIMENTAL/RANDOMIZED CONTROLLED TRIAL RESEARCH METHOD

The holistic view of the true experimental/randomized controlled trial research method that provides a context for our discussion throughout most of this chapter is succinctly displayed by the schematic illustration provided in Figure 3-1. This figure reflects only select features of, as well as a slight modification in, the childbirth study by Chang et al. (2002) to allow a panoramic view of the research

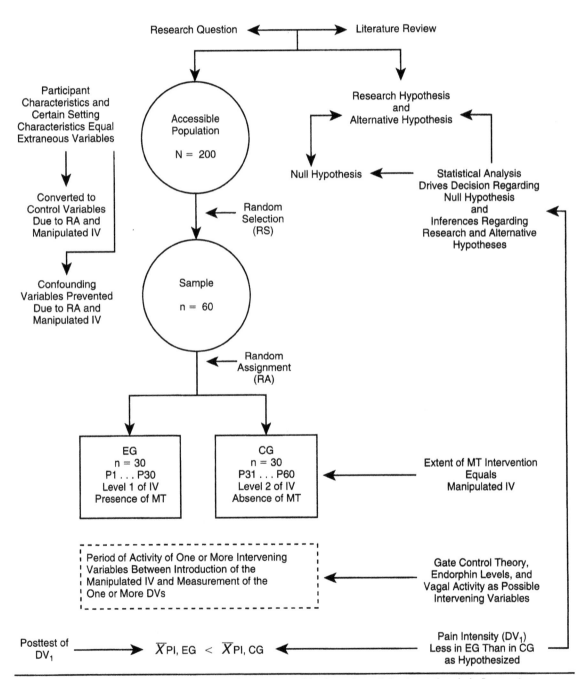

FIGURE 3-1 ■ Schematic illustration of true experimental/randomized controlled trial research method reflecting only select features of and a slight modification in the Chang et al. (2002) study.

process that we have examined thus far, which has involved a sequential and linear progression of certain concepts, principles, and procedures.

Specifically, the progression reflected in this schematic begins with the simultaneous interplay between formulating the research question and reviewing the professional literature. This interplay becomes the basis for initiating the sequence of research procedures that begins with the accessible population (the slight modification in the actual study) and continues to the eventual decision to reject the null hypothesis regarding the DV of pain intensity. The interplay between the research question and the literature review is also the basis for the researchers formulating the research hypothesis at the outset of the study as well as the implied null and alternative hypotheses that follow.

OVERVIEW OF MEASUREMENT AND STATISTICS AS RESEARCH TOOLS

Before proceeding with this overview of measurement and statistics, please recall that Appendix D to this book addresses in greater detail both measurement and statistics as critical tools in the research process. The intent in this section is to provide you with only a brief coverage of certain themes in measurement and statistics that are appropriate at this point in our journey to understand the research process.

THE NECESSITY OF VALID AND RELIABLE MEASURING INSTRUMENTS

At the very least, any study will involve the measurement of the DV. Several characteristics of any measuring instrument must be taken into account for research projects to generate trusted data. Two of the most critical characteristics (also known as psychometric or technical characteristics) of any measuring instrument are its validity and reliability.

The *validity* of an instrument refers to the extent to which the instrument is actually measuring what it claims to be measuring. Stated another way, validity refers to the degree to which an instrument is doing what it claims or purports to be doing. Because different instruments may have different purposes and, therefore, different claims as to what they are doing, various types of validity may need to be considered.

An instrument's **reliability (of measurement)** pertains to the consistency of measurement that the instrument is demonstrating. Here, too, consistency

of measurement might be viewed in different contexts. For example, we might consider the consistency of measurement of an entire instrument across two or more points in time. Also, we might consider the consistency of measurement internal to the instrument itself as we examine the responses of participants across the initial, middle, and concluding sections of the instrument. From different perspectives, then, researchers must ensure that the measurement tools being used to collect data on a variable of interest are doing so in a consistent fashion. Otherwise, all of the subsequent statistical analyses of the data will be seriously compromised.

These two technical characteristics of measuring instruments are not completely independent of each other, nor fully related. Reliability is a prerequisite for validity (in other words, an instrument cannot be valid unless it is reliable). This is the case because if an instrument is inconsistently measuring a variable, then the numbers generated have no real meaning in terms of what they represent. Accordingly, we cannot have any confidence regarding what the instrument is measuring. Again, reliability is a prerequisite for validity. Or, stated another way, validity guarantees reliability.

On the other hand, it is not necessary for an instrument to be valid in order for it to be reliable. As an illustration, someone could measure your height and claim that it is a measure of your blood pressure. Even if the measurement of your height were consistent (reliable), it would not follow that the measurement effort is valid (as obviously it is not). Reliability does not guarantee validity.

MEASUREMENT SCALE AND RESEARCH STRATEGY, METHOD, AND DESIGN AS CRITICAL DETERMINANTS OF STATISTICAL USAGE

The selection of the appropriate statistical technique for analyzing data that have been collected on a given variable (for example, a DV) is dependent on specific criteria. Though not a complete discussion at this point, we can identify certain considerations or **determinants of statistical usage** that must be taken into account when determining which statistical technique should be used.

One such criterion is the measurement scale on which your DV has been documented. As elaborated on in Appendix D, the nominal and ordinal scales would call for a nonparametric statistical technique to be used. If the DV has been measured on the interval or ratio scale, however, then a statistical technique from the parametric statistical family would most likely be appropriate. Other criteria that would come into play in choosing an appropriate statistical technique for analyzing your data include such factors as the research strategy used as well as the research method and its affiliated research design.

Again, Appendix D provides a more detailed discussion of these themes as well as several other factors that must be considered in making a justifiable selection of the best statistical technique for analyzing your data.

DISTINCTIONS BETWEEN DESCRIPTIVE STATISTICS AND INFERENTIAL STATISTICS

Statistics is an area of applied mathematics that is a critical tool for researchers in the effort to make data that have been collected on variables in a research study both manageable and meaningful. Statistics can be thought of as being divided into two major categories, or "families," of techniques: descriptive statistics and inferential statistics.

Descriptive statistics refers to that family of quantitative techniques that allows us to characterize, portray, or literally describe a data set in succinct and economical ways. Subdivisions within descriptive statistics include such clusters of techniques as graphical techniques, measures of central tendency, measures of variability, and possibly correlational techniques. Familiar illustrations from each of these four subdivisions, respectively, might include pie charts, the arithmetic average or mean, the range of scores, and a correlation coefficient.

Inferential statistics refers to that family of quantitative techniques that primarily allows us not only to test hypotheses in a study but also to estimate values in a population from which a sample has been derived and on which data have been generated. Inferential statistics can be subdivided into two clusters of techniques known as parametric statistics and nonparametric statistics. A partial distinction between these two subdivisions was made in the preceding section of this chapter, along with more detailed coverage in Appendix D.

MAJOR ETHICAL CONSIDERATIONS PREVALENT IN BEHAVIORAL SCIENCE AND HEALTH SCIENCE RESEARCH

Our brief look at the Chang et al. (2002) study throughout most of this chapter could have caused you to reflect on some of the ethical considerations that may have arisen prior to, during, and after the actual study.

For example, what kinds of collegial input and supervision were the researchers provided both before and during the study with respect to the study's design as well as the measures taken to protect the participants during the conduct of the study? Was there any type of institutional review of the study's proposal in advance of its being implemented? What types of information regarding the study were provided to the participants in advance of their actual involvement in the investigation? What type of consent was received from the participants prior to their admission to the study? Did the participants have the option to discontinue their involvement at any time and without prejudice? Were there any questions regarding the confidentiality of the data collected on the several variables for each participant? Also, what would have been your thoughts and feelings if you or a family member were assigned to the control group and, in effect, not provided with the massage intervention? And were you curious as to whether or not the study's results were shared with the participants afterward?

These are just a few of several important concerns that relate to the ethical conduct of research. Issues pertaining to the role of an **institutional review board** (IRB) in granting approval for the study to be conducted would certainly have encompassed most if not all of the concerns expressed in the preceding paragraph. Informed consent, confidentiality, latitude to exit the study at any time without prejudice, entitlement of the control group participants to the experimental level of the IV, and debriefing are among an array of ethical issues that researchers must face responsibly. This is essential because the advancement of science must not occur at the expense of the safety and well-being of research participants.

Appendix B provides considerably more detailed coverage of ethical principles governing research in the behavioral and health sciences. Furthermore, subsequent chapters will certainly acknowledge and discuss various ethical concerns as they relate to conducting research with the protection of research participants foremost in mind.

WHERE DO WE GO FROM HERE?

A MORE FOCUSED VIEW OF THE TRUE EXPERIMENTAL/RANDOMIZED CONTROLLED TRIAL RESEARCH METHOD

Our use of the Chang et al. (2002) study's abstract and the discussion it provoked was intended to introduce you to several of the basic concepts, principles, and procedures that define the true experimental research process. With that overview completed, we are now in a better position to delve more deeply into the nature of the true experimental/randomized controlled trial research method and its favored place in the research continuum.

CONCEPTS, PRINCIPLES, AND PROCEDURES CONSIDERED IN DETAIL

Chapter 4 is actually an extension of this chapter in that many of the topics we have addressed here are revisited, but with somewhat more elaboration and in greater detail. Particular attention will be given to clarifying where, how, and why the true experimental/randomized controlled trial research method is located in the difference-oriented research strategy that is, in turn, part of the quantitative research category.

The latter part of the upcoming chapter will provide in its entirety a published study illustrating, once again, the true experimental/randomized controlled trial research method. This will give us the opportunity to analyze in somewhat greater detail the concepts, principles, and procedures that have already been introduced. This exercise will provide a basis for you to complete—independently and at a later time—a similar critique not only of a comparable study of your choosing but also of studies that represent variations from the highly regarded true experimental/randomized controlled trial.

REFERENCES

Chang, M. Y., Wang, S. Y., & Chen, C. H. (2002). Effects of massage on pain and anxiety during labour: A randomized controlled trial in Taiwan. *Journal of Advanced Nursing, 38*(1), 68–73.

Cherkin, D. C., Eisenberg, D., Sherman, K. J., Barlow, W., Kaptchuk, T. J., Street, J., et al. (2001). Randomized trial comparing traditional Chinese medical acupuncture, therapeutic massage, and self-care education for chronic low back pain. *Archives of Internal Medicine, 161*, 1081–1088.

Field, T. M. (2000). *Touch therapy.* New York: Churchill Livingstone.

Harris, S. (1991). *"You want proof? I'll give you proof!": More cartoons from Sidney Harris.* New York: W. H. Freeman.

Hernandez-Reif, M., Dieter, J., Field, T., Swerdlow, B., & Diego, M. (1998). Migraine headaches are reduced by massage therapy. *International Journal of Neuroscience, 96*, 1–11.

ADDITIONAL RECOMMENDED RESOURCES

Lilienfeld, A. M. (1982). *Ceteris paribus*: The evolution of the clinical trial. *Bulletin of the History of Medicine, 56*, 1–18.

Mathai, S., Fernandez, A., Mondkar, J., & Kanbur, W. (2001). Effects of tactile-kinesthetic stimulation in preterms: A controlled trial. *Indian Pediatrics, 38*, 1091–1098.

Moher, D., Jadad, A. R., Nichol, G., Penman, M., Tugwell, P., & Walsh, S. (1995). Assessing the quality of randomized controlled trials: An annotated bibliography of scales and checklists. *Controlled Clinical Trials, 16*, 62–73.

Moher, D., Jadad, A. R., & Tugwell, P. (1996). Assessing the quality of randomized controlled trials: Current issues and future directions. *International Journal of Technology Assessment in Health Care, 12*(2), 195–208.

Sackett, D. L., & Wennberg, J. E. (1997). Choosing the best research design for each question. *BMJ, 315*(7123), 1636.

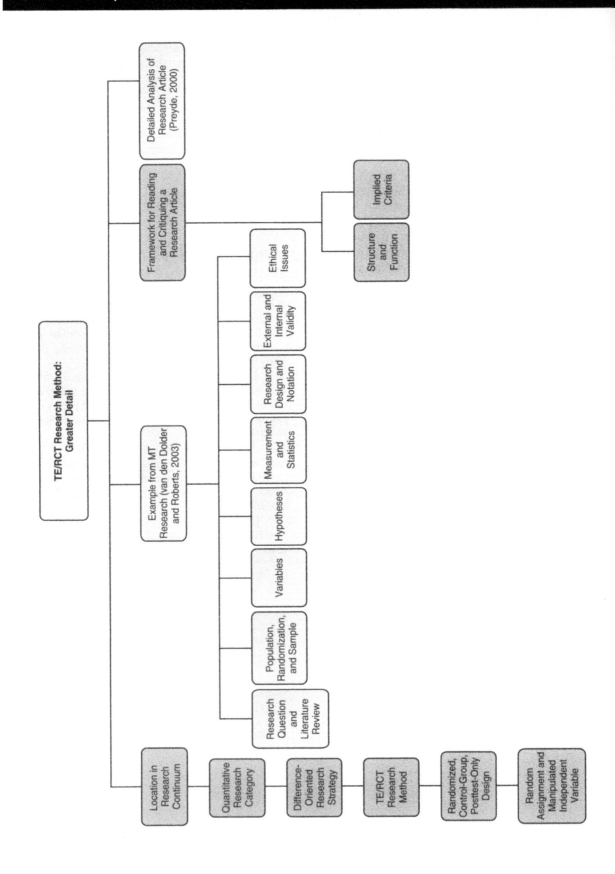

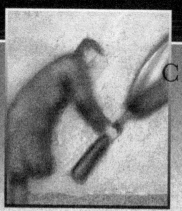

CHAPTER

4

A MORE FOCUSED VIEW OF THE TRUE EXPERIMENTAL/ RANDOMIZED CONTROLLED TRIAL RESEARCH METHOD

OUTLINE

OBJECTIVES

Upon completion of this chapter, the reader will have the information necessary to perform the following tasks:

1 Locate the true experimental/randomized controlled trial (RCT) research method, as illustrated by the Chang, Wang, and Chen (2002) study, in the research category-to-procedures continuum by identifying the research category, strategy, design, and two most critical procedures affiliated with this method.

2 Working from the example provided by the study by van den Dolder and Roberts (2003), discuss the following features of that study in the context of its representing a true experimental/RCT research method:
  a. research question and literature review
  b. population, randomization, and sample
  c. variables from a research design perspective
  d. hypotheses and their relationship to the population and sample
  e. measurement procedures and statistical analyses
  f. research design and notation
  g. external validity and internal validity
  h. major ethical considerations

3 Explain how a research article's structure and function are analogous to the concepts of anatomy and physiology.

4 Identify and discuss the six sections that define the structure of a research article as well as the subsections included in each section.

5 For each of the six sections of a research article as well as their respective subsections, identify and explain the function served by each.

Abstract page
Blinded (or masked)
Concluding section
Criteria for critiquing a research article
Difference-oriented research strategy
Discussion section
General literature review subsection
Global research hypothesis
Equivalent groups
Inclusion and exclusion criteria
Instrumentation subsection
Introductory section
Method section

Null hypothesis significance testing
Participants and sampling procedures
   subsection
Preliminary section
Purpose statement subsection
Quantitative research category
Randomized, control-group, posttest-only
   research design
Randomized, control-group, pretest-posttest
   research design
Rationale for research hypothesis
   subsection
References

Research article function ("physiology")
Research article structure ("anatomy")
Research category-to-procedures continuum
Research design notation
Research method and design subsection
Results section
Specific literature review subsection
Statement of research hypothesis subsection
Title page
True experimental or randomized controlled
   trial (RCT) research method
Variables from a research design perspective
Variables subsection

6 Provided with a list of the criteria for critiquing each of the six sections of a research article, explain why each criterion or standard represents a basis for analyzing its associated section of the article.

7 Working with the complete text of the research article by Preyde (2000), critique each of the major sections of that research report using the 29 criteria or standards identified in this chapter.

8 Explain how the issues discussed in this chapter provide a foundation for moving on to a more expanded view of the quantitative research category in Part Three of this book.

9 List the three research strategies that constitute the quantitative research category that will be developed more fully in Part Three of this book.

WHERE HAVE WE BEEN AND WHERE ARE WE NOW? THE CONNECTION

In the previous chapter, we overviewed one of the most highly respected research designs known as the randomized, control-group, posttest-only design. This research design represents a fundamental way in which the **true experimental or randomized controlled trial (RCT) research method** can be implemented. We explored the reasons why this research method is considered to be a member of the **difference-oriented research strategy** family that, in turn, belongs to the **quantitative research category**. An illustrative excerpt of an abstract from a published study that used this particular research method provided us with a context for considering the various research procedures that came into play. Figure 3-1 attempted a panoramic view of the sequence of those research procedures actually used, or at least relevant to, the illustrated study.

This chapter likewise elaborates on the true experimental/RCT research method by once again appealing to an excerpted abstract of a published research study (van den Dolder & Roberts, 2003). A review of this study's research procedures allows us to consider, at a somewhat deeper level than before, a randomized controlled trial's critical reliance on two important features: (a) the random assignment of participants to the study's two or more comparison groups and (b) an independent variable that allows for the manipulation of its two or more levels—the study's comparison groups—if indeed the potential for cause-and-effect conclusions

- **Research Category:** *Quantitative*
  - • **Research Strategy:** Difference-Oriented
    - • • **Research Method:** True Experimental/RCT
      - • • • **Research Design:** Randomized, Control-Group, Posttest-Only
        - • • • • **Research Procedures (four most defining procedures):** Random Assignment, EG and CG, Manipulated IV, and Posttest

FIGURE 4-1 ■ Research category-to-procedures continuum that locates the Chang et al. (2002) study.

is to be ensured. Finally, a published research article (Preyde, 2000) in its entirety, positioned in the latter part of this chapter, gives us the opportunity to critique a complete study.

LOCATING THE TRUE EXPERIMENTAL/RCT RESEARCH METHOD IN THE RESEARCH CATEGORY-TO-PROCEDURES CONTINUUM

Building on Figure 1-4, we can trace the progression of our discussion so far by once again studying the **research category-to-procedures continuum**, which starts at the most general level of research category and ends at the most specific level of research procedures.

Box 3-1 (Chang et al., 2002) was used in the preceding chapter to show a progression from general to specific that is displayed in Figure 4-1.

We can locate this earlier study on childbirth in the research continuum and label it as (a) belonging to the quantitative research category, (b) employing

a difference-oriented research strategy, (c) being implemented by way of a true experimental/RCT research method, (d) taking the form of a **randomized, control-group, posttest-only research design**, and (e) including the random assignment and manipulated independent variable (IV) research procedures that are so critical to defining this method as highly valued due to its potential for cause-and-effect conclusions.

THE TRUE EXPERIMENTAL/RCT RESEARCH METHOD: A CLOSER LOOK

AN EXAMPLE FROM THE MASSAGE THERAPY RESEARCH LITERATURE

In a manner similar to what we did in Chapter 3, Box 4-1 provides the published abstract of a study conducted by van den Dolder and Roberts (2003) that investigated the effectiveness of soft tissue massage in the treatment of shoulder pain. Following this abstract is a discussion of the study's various features

---

BOX 4-1   EXCERPT FROM ABSTRACT FOR A STUDY ILLUSTRATING A RANDOMIZED CONTROLLED TRIAL CONDUCTED BY VAN DEN DOLDER AND ROBERTS (2003) THAT INVESTIGATED THE EFFECTIVENESS OF SOFT TISSUE MASSAGE IN THE TREATMENT OF SHOULDER PAIN

The purpose of this single blinded randomised controlled trial was to investigate the effects of soft tissue massage on range of motion, reported pain and reported function in patients with shoulder pain. Twenty-nine patients referred to physiotherapy for shoulder pain were randomly assigned to a treatment group that received six treatments of soft tissue massage around the shoulder (n = 15) or to a control group that received no treatment while on the waiting list for two weeks (n = 14). Measurements were taken both before and after the experimental period by a blinded assessor. Active range of motion was measured for flexion, abduction and hand-behind-back movements. Pain was assessed with the Short Form McGill Pain Questionnaire (SFMPQ) and functional ability was assessed with the Patient Specific Functional Disability Measure (PSFDM). The treatment group showed significant improvements in range of motion compared with the control group for abduction (mean 42.2 degrees, 95% CI 24.1 to 60.4 degrees), flexion (mean 22.6 degrees, 95% CI 12.4 to 32.8 degrees) and hand-behind-back (mean 11.0 cm improvement, 95% CI 6.3 to 15.6 em). Massage reduced pain as reported on the descriptive section of the SFMPQ by a mean of 4.9 points (95% CI 2.5 to 7.2 points) and on the visual analogue scale by an average of 26.5 mm (95% CI 5.3 to 47.6 mm), and it improved reported function on the PSFDM by a mean of 8.6 points (95% CI 4.9 to 12.3 points). We conclude that soft tissue massage around the shoulder is effective in improving range of motion, pain and function in patients with shoulder pain. The mechanisms behind these effects remain unclear.

Key words: Massage; pain; physical therapy; shoulder

From Van den Dolder, P. A., & Roberts, D. L. (2003). A trial into the effectiveness of soft tissue massage in the treatment of shoulder pain. *Australian Journal of Physiotherapy, 49*(3), 183–188.

with, once again, a particular emphasis on the use of random assignment and a manipulated IV. When appropriate, additional information not explicitly contained in the abstract is identified and discussed.

RESEARCH QUESTION AND LITERATURE REVIEW: THE JOINT CATALYSTS FOR DECISIONS REGARDING THE RESEARCH CATEGORY-TO-PROCEDURES CONTINUUM

In this study by van den Dolder and Roberts (2003), the implied research question is the following: What are the effects of soft tissue massage on active range of motion (ROM), pain, and functional ability in treating shoulder pain? More specifically, is there a statistically significant difference between participants in an experimental group receiving soft tissue massage for shoulder pain and those in a wait-list control group not receiving the massage intervention relative to active ROM, pain, and functional ability? Regarding the literature review, the 33 citations that appear in the complete research report itself position this investigation in the context of earlier research efforts that involved similar interests.

The implied research question in particular indicates that we are dealing with a difference-oriented research strategy that is included in the quantitative research category. This is because we are essentially asking if there is a significant difference between two levels of a manipulated IV relative to three different dependent variables (DVs) for the participants involved. Insight into the issues of research method, research design, and definitive research procedures awaits a later discussion of further information provided in the abstract.

POPULATION, RANDOMIZATION, AND SAMPLE: ENSURING REPRESENTATIVENESS AND EQUIVALENCE

This study's participants include a total of 29 patients between the ages of 18 and 80 who were referred to physiotherapy for shoulder pain. The participants also are identified as being able to understand English. Other inclusion criteria for participation in the study are not identified. Exclusion criteria, however, are acknowledged and operationalized in terms of (a) certain descriptive features of the origin and nature of the shoulder pain experienced and (b) the degree of palpable tenderness present.

Both the study's abstract and the body of the report are silent regarding the actual size of the larger set of potential participants who might

have been originally referred and considered with respect to the **inclusion and exclusion criteria**. Consequently, there is no discussion of what we might identify as the accessible population's size and characteristics. The 29 patients who were referred and who met the inclusion criteria, therefore, constitute the sample for this study. There is no way of knowing to what extent the sample of 29 participants is truly representative of the actual larger set or group or accessible population of which the sample is a subset. This is due to the absence of randomly selecting participants from a clearly defined accessible population when obtaining the study's sample. This feature of the study eventually presents some limitations regarding the external validity or generalizability of the study's findings.

The study's abstract does specify that the 29 participants were randomly assigned to a treatment or experimental group (n = 15), where they received six treatments of soft tissue massage around the shoulder, or to a control group (n = 14), where they did not receive the treatment but instead were placed on a waiting list for the two-week duration of the study. The use of random assignment, then, did afford a degree of control in the study. This was the case because the random assignment procedure allowed the researchers to assume with some confidence that the two comparison groups were in all likelihood equivalent on extraneous variables that otherwise might eventually obfuscate, confuse, or confound the interpretation of the study once completed.

This research procedure of randomly assigning participants to comparison groups elevated the internal validity of the study. This was the case because the two groups could be viewed as being equivalent on all factors or variables other than the specific variable on which they were operationally defined as differing, namely, the manipulated IV. The manipulated IV here is degree of soft tissue massage intervention, with the first level of the IV involving the presence of soft tissue massage (the experimental group [EG]) and the second level involving the absence of the treatment (the wait-list control group [CG]). Designed in such a manner, this study allowed the researchers eventually to view as tenable the manipulated IV as the likely cause of any differences between the two groups on one or more of the DVs.

VARIABLES FROM A RESEARCH DESIGN PERSPECTIVE: COVERING ALL BASES

The principal focus of this study is on the relationship between the manipulated IV of degree of soft tissue massage intervention and each of the three DVs: active ROM, pain, and functional ability.

As indicated earlier, the absence of random selection of sample participants from a known accessible population compromises the external validity or generalizability of the study. The use of random assignment of the 29 participants to the experimental and control groups, however, does transform the study's extraneous variables into control variables.

More specifically, other than the manipulated IV and the DVs, those **variables from a research design perspective** that relate to person-specific features of the participants as well as the situation-specific aspects of the study's setting—namely, the extraneous variables—are viewed as equally present in the two comparison groups due to random assignment. For this reason, these original extraneous variables are now considered to be control variables because they are viewed as *not* being *unequally* present in the two comparison groups. They are *controlled* in that we can assume that whatever differences eventually occur between the two groups on the DVs cannot be attributed to any earlier factors on which the two groups were believed to be equivalent. This assumption of starting out with **equivalent groups** in place prior to the introduction of the manipulated IV sets the stage for eventually attributing whatever differences do occur on the DVs back to the manipulated IV, again, the only earlier variable on which the groups differed.

Regarding the issue of intervening variable(s), the abstract explicitly states that the mechanisms underlying the effects observed in the study are unclear. The discussion section of the complete research report, however, does engage in a commendable effort at speculating on several possible explanations for the relationship uncovered between the study's manipulated IV and the three DVs. Perhaps the abstract could have been more descriptive in at least acknowledging succinctly those mechanisms that potentially might inform our understanding of the study's dynamics.

HYPOTHESES AS STATEMENTS ABOUT THE CHARACTERISTICS OF OUR POPULATION AND SAMPLE

Though not explicitly stated in the abstract or the body of the report, the research hypothesis implied in this study is as follows: Regarding patients in the study's sample suffering with shoulder pain, there will be a statistically significant difference between those in an experimental group receiving soft tissue massage and those in a wait-list control group not receiving massage relative to active ROM, pain, and functional ability. More specifically, participants in the experimental group receiving soft tissue massage will demonstrate significantly greater active range of motion, less pain, and greater functional ability than will those participants in the wait-list control group not receiving the soft tissue massage.

Actually, this **global research hypothesis** contains three individual research hypotheses, each pertaining to one of the three DVs. The notation conventionally used in expressing each of these hypotheses is as follows:

$$H_{R1}: \bar{X}_{AROM, EG} > \bar{X}_{AROM, CG}$$
$$H_{R2}: \bar{X}_{P, EG} < \bar{X}_{P, CG}$$
$$H_{R3}: \bar{X}_{FA, EG} > \bar{X}_{FA, CG}$$

These three individual research hypotheses are understood to be specific to the actual sample of 29 participants engaged in the study and, in effect, speak to certain characteristics—or statistics—of the sample. The first research hypothesis, for example, addresses the average or mean (symbolized by $\bar{X}$ and read as X bar) active ROM characteristic (i.e., statistic) observed in the two comparison groups constituting the sample. The second research hypothesis speaks to the characteristic or statistic of the mean ($\bar{X}$) pain level existing in the sample, and so forth.

The null or statistical hypothesis, likewise, is only implied in this research report as well and, in its "global" form, reads as follows: Regarding patients suffering with shoulder pain in the population from which the study's sample was derived, there will be no statistically significant difference between those in an experimental group receiving soft tissue massage and those in a wait-list control group not receiving massage relative to active range of motion, pain, and functional ability.

This global null hypothesis statement would actually be operationalized and tested statistically in the context of three individual "null" statements, with each individual null hypothesis obviously pertaining to one of the three DVs. Illustrations of these three null hypotheses, with the only distinguishing feature being the DV identified, are as follows:

$$H_{01}: \mu_{AROM, EG} = \mu_{AROM, CG}$$
$$H_{02}: \mu_{P, EG} = \mu_{P, CG}$$
$$H_{03}: \mu_{FA, EG} = \mu_{FA, CG}$$

These three individual null hypotheses are understood to be specific to the population of potential study participants that exists and from which the sample of 29 participants was taken. Furthermore, these three null hypotheses speak to certain characteristics—or parameters—of the population. The first null hypothesis addresses the average or mean (symbolized by the lower case Greek letter μ, read mu) active ROM characteristic (i.e., parameter) that exists in the population of all potential study participants from which the sample was derived. The second null hypothesis speaks to the characteristic or parameter of the mean (μ) pain level existing in the population of participants, and so forth.

The alternative hypothesis, symbolized by either H_1 or H_A, is implied in this study's report as well and in its "global" form reads as follows: Regarding patients suffering with shoulder pain in the population from which the study's sample was derived, there will be a statistically significant difference between those in the experimental group receiving soft tissue massage and those in the wait-list control group not receiving massage relative to active range of motion, pain, and functional ability. More specifically, participants in the experimental group receiving soft tissue massage will demonstrate significantly greater active ROM, less pain, and greater functional ability than will those participants in the wait-list control group not receiving the soft tissue massage.

This global alternative hypothesis, likewise, actually contains three individual alternative hypotheses, with each referring to one of the three DVs. The notation that is customary in stating each of these three individual alternative hypotheses is as follows:

$$H_{A1}: \mu_{AROM, EG} > \mu_{AROM, CG}$$
$$H_{A2}: \mu_{P, EG} < \mu_{P, CG}$$
$$H_{A3}: \mu_{FA, EG} > \mu_{FA, CG}$$

As was the case with the three individual null or statistical hypotheses, these three individual alternative hypotheses are understood to be specific to the population of potential study participants that exists and from which our sample of 29 participants was derived. These three alternative hypotheses, furthermore, address certain characteristics—or parameters—of the population. The first alternative hypothesis, for example, speaks to the average or mean (again symbolized by the lower case Greek letter μ) active range of motion characteristic (i.e., parameter) that exists in the population of all potential study participants from which the

sample was taken. The second alternative hypothesis addresses the characteristic or parameter of the mean (μ) pain level existing in the population of participants, and so forth.

MEASUREMENT PROCEDURES AND STATISTICAL ANALYSES AS CRITICAL RESEARCH TOOLS

The study's abstract indicates that participants in both the experimental group and the wait-list control group were tested on each of the three DVs both *before* and *after* the experimental period by an assessor who was blinded as to each participant's group membership. In the case of the experimental group, participants were posttested on completion of their six treatment sessions, which spanned the experimental period of two weeks. Participants in the wait-list control group were likewise posttested following their two weeks on the waiting list. Statistical analyses indicated that the experimental group demonstrated greater active range of motion, less pain intensity, and greater functional ability than did the wait-list control group.

Inherent in what has just been summarized about the study are several critical points that need explanation. All 29 participants, regardless of their comparison group membership, were pretested on the three DVs before the actual start of the study's experimental period and posttested on the same variables at the conclusion of the two-week experimental period. This has implications for the nature of the research design that was used and will be elaborated on extensively in a subsequent section.

The abstract also notes that the pretesting and posttesting were performed by an assessor who was **blinded (or masked)** as to the group membership of each participant. This is a standard procedure whereby the research team member responsible for collecting and analyzing the data generated on the study's variables is not privy to participant membership. This ensures a certain degree of objectivity and absence of bias in the study that otherwise might be compromised if group affiliations were known by the assessor.

On yet another aspect of the study, the use of a wait-list control group ensured that for the duration of the study, those participants who met the inclusion criteria and were being compared to the experimental group on the three DVs did not receive the experimental treatment. Instead, they were quite literally on a list awaiting their involvement with the soft tissue massage treatment once the study was completed. This made possible the availability of a group of participants for comparison purposes to the experimental group, but it did not deprive these subjects of the eventual potential benefit to be derived from the soft tissue massage. This type of *wait-list control group* is a very attractive alternative to either (a) a control group for which no intervention is being provided—neither during nor after the experimental period—or (b) a control group that is receiving a recognized standard treatment alone while the experimental group is receiving both the standard treatment and some additional intervention that defines the experimental level of the manipulated IV. It is important to note here that the control group participants do not receive the experimental treatment in either the *no treatment control group* or the *standard treatment control group*, even once the study is completed.

Although discussed in detail later, still another type of control group that is sometimes appealed to is the *sham placebo control group*. This alternative to the three types of control groups mentioned in the preceding paragraph is one wherein a control group receives a type of intervention or treatment that simply mimics the attention being given to the experimental group's participants, yet the sham intervention is inert or at least inconsequential by design. A later discussion in this chapter of a study by Preyde (2000) provides an excellent example of a sham placebo control group in use.

The statistical analyses conducted on the study's data sets reveal statistically significant results favoring the experimental group over the control group on each of the three DVs. The results section of the report provides detailed information representing the quantitative basis for this conclusion. Essentially, the meaning here is that the results generated in the study were of such a nature that—if indeed the null hypotheses are valid—then the probability is extremely small that the actual results obtained could have happened by chance alone. And because the obtained results could have occurred by chance alone to such a small degree, it becomes more likely or tenable that the observed results are indeed attributable to something other than chance—some

*non*chance reality—namely, the reality of a meaningful and significant relationship between soft tissue massage and the desired effects on active range of motion, pain intensity, and functional ability. Translated, the study's statistical analyses indicate a statistically significant relationship between the study's manipulated IV and each one of the three DVs.

RESEARCH DESIGN AND ITS NOTATION

The preceding discussions regarding the study's use of (a) random assignment, (b) a manipulated IV encompassing an experimental group and a wait-list control group, and (c) both the pretesting and posttesting of participants on each of the three DVs allow us to identify the nature of the research design that was used.

Specifically, this design is labeled a **randomized, control-group, pretest-posttest research design**. Due to the presence of both random assignment and a manipulated IV as defining research procedures, the study made use of a true experimental/RCT research method. This method was used as one way to implement a difference-oriented research strategy. Everything we have just noted about procedures, design, method, and strategy falls under the rubric or label of quantitative research category. Accordingly, the research design here is represented by using the following **research design notation**:

$$RA \quad EG \quad O_{Pre} \quad X \quad O_{Post}$$
$$RA \quad CG \quad O_{Pre} \quad \bullet \quad O_{Post}$$

Furthermore, Figure 4-2 shows the complete progression from research category to research procedures that defines the nature of the study by van den Dolder and Roberts (2003).

ISSUES OF EXTERNAL VALIDITY AND INTERNAL VALIDITY: THE LINKAGE TO RANDOMIZATION AND A MANIPULATED INDEPENDENT VARIABLE

Our earlier discussions in the previous chapter of external validity and internal validity should serve

- **Research Category:** *Quantitative*
  - **Research Strategy:** Difference-Oriented
    - **Research Method:** True Experimental/RCT
      - **Research Design:** Randomized, Control-Group, Pretest-Posttest
        - **Research Procedures (five most defining procedures):** Random Assignment, EG and CG, Pretest, Manipulated IV, and Posttest

FIGURE 4-2 ■ Research category-to-procedures continuum that locates the van den Dolder and Roberts (2003) study.

us well now as we reflect on these two features in the study by van den Dolder and Roberts (2003).

As we observed in an earlier section of this chapter, this study did not involve the random selection of participants from a known accessible population. Consequently, we do not know the actual size of the larger set of potential participants who might have been originally referred for treatment of shoulder pain and, in turn, whose participation would have been considered by the researchers with respect to the study's inclusion and exclusion criteria. The end result of the absence of random selection is that the study's ability to generalize from the sample back to its accessible population is seriously compromised. This is another way of saying that the external validity of this study is lacking.

Random assignment of participants to the two comparison groups, however, is indeed a critical feature of the study. Because the researchers used this aspect of randomization, along with the presence of a manipulated IV, we can say that the internal validity of the study is enhanced. In turn, this makes the statement of cause-and-effect conclusions at least somewhat possible.

MAJOR ETHICAL CONSIDERATIONS IN RESEARCH: AN EVER-PRESENT CONCERN FROM BEGINNING TO END IN THE RESEARCH PROCESS

The study by van den Dolder and Roberts (2003) exemplifies several features that accommodate certain ethical mandates inherent in any scientific investigation involving human participants. In sequential order as the study unfolded, we learned initially that potential participants were referred to a hospital for management of shoulder pain over a period of four months. Also, the researchers spelled out certain inclusion and exclusion criteria as a standard way of consistently monitoring exactly which prospective participants would be selected.

The complete report of the study indicates that the Human Ethics Committee at the hospital where the study was conducted did indeed review and approve the research protocol in advance of its implementation. The generic name for such a committee across many scientific disciplines and professions is *institutional review board* (IRB). Although the study's report does not explicitly acknowledge the issues of informed consent, confidentiality, and debriefing after the study is completed, we can assume that these ethical safeguards were in place given the approval received from the hospital's IRB.

Another ethical aspect of the study alluded to earlier is that of the pretesting and posttesting conducted by a research team member who was blinded (or masked) with respect to participants' affiliations with the comparison groups. This was done to ensure an objective and unbiased sequence of measurement and statistical analysis procedures so that the integrity of the study would not be compromised.

The integrity of the study was likewise protected by the researchers' decision to use a wait-list control group so that eventually all participants in the study would be privy to the potential benefits that might accrue from the soft tissue massage intervention.

As a final point and reminder here, Appendix B discusses in considerable detail these and related ethical principles governing research in the various behavioral and health sciences.

A FRAMEWORK FOR READING A RESEARCH ARTICLE: STRUCTURE, FUNCTION, AND IMPLIED CRITERIA FOR EVALUATION

STRUCTURE AND FUNCTION: AS IN THE RESEARCH REPORT'S "ANATOMY" AND "PHYSIOLOGY"

The **research article structure or "anatomy"** of an empirical research article is a standard feature of this form of scientific or technical writing. Because the intent is that of enhancing communication among professionals across various disciplines and professions, you would expect that the sections and subsections that constitute a research report are not left to the preferences or idiosyncrasies of individual researchers.

The various sections and subsections that guide the structure of the research report are there for the express purpose of accomplishing certain functions that represent the **research article function or "physiology"** of the research report.

The combination, then, of a research article's structure and function sets the stage for our being able to identify several criteria or standards that we might use to determine if a research report is providing appropriate information. The availability of appropriate information in a report allows us to evaluate or assess the merit of the research effort regarding its potential for advancing our knowledge base and, in turn, advancing the evidence-based practice we provide for our clients.

The following parts of this section provide an overview of the six major sections and their

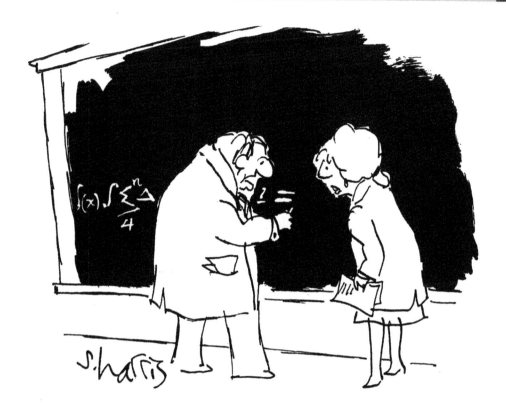

"This is the part I always hate."

HUMOR BREAK ■ Embrace your study's results—even if contrary to your hypothesis! (From Harris S, [1992]. *Chalk up another one: The best of Sidney Harris.* New Brunswick, NJ: Rutgers University Press.)

corresponding subsections that constitute a research article. Appendix C provides a more detailed discussion of these and related topics.

Preliminary Section: Title and Abstract

The **preliminary section** of the research article contains the **title page** and **abstract page** of the study. Although fairly self-explanatory, one has to be cautious to formulate a study's title in such a way that a potential reader—perhaps scanning a listing of studies by bibliographic citation only—can accurately determine from the title such information as the type of study being reported, the major variables involved, and the participants who were the focal point of the researcher's efforts.

Regarding the report's abstract or summary, the article's author is obligated to synthesize as efficiently and effectively as possible the main body of the report (i.e., the study's introduction, method, results, and discussion sections). If successfully written, then the reader should have a precise idea as to the actual functions that the study accomplished. This would then allow the reader to decide whether or not to read the report in its entirety.

Introductory Section

The article's **introductory section** provides the context within which the remainder of the report is to be considered. Specifically, the introductory section spans the following five subsections or areas: (a) general literature review, (b) specific literature review, (c) purpose statement identifying the research question, (d) rationale for the study's research hypothesis, and (e) statement of the research hypothesis.

The **general literature review subsection** identifies the broader context of the study's major research problem area. The appeal here is at a general level to those earlier researchers and authors who have contributed to the research problem area. Following this overview, the **specific literature review subsection** provides a more detailed treatment of related sources in the professional literature. This subsection allows the reader to become considerably more familiar with the earlier literature that informs the study being reported. Both of these subsections serve a dual purpose: (a) to establish the credibility of the study's authors in the mind of the reader regarding their familiarity with the existing sources of information in the research problem area and (b) to inform the reader of pertinent information and insight that you should have in order to better comprehend the research report at hand.

The next area covered in the introduction is the study's **purpose statement subsection**, which identifies the research question. At the very least the research question must be implied, although an explicit formulation of the research question is considerably more preferred. This subsection communicates to the reader what is truly the starting point in the study. This is because any research endeavor bases its many decisions precisely on the research question that represents the reason or purpose for the study being conducted in the first place. In considering a research question, you need to keep foremost in mind that it is never formulated in a vacuum. The researcher must have some degree of familiarity with the relevant literature in order to identify the question. At the same time, though, the researcher must at least have the beginnings of a research question in place to know exactly where in the literature one has to search.

The fourth subsection in the introduction, the **rationale for research hypothesis subsection**, relies on—and perhaps might even extend—the earlier subsections that dealt with the literature review. A study's authors must rely on the available research literature in a given problem area to acknowledge the rationale or justification for what becomes the study's research hypothesis. The research hypothesis, again, is basically the predicted answer to the study's research question. It is *not* an educated guess. It is a predicted answer to the research question that is informed or justified primarily by concepts, theories, and/or existing empirical research contained in the professional literature. The rationale for the research hypothesis, then, should be presented immediately prior to the actual statement of the hypothesis. In this way, a context is already in place that clarifies the rationale for, or reasons why, the researchers are predicting a certain answer to the study's question. Although the rationale is usually only implied, a more preferred approach is for it to be identified explicitly for the benefit of the reader.

The final area in the introduction is the **statement of research hypothesis subsection**. Unfortunately, far too many authors fail to provide an explicit statement of what they anticipate—with justification—will be the outcome of the study (i.e., the answer to the study's research question). Instead, the tendency is to allow the research hypothesis to simply be implied. The major advantage to an explicit statement of the hypothesis is that it alerts the reader to several critical features of the study, not the least of which include the following: the research category, strategy, and method used; the variables investigated and their predicted relationship; the participants studied; and the context or setting of the study. Knowledge of a study's research hypothesis sets the stage for a more informed consideration of the study's methodology, which is the next major section in a research article.

Method Section

Just as the name suggests, the **method section** of the research report provides a detailed account of the methodology used in carrying out the study. It identifies the various research procedures used at different stages of the study and operationalizes them at such a specific level that one could replicate the study if so desired. This section also gives the reader as complete a basis as possible for determining if the implementation of the study justifies, or compromises, in any way the results and conclusions reached.

To accomplish these tasks, the method section must speak to the issues of participants and how they were derived, instruments used for measuring variables, and procedures by which the study was actually implemented. Accordingly, standard subsections that constitute the method section are as follows: (a) participants and sampling procedures, (b) research method and design, (c) variables, and (d) instrumentation. This list of four specific subsections provides ample opportunity for an author to specify precisely what was done in carrying out the study. As a word of caution, though, you may notice across different studies some slight variations in the manner in which these subsections are labeled. The important point here, however, is that this section address the themes of participants, measuring instruments, and procedures.

The first area, typically labeled the **participants and sampling procedures subsection**, identifies the characteristics of the participants used in the study as well as the activities used in selecting and assigning them. The researchers identify and justify inclusion criteria and exclusion criteria used as the bases for determining who would and would not qualify as study participants. Researchers also rely on this subsection to provide information regarding the power analysis used to determine the optimal sample size for a given study. Additionally, researchers must acknowledge here the extent to which the random selection of sample participants from an accessible population was used as well as the random assignment of subjects to comparison groups. If the researchers used procedures other than random selection and random assignment, then they must specify the alternatives employed. These issues are critical given the nature of what we have already seen about the bases for, and importance of, a study's external and internal validity. Finally, this subsection should specify the ethical provisions taken in the study to ensure participant protection, the overall integrity of the study, and prior approval from the appropriate IRB.

The second subsection is labeled the **research method and design subsection**. The focus on these two intermediate points in our research continuum is strategic because it allows the reader to recognize the research category, strategy, and procedures that, by implication, the researchers used in the study. Here, too, there are implications regarding both the external and internal validity of the study.

The third subsection, the **variables subsection**, addresses the variables investigated in the study. Although the variables are previously mentioned in the report, the important feature here is that the researchers operationalize the variables as specifically as possible. This subsection is where a reader would acquire all of the details as to how the researchers identified, defined, characterized, controlled, manipulated, or measured the study's variables.

The final part of the method section is the **instrumentation subsection**. Although the reference here is primarily to measuring instruments used to generate data—numerical and/or verbal—this subsection may also refer to a type/model of equipment or apparatus that played a role in the study. Technical characteristics such as the validity and reliability of instruments are crucial and, therefore, prominent features of the information provided in this subsection.

Results Section

As indicated, the **results section** provides the reader with a full accounting of the outcomes or results of the data analysis performed in the study. This is accomplished mainly by a disclosure of the descriptive and/or inferential statistical techniques used in analyzing the study's data, the results of the analysis, and their interpretation. This section is also where the researchers acknowledge—usually by implication—the study's null or statistical hypothesis, along with their explicit decision to reject or fail to reject it. Based on the decision regarding the null hypothesis, the researchers then develop the inferences to be made regarding the alternative and research hypotheses.

This section also provides the opportunity for the researchers to specify other statistical findings beyond hypothesis testing if the study provided for such. For example, the establishment of confidence intervals and the citing of effect sizes may appear here in an attempt to augment traditional **null hypothesis significance testing** (NHST).

Discussion Section

The fourth and final section of the report's main body is the **discussion section**, the examination of the study's findings. This provides the researchers with the opportunity to (a) reflect on the manner in which the study was conducted, inclusive of its limitations and delimitations (boundaries), (b) elaborate on the interpretation of the study's findings that was begun in the results section, (c) acknowledge the significance of the study's results as well as their relationship to earlier research findings in the problem area investigated, (d) theorize as to why the results were forthcoming (i.e., which intervening variables might have come into play during the conduct of the study), and (e) suggest recommended areas of further research that would be logical sequels to the study.

Concluding Section: References and Beyond

The **concluding section** of the research report begins with a listing of the bibliographic citations for each of the sources actually cited in the research report. This listing constitutes the **references**, and is very important not only in terms of giving detailed credit to sources used in the study, but also providing the reader with the necessary information for accessing the sources cited. Beyond this listing, it is not uncommon for a research report to include additional information such as appendixes, author notes, and footnotes.

IMPLIED CRITERIA FOR CRITIQUING A RESEARCH ARTICLE: REFLECTIONS OF STRUCTURE AND FUNCTION

The structure and function of the sections and subsections constituting a research report provide the foundation for us to identify certain criteria or standards that can be used to critique or evaluate the merits of a report. Additionally, such an approach gives us an organizational framework for systematically working through the process of reflecting on a study report's contents. The following, therefore, provides a comprehensive listing of specific questions that are relevant to evaluating the designated sections and subsections of a research article. It is important to note that this particular listing of **criteria for critiquing a research article** is geared primarily, though not exclusively, to those types of studies that we have seen thus far, namely, studies that fall into the research continuum at the following two points: quantitative research category and difference-oriented research strategy.

Preliminary Section

1. Does the *title* of the study provide a basis for identifying the *type of study*, *major variables*, and *participants*?
2. Does the *abstract* synthesize the main body of the report (i.e., the introduction, method, results, and discussion) with a particular focus on the *research question, research hypothesis, participants, research method and design, major variables, instruments, statistical techniques, principal findings*, and *conclusions*?

Introductory Section

3. Is the reader introduced to the *relevant professional literature* bearing on the study being reported by way of a *general overview of the research problem area* as well as a more *specific coverage of individual studies*?
4. Is the purpose of the study identified by way of the *research question* being formulated at an *operational level*?
5. Is a *rationale or justification*, based on various features of the professional literature, presented as a context or framework for the study's *research hypothesis*?
6. Do the authors state the study's *research hypothesis* in such a way that the predicted answer to the study's research question is clear and unambiguous?

Method Section

7. Are the study's *participants* clearly characterized along with the *inclusion and exclusion criteria* used for identifying them?
8. Did the researchers justify the *number of participants* constituting the sample size by way of a *power analysis*?
9. Was an *accessible population* of potential participants acknowledged along with an indication of *how the sample was derived* from such a population, be it through random selection or some other procedure?
10. Did the authors specify the manner in which the participants were *assigned* to the two or more comparison groups, be it through random assignment or some other means?
11. Was any clarification provided as to how the *ethical aspects* of the study were governed, particularly in reference to the protection of the participants, the overall integrity of the research, and the earlier approval of the study by an IRB?
12. Was the nature of the research effort adequately characterized in terms of its position in the research continuum (i.e., its position regarding *research category, strategy, method, design, and defining procedures*)?
13. Were the study's *variables operationalized* in a comprehensive fashion so that their manipulation or measurement could be replicated?
14. Did the authors clearly specify the *equipment or instruments* used in the study for variable manipulation or measurement purposes, along with a documentation of the technical characteristic of such including validity and reliability?

Results Section

15. Were the *data analysis techniques* used in the study identified and justified?
16. Were the results of the study communicated by an appeal to *descriptive and/or inferential statistics* consistent with the nature of the research question as well as the research method and measurement scales used?
17. Were the results of the data analysis related to an appropriate *decision* regarding the study's *null or statistical hypothesis*?
18. Was the decision regarding the null hypothesis acknowledged as a basis for inferring decisions concerning the *alternative and research hypotheses*?

19. If hypothesis testing was performed, were the analyses augmented with other statistical techniques such as *confidence interval estimation* or *effect size calculations*?

20. Were *tables and figures* appropriately used so as to render the data analyses more comprehensible?

Discussion Section

21. Did the researchers reflect on the manner in which the study was designed and conducted regarding any *limitations and/or delimitations* (i.e., intentional or unintentional boundaries)?

22. Did the authors *elaborate* on the *interpretation of the study's findings* beyond the interpretation that was begun in the results section?

23. Did the researchers address the *significance* of the study and its findings, particularly as they relate to earlier studies in the problem area investigated?

24. Did the discussion section address possible *intervening variables* in the study that might explain why the results obtained were indeed forthcoming?

25. Were *recommendations* suggested to the reader regarding needed follow-up studies that might replicate, fully or partially, or at least augment, the study?

Concluding Section

26. Does the list of *references* accurately reflect each of the sources cited in the research report, with a consistent bibliographic citation style used?

27. Does the research report contain any *appendixes* that augment in greater detail information provided earlier in the article?

28. Is there any information in the form of *author notes* providing insight regarding funding support for the study, contact directives for communicating with the authors as a follow up, or collegial assistance in completing the study?

29. Are any *footnotes* provided that elaborate on one or more aspects of the study that would have been misplaced or distracting if they had been embedded in the main body of the report?

ILLUSTRATION OF THE TRUE EXPERIMENTAL/RCT RESEARCH METHOD: AN ANALYSIS OF A COMPLETE RESEARCH ARTICLE

Box 4-2 provides, in its entirety, a research article by Preyde (2000) that represents an RCT study of the effectiveness of massage therapy for subacute low-back pain. This study lends itself to the type of critique or evaluation that we have been building to thus far in this book.

BOX 4-2   EFFECTIVENESS OF MASSAGE THERAPY FOR SUBACUTE LOW-BACK PAIN: A RANDOMIZED CONTROLLED TRIAL

*Michele Preyde**

Abstract

Background: *The effectiveness of massage therapy for low-back pain has not been documented. This randomized controlled trial compared comprehensive massage therapy (soft-tissue manipulation, remedial exercise and posture education), 2 components of massage therapy and placebo in the treatment of subacute (between 1 week and 8 months) low-back pain.*

Methods: *Subjects with subacute low-back pain were randomly assigned to 1 of 4 groups: comprehensive massage therapy (n = 25), soft-tissue manipulation only (n = 25), remedial exercise with posture education only (n = 22) or a placebo of sham laser therapy (n = 26). Each subject received 6 treatments within approximately 1 month. Outcome measures obtained at baseline, after treatment and at 1-month follow-up consisted of the Roland Disability Questionnaire (RDQ), the McGill Pain Questionnaire (PPI and PRI), the State Anxiety Index and the Modified Schober test (lumbar range of motion).*

Results: *Of the 107 subjects who passed screening, 98 (92%) completed post-treatment tests and 91 (85%) completed follow-up tests. Statistically significant differences were noted after treatment and at follow-up. The comprehensive massage therapy group had improved function (mean RDQ score 1.54 v. 2.86–6.5, p < 0.001), less intense pain (mean PPI score 0.42 v. 1.18–1.75, p < 0.001) and a decrease in the quality of pain (mean PRI score 2.29 v. 4.55–7.71, p = 0.006) compared with the other 3 groups. Clinical significance was evident for the comprehensive massage therapy group and the soft-tissue manipulation group on the measure of function. At 1-month follow-up 63% of subjects in the comprehensive massage therapy group reported no pain as compared with 27% of the soft-tissue manipulation group, 14% of the remedial exercise group and 0% of the sham laser therapy group.*

*Michele Preyde is a PhD student in the Faculty of Social Work, University of Toronto, and a member of the college of Massage Therapists of Ontario, Toronto, Ont.
CMAJ 2000;162(13):1815-20

Continued

BOX 4-2   EFFECTIVENESS OF MASSAGE THERAPY FOR SUBACUTE LOW-BACK PAIN: A RANDOMIZED CONTROLLED TRIAL—CONT'D

Interpretation: *Patients with subacute low-back pain were shown to benefit from massage therapy, as regulated by the College of Massage Therapists of Ontario and delivered by experienced massage therapists.*

Low-back pain affects a considerable proportion of the population.[1,2] In a methodological review of prevalence studies of low-back pain,[3] a mean point prevalence of 19.2% and a mean 1-year prevalence of 32.7% were estimated. Research on the effectiveness of treatment of subacute low-back pain has yielded inconsistent results,[4-6] and studies often contain methodological flaws[6-9] such as inadequate randomization procedures and lack of a placebo control. Flaws in studies employing massage include not using a registered massage therapist and making no attempt to ensure fidelity to a treatment model.[8] Researchers have compared massage to other treatments of low-back pain but have used nonspecific massage as a control.[9] No studies were found that specifically evaluated massage therapy as a treatment for low-back pain.

This study compared the effectiveness of comprehensive massage therapy, 2 separate components of massage therapy (soft-tissue manipulation and remedial exercise with posture education) and a placebo of sham laser therapy for the treatment of subacute low-back pain. Outcome measures were function, pain, anxiety and lumbar range of motion.

Methods

This study was conducted at the Health and Performance Centre, University of Guelph, Guelph, Ont., which offers multidisciplinary services such as sports medicine, physiotherapy and chiropractic manipulation. Treatments were provided and outcome measures were obtained at this centre. Ethics approval was obtained from the University of Guelph Ethics Review Committee, and all subjects gave informed consent.

Subjects were recruited through university email, flyers sent to family physicians and advertisements in the local newspapers between November 1998 and July 1999. Potential subjects aged 18 to 81 years were screened by telephone according to the following criteria: existence of subacute (between 1 week and 8 months) low-back pain; absence of significant pathology, such as bone fracture, nerve damage or severe psychiatric condition, including clinical depression as determined by a physician; no pregnancy; and stable health. The screening process relied on self-reported criteria plus information concerning the existence of medical conditions, medication use and the possibility of serious injury. Any doubt of appropriateness for inclusion was verified by the potential subject's physician. Having a history or previous episode of low-back pain and a positive radiograph finding of mild pathology were not reasons for exclusion.

Subjects were randomly assigned with the use of a random-numbers table to 1 of 4 groups: comprehensive massage therapy (soft-tissue manipulation, remedial exercise and posture education), soft-tissue manipulation only, remedial exercise with posture education only or a placebo of sham laser treatment. Upon arrival for the first appointment, patient characteristics and health information, informed consent and baseline measures (function, pain, anxiety and lumbar range of motion) were recorded. All subjects received 6 treatments within about 1 month. Post-treatment measures were obtained after 1 month of treatment, and follow-up measures were obtained 1 month after treatment ended. Subjects were asked not to seek additional therapy for their backs for the 2 months that they were involved in the study. The 6 subjects (1 in the comprehensive massage therapy group, 2 in the soft-tissue manipulation group, 1 in the remedial exercise group and 2 in the sham laser group) who reported that they took acetaminophen or anti-inflammatory medication for back pain were asked to refrain from doing so on test days until they had completed all the outcome measures.

Treatment Variables

For subjects in the comprehensive massage therapy group various soft-tissue manipulation techniques such as friction, trigger points and neuromuscular therapy were used to promote circulation and relaxation of spasm or tension. The exact soft tissue that the subject described as the source of pain was located and treated with the specific technique indicated for the specific condition of the soft tissue (e.g., friction for fibrous tissue and gentle trigger points for muscle spasm). The duration of the soft-tissue manipulation was between 30 and 35 minutes. For each treatment, stretching exercises for the trunk, hips and thighs, including flexion and modified extension, were taught and reviewed to ensure proper mechanics. Stretches were to be within a pain-free range, held for about 30 seconds in a relaxed manner, and performed twice on one occasion per day for the related areas and more frequently for the affected areas. Subjects were encouraged to engage in general strengthening or mobility exercises such as walking, swimming or aerobics and to build overall fitness progressively. Compliance was recorded; 6 subjects (3 from the comprehensive massage therapy group and 3 from the remedial exercise group) had low compliance with performing the remedial exercise on their own. Education of posture and body mechanics, particularly as they related to work and daily activities, was provided. The exercise and education segment took about 15-20 minutes.

Subjects in the soft-tissue manipulation group received the same soft-tissue manipulation as the subjects in the comprehensive massage therapy group and no other treatment. Those in the remedial exercise group received the same exercise and education components of treatment as subjects in the comprehensive massage therapy group. The control group received sham low-level laser (infrared) therapy. The laser was set up to look as if it was functioning but was not. The subject was "treated" lying on his or her side with proper support to permit relaxation. The instrument was held on the area of complaint by the treatment provider, so the subject was attended for the duration of the session (about 20 minutes) to control for the effects of interpersonal contact and support.

Two treatment providers were hired to deliver treatments, but it became necessary for the principle investigator, who is also a registered massage therapist, to provide treatment when the other providers experienced personal distress (e.g., death of a family member). The 2 providers hired for this study underwent training to enhance treatment delivery and similarity of delivery techniques; they also underwent process checks. Two of the treatment providers were massage therapists with more than 10 years' experience each; they provided treatment for the comprehensive massage therapy and soft-tissue manipulation groups. The third was a certified personal trainer and certified weight-trainer supervisor who, with one of the massage therapists, provided treatment for the remedial exercise and sham laser groups. The one objective measure, the range of motion test, was conducted by 3 physiotherapists who were blind to which group each subject was allocated.

Outcome Measures

Two primary outcome measures were functionality and pain relief. The Roland Disability Questionnaire[10] (RDQ), an adaptation of the Sickness Impact Profile, was used to measure subjects' level of functioning when performing daily tasks. Scores can range from 0 to 24 based on responses to 24 questions to which subjects answer Yes or No. A score of 14 or more is considered a poor outcome.[10] This questionnaire has shown reliability, validity and sensitivity[10,11] and has been used in trials of the treatment of low-back pain.[6,12,13]

The McGill Pain Questionnaire[14] consists of 2 indexes. The Present Pain Index (PPI) measures intensity of pain; the score ranges from 0 (no pain) to 5 (excruciating pain). The Pain Rating Index (PRI) measures quality of pain and is the sum total of 79 qualitative words the subject chooses to describe the pain. These indexes have shown reliability and validity.[15-17]

Two secondary outcome measures were anxiety and lumbar range of motion. The State Anxiety Index[18,19] (SAI) comprises separate self-report scales to measure state (at this moment) anxiety. Scores can range from 20 (minimal anxiety) to 80 (maximum). The norms of state anxiety for working adults are considered to be 35.7 (standard deviation [SD] 10.4) for men and 35.2 (SD 10.6) for women. This index has shown reliability, validity and internal consistency[18,19] and has been widely used in research[20] in a variety of disciplines including psychology and medicine.[21,22]

Lumbar range of motion was measured with the Modified Schober test,[23] and the norm is about 7 cm (SD 1.2).[24] It has shown intraobserver ($r = 0.99$) and interobserver ($r = 0.97$) reliability[25] and has been used in studies of the effectiveness of treatment for subacute low-back pain.[4,12]

With a level of significance of 0.05 and a power of 0.80, minimum samples of 20 subjects per group[26] were required to detect a proportional reduction of pain of 50%. Outcome data were analysed by intention to treat and group means compared with ANOVA, and subsequently Scheffé (post hoc). Minimal, insignificant differences between groups at baseline with near normal distributions permitted analysis without adjustment.

Results

Of the 165 potential subjects who responded to the advertisements, 107 (65%) met the inclusion criteria. Potential subjects were most commonly excluded because their low-back pain was beyond the 8-month subacute cut-off (15 subjects), they were not currently experiencing low-back pain (13), or they indicated a diagnosis of complex health problems such as multiple sclerosis (9).

Of the 107 subjects who met the inclusion criteria (Table 1), 5 dropped out before treatment (3 before randomization, 1 from the comprehensive massage therapy group and 1 from the remedial exercise group), and 4 subjects dropped out before the end of the treatment (2 from the soft-tissue

TABLE I   **PROFILE OF STUDY OF EFFECTIVENESS OF MASSAGE THERAPY FOR SUBACUTE LOW-BACK PAIN INVOLVING 104 SUBJECTS WHO MET THE ELIGIBILITY CRITERIA AND WERE RANDOMLY ASSIGNED TO 1 OF 4 TREATMENT GROUPS**

	TREATMENT GROUP, NO. OF SUBJECTS			
STAGE OF TRIAL	COMPREHENSIVE MASSAGE THERAPY	SOFT-TISSUE MANIPULATION	REMEDIAL EXERCISE AND POSTURE EDUCATION	PLACEBO (SHAM LASER TREATMENT)
Randomly assigned to group but did not receive treatment	1	0	1	0
Started but did not complete treatment	0	2	1	1
Received and completed treatment*	25	25	22	26
Withdrawn and lost to follow-up†	1	3	1	2
Completed trial‡	24	22	21	24

*Completed treatment and completed post-treatment tests.
†Completed treatment and completed post-treatment tests but not follow-up tests.
‡Completed treatment, completed post-treatment tests and follow-up tests.

Continued

BOX 4-2 EFFECTIVENESS OF MASSAGE THERAPY FOR SUBACUTE LOW-BACK PAIN: A RANDOMIZED CONTROLLED TRIAL—CONT'D

manipulation group, 1 from the remedial exercise group and 1 from the sham laser group). These 4 subjects appeared typical at baseline. Because each group experienced a similar number of dropouts and results are based on comparisons of group means, these 4 subjects were excluded from analysis. One subject dropped out because she experienced a motor vehicle accident after screening, 5 dropped out because they were "too busy" and 3 subjects could not give a clear reason.

Ninety-eight subjects (92%) completed the treatment: 25 received comprehensive massage therapy, 25 soft-tissue manipulation, 22 remedial exercise and 26 sham laser treatment. Follow-up measures were completed by 91 subjects (85%).

The 4 treatment groups exhibited similar demographic characteristics (Table 2). The mean age of all subjects was 46 years, most (68%) were married or in a relationship with a partner, and most (70%) had at least a college education. The mean body mass index (kg/m^2) was 25.5, which is considered overweight.[27] Previous episodes of low-back pain were experienced by 60% of the subjects, and the average duration of the present episode of pain was greater than 3 months. The most common reasons for low-back pain were identified by the subjects as bending or lifting injuries, work-related mild strains, sports injuries and unknown. There were no significant differences between the groups at baseline.

TABLE 2 BASELINE CHARACTERISTICS OF SUBJECTS WHO RECEIVED TREATMENT

| | TREATMENT GROUP | | | |
CHARACTERISTIC	COMPREHENSIVE MASSAGE THERAPY $n = 25$	SOFT-TISSUE MANIPULATION $n = 25$	REMEDIAL EXERCISE AND EDUCATION $n = 22$	PLACEBO (SHAM LASER TREATMENT) $n = 26$
Mean age, yr	47.9 (16.2)*	46.5 (18.4)	48.4 (12.9)	41.9 (16.6)[†]
Female, %	56	56	41	54[†]
Relationship status, %				
Partnered or married	68	64	73	69[†]
Single, divorced or widowed	32	36	27	31[†]
Education, %				
High school or less	36	32	27	23
College	20	24	27	20
University	44	44	45	57
Mean body mass index (kg/m^2)	25.0 (4.1)	25.5 (3.8)	26.5 (3.5)	25.0 (2.6)[†]
Occupational activity, %				
Not working or retired	32	28	27	15
Student	4	16	9	15
At desk mainly	12	24	9	19
At desk and movement	36	16	27	27
Physical labour	16	16	27	23
Duration of LBP, wk	12.0 (9.1)	14.8 (8.2)	13.2 (11.1)	13.3 (8.8)[†]
Previous episode of LBP, %	68	56	68	50[†]
Problem, %				
Not known	20	8	9	19
Mild strain (overworked)	8	40	14	35
Sports injury	16	12	18	12
Bending or lifting injury	36	28	45	27
Fall or accident	12	8	9	0
Stress related	8	4	5	8
Outcome measures[‡]				
RDQ score	8.3 (4.2)	8.6 (4.4)	7.2 (5.2)	7.2 (4.2)[†]
PPI score	2.4 (0.8)	2.2 (0.8)	2.2 (0.7)	2.0 (0.7)[†]
PRI score	12.3 (5.0)	10.6 (5.8)	10.2 (6.4)	11.1 (5.5)[†]

BOX 4-2   **EFFECTIVENESS OF MASSAGE THERAPY FOR SUBACUTE LOW-BACK PAIN: A RANDOMIZED CONTROLLED TRIAL — CONT'D**

State Anxiety Index score	31.8 (9.8)	37.3 (10.3)	32.6 (7.5)	34.1 (8.4)[†]
Modified Schober test, cm	5.6 (1.3)	5.2 (1.8)	5.3 (1.1)	5.5 (1.2)[†]

Note: SD = standard deviation, LBP = low-back pain, RDQ = Roland Disability Questionnaire, PPI = Present Pain Index, PRI = Pain Rating Index.

*Figures represent mean (and SD), unless stated to be a percentage of the group.

[†]No significant difference between groups.

[‡]RDQ (score range 0–24) measures function (a lower score indicates less dysfunction); PPI (score range 0–5) measures intensity of pain (a lower score indicates less intensity); PRI (score range 0–79) measures quality of pain (a lower score indicates fewer qualitative symptoms); State Anxiety Index (score range 20–80) measures level of anxiety experienced at this moment (a lower score indicates less anxiety); modified Schober test measures lumbar range of motion in centimetres.

The post-treatment and follow-up outcome measures appear in Table 3. Statistically significant differences were found between the groups on self-reported measures of function, pain and state anxiety. There was no difference between the groups in lumbar range of motion.

Post hoc testing (Scheffé, significance at $p < 0.05$) for post-treatment scores indicated that the comprehensive massage therapy group had significantly better scores than the remedial exercise and sham laser groups on measures of function (RDQ), intensity of pain (PPI) and quality of

TABLE 3   **OUTCOME DATA**

VARIABLE	COMPREHENSIVE MASSAGE THERAPY MEAN (AND 95% CI)	SD	SOFT-TISSUE MANIPULATION MEAN (AND 95% CI)	SD	REMEDIAL EXERCISE AND POSTURE EDUCATION MEAN (AND 95% CI)	SD	PLACEBO (SHAM LASER TREATMENT) MEAN (AND 95% CI)	SD	P VALUE
Primary outcomes									
Post treatment	n = 25		n = 25		n = 22		n = 26		
RDQ score	2.36 (1.2–3.5)	2.8	3.44 (2.3–4.6)	2.8	6.82 (4.3–9.3)	5.6	6.85 (5.4–8.2)	3.5	< 0.001
PPI score	0.44 (0.17–0.71)	0.6	1.04 (0.76–1.3)	0.7	1.64 (1.3–2)	0.8	1.65 (1.3–2)	0.8	< 0.001
PRI score	2.92 (1.5–4.3)	3.4	5.24 (2.9–7.6)	5.7	7.91 (5.2–10.6)	6.1	8.31 (6.1–10.5)	5.4	0.001
Follow-up (1 mo)	n = 24		n = 22		n = 21		n = 24		
RDQ score	1.54 (0.69–2.4)	2.0	2.86 (1.5–4.2)	3.1	5.71 (3.5–7.9)	4.8	6.50 (4.7–8.3)	4.2	< 0.001
PPI score	0.42 (0.17–0.66)	0.6	1.18 (0.52–1.8)	1.5	1.33 (0.97–1.7)	0.8	1.75 (1.5–2)	0.6	< 0.001
PRI score	2.29 (0.5–4.0)	4.2	4.55 (2.0–7.1)	5.7	5.19 (3.3–7.1)	4.3	7.71 (5.2–10.3)	6.0	0.006
Secondary outcomes									
Post treatment	n = 25		n = 25		n = 22		n = 26		
State Anxiety Index score	23.96 (22.4–25.5)	3.8	28.96 (25.5–32.4)	8.4	30.91 (27.9–34.0)	6.9	32.54 (29.4–35.7)	7.8	< 0.001
Modified Schober test, cm	6.36 (5.8–6.9)	1.2	5.87 (5.2–6.5)*	1.5	5.86 (5.3–6.4)	1.3	5.98 (5.5–6.5)	1.2	0.51
Follow-up (1 mo)	n = 24		n = 22		n = 21		n = 24		
State Anxiety Index score	23.79 (22.2–25.4)	3.8	30.73 (26.4–35.1)	9.8	28.81 (25.6–32)	7.1	32.63 (29.5–35.7)	7.4	< 0.001
Modified Schober test, cm	6.47 (6.0–7.0)	1.2	5.93 (5.3–6.6)[†]	1.4	5.39 (4.8–6.0)[†]	1.4	5.50 (4.8–6.1)	1.5	0.04

Note: CI = confidence interval.

*n = 24.

[†]n = 20. Some range of motion tests were missed because of scheduling difficulties.

Continued

pain (PRI) and significantly better scores than the soft-tissue manipulation group on the PPI. At follow-up the comprehensive massage therapy group continued to have significantly improved scores over the sham laser group on the RDQ, PPI and PRI and had significantly better scores than the remedial exercise group on the RDQ and PPI.

At the end of treatment the soft-tissue manipulation group had significantly better scores than the remedial exercise and sham laser groups on the RDQ and significantly better scores than the sham laser group on the PPI. At follow-up the soft-tissue manipulation group was not distinguishable from the exercise group; both group means were statistically better than the mean for the sham laser group on the RDQ.

At the end of treatment and at follow-up the comprehensive massage therapy group had significantly better scores than the sham laser group on state anxiety, whereas no other group did. The mean scores on the pain indexes for all of the groups was lower at the end of treatment than at baseline. All subjects' reported levels of pain in the comprehensive massage therapy group decreased in intensity from baseline to post treatment, which did not occur in any other group. At the 1-month follow-up, 63% of the subjects in the comprehensive massage therapy group reported no pain, as compared with 27% in the soft-tissue manipulation group, 14% in the exercise group and 0% in the sham laser group.

Interpretation

A difference in RDQ scores of 2.5 has been considered to be minimally important in terms of clinical effects.[28] When this criterion was applied to the outcome measures at follow-up in the present study, clinical significance was demonstrated in the comprehensive massage therapy group in comparison with the remedial exercise group (difference 4.2) and the sham laser group (difference 5.0). Clinical significance was also evident in the soft-tissue manipulation group at follow-up in comparison with the exercise group (difference 2.8) and the sham laser group (difference 3.6). Both the comprehensive massage therapy group and the soft-tissue manipulation group showed clinical significance for the improvement of function.

Self-reported levels of function and pain (intensity and quality) improved the most for patients with subacute low-back pain who had comprehensive massage therapy administered by experienced massage therapists. Soft-tissue manipulation was shown to have some benefit after treatment, but by follow-up there was no statistical difference between the soft-tissue manipulation group and the remedial exercise group. Comprehensive massage therapy was shown in this study to maintain statistical significance over the sham laser group on all 3 outcome measures and over the exercise group on 2 outcome measures. This did not occur for any other group. However, at follow-up there were no statistical differences between the comprehensive massage therapy group and the soft-tissue manipulation group. Soft-tissue manipulations were shown to have considerable benefit, and the addition of remedial exercise and posture education was shown to improve the clinical results moderately. Comprehensive massage therapy seemed to have the greatest impact on pain scores but was only marginally better than soft-tissue manipulation alone for improving function.

The cost of treatment per subject in the comprehensive massage therapy group was $300 (6 sessions at $50 per treatment) and $240 for the soft-tissue manipulation group. The estimated cost of treatment per subject in the remedial exercise and sham laser groups was $90. Thus, comprehensive massage therapy had the most benefit but cost $60 more per subject than soft-tissue manipulation alone.

Limitations of the study included the use of a single setting, the use of a specific form of massage therapy provided by only 2 massage therapists, unmeasured provider effects on the validity of outcome measures and the confines of the protocol (e.g., a set number of treatments regardless of the severity or complexity of the problem and short-term follow-up). The treatment was provided by therapists with clinical experience and continuing education that focused on physiology. It is likely that massage therapists with similar education and training based on physiology, as opposed to reflexology or craniosacral therapy, would provide similar treatment. Only in British Columbia and Ontario is massage therapy regulated, although most other provinces, except Quebec, have similar training.

This is the first randomized controlled trial of the effectiveness of massage therapy for subacute low-back pain. Replication of this study, comparisons with other forms of treatment and external evaluation are required to help ascertain which types of low-back problems with which types of complicating factors (e.g., levels of stress and activity) will respond best to massage therapy. Massage therapy that is based on physiology and emphasizes the soft-tissue manipulation component of treatment was found to be effective in the nonpharmacological management of subacute low-back pain.

A special thanks is extended to Kevin Gorey, research adviser at the University of Windsor, Windsor, Ont. Gratefully acknowledged are Cyndy McLean, Centre Coordinator, and Terry Graham, Professor, University of Guelph, Guelph, Ont., for their support of the project. This project was funded by the College of Massage Therapists of Ontario (CMTO).
Competing interests: None declared.

BOX 4-2	EFFECTIVENESS OF MASSAGE THERAPY FOR SUBACUTE LOW-BACK PAIN: A RANDOMIZED CONTROLLED TRIAL — CONT'D

References

1. Sternbach RA. Survey of pain in the United States: the Nuprin pain report. *Clin J Pain* 1986;2:49-53.
2. Andersson GBJ. The epidemiology of spinal disorders. In: Fryomyer JW, editor. *The adult spine: principles and practice.* New York: Raven Press; 1991. p. 107-46.
3. Loney PL, Stratford PW. The prevalence of low back pain in adults: a methodological review of the literature. *Phys Ther* 1999;79:384-96.
4. Pope MH, Phillips RB, Haugh LD, Hsieh CJ, MacDonald L, Haldeman S. A prospective randomized three-week trial of spinal manipulation, transcutaneous muscle stimulation, massage and corset in the treatment of subacute low back pain. *Spine* 1994;19:2571-7.
5. Koes BW, Assendelft WJ, van der Heijden GJ, Bouter LM. Spinal manipulation for low back pain. An updated systematic review of randomized controlled clinical trials. *Spine* 1996;21:2860-71.
6. Cherkin DC, Deyo RA, Battie M, Street J, Barlow W. A comparison of physical therapy, chiropractic manipulation, and provision of an educational booklet for the treatment of patients with low back pain. *N Engl J Med* 1998;339:1021-9.
7. Van Tulder MW, Koes BW, Bouter LM. Conservative treatment of acute and chronic nonspecific low back pain. A systematic review of randomized controlled trials of the most common interventions. *Spine* 1997;22:2128-56.
8. Crawley N. A critique of the methodology of research studies evaluating massage. *Eur J Cancer Care (Engl)* 1997;6:23-31.
9. Ernst E. Massage therapy for low back pain: a systematic review. *J Pain Symptom Manage* 1999;17:65-9.
10. Roland M, Morris R. A study of the natural history of back pain. Part I: development of a reliable and sensitive measure of disability in low-back pain. *Spine* 1983;8:141-4.
11. Deyo RA. Measuring the functional status of patients with low back pain. *Arch Phys Med Rehabil* 1988;69:1044-53.
12. Hsieh CJ, Phillips RB, Adams AH, Pope MH. Functional outcomes of low back pain: comparison of four treatment groups in a randomized controlled trial. *J Manipulative Physiol Ther* 1992;15:4-9.
13. Hadler NM, Curtis P, Gillings DB, Stinnett S. Benefit of spinal manipulation as adjunctive therapy for acute low back pain: a stratified controlled trial. *Spine* 1987;12:703-6.
14. Melzack R. The McGill pain questionnaire: major properties and scoring methods. *Pain* 975;1:277-99.
15. Melzack R, Vetere P, Finch L. Transcutaneous electrical nerve stimulation for low back pain. *Phys Ther* 1983;63:489-93.
16. Prieto EJ, Hopson L, Bradley LA, Byrne M, Geisinger KF, Midax D, et al. The language of low back pain: factor structure of the McGill Pain Questionnaire. *Pain* 1980;8:11-9.
17. McCreary C, Turner J, Dawson E. Principal dimensions of the pain experience and psychological disturbance in chronic low back pain patients. *Pain* 1981;11: 85-92.
18. Spielberger CD, Gorusch RL, Lushene RE. *Manual for the State-Trait Anxiety Inventory.* Palo Alto (CA): Consulting Psychologists Press; 1970.
19. Spielberger CD. *State-Trait Anxiety Inventory for adults.* Palo Alto (CA): Mind Gardens; 1983.
20. Spielberger CD. *State-Trait Anxiety Inventory: a comprehensive bibliography.* 2nd ed. Palo Alto (CA): Consulting Psychologists Press; 1989.
21. Blanchard EB, Andrasik F, Neff DF, Arena JG, Ahles TA, Jurish SE, et al. Biofeedback and relaxation training with three kinds of headache: treatment effects and their prediction. *J Consult Clin Psychol* 1982;50:562-75.
22. Hart JD. Failure to complete treatment for headache: a multiple regression analysis. *J Consult Clin Psychol* 1982;50:781-2.
23. Moll JMH, Wright W. Normal range of spinal mobility. *Ann Rheum Dis* 1971;30:381-6.
24. Hyytiainen K, Salminen JJ, Suvitie T, Wickstrom G, Pentti J. Reproducibility of nine tests to measure spinal mobility and trunk muscle strength. *Scand J Rehabil Med* 1991;23:3-10.
25. Jenkinson TR, Mallorie PA, Whitelock HC, Kennedy LG, Garrett SL, Calin A. Defining spinal mobility in ankylosing spondylitis. *J Rheumatol* 1994; 21:1694-8.
26. Fleiss JL. *Statistical methods for rates and proportions.* 2nd ed. Toronto: John Wiley & Sons; 1981.
27. Bray GA. Definitions, measurements and classification of the syndromes of obesity. *Int J Obes* 1978;2:99-112.
28. Patrick DL, Deyo RA, Atlas SJ, Singer DE, Chapin A, Keller RB. Assessing health-related quality of life in patients with sciatica. *Spine* 1995;20:1899-908.

Reprint requests to: Michele Preyde, Faculty of Social Work, University of Toronto, 246 Bloor St. W, Toronto ON M5S 1A1.

From Preyde, M. (2000). Effectiveness of massage therapy for subacute low-back pain: A randomized controlled trial. *Canadian Medical Association Journal, 162*(13), 1815-1820.

Based on your reading of the Preyde (2000) study (Box 4-2), let us now proceed with our critique of the research article. In so doing, we will rely on the earlier listing of 29 questions that represent the various criteria or standards that should be helpful as we work our way through the article. Let the games begin!

Preliminary Section

1. Does the *title* of the study provide a basis for identifying the *type of study*, *major variables*, and *participants*?

To a large extent, the title does accomplish what it should. We can infer from the title that this study is classified as follows: it falls in the quantitative research category, entails a difference-oriented research strategy, and uses a true experimental/RCT research method. The IV apparently is a manipulated one that involves some type of massage therapy intervention. We can also surmise that pain intensity is a dependent variable measured in the study. Finally, the participants are individuals suffering from subacute low-back pain.

2. Does the *abstract* synthesize the main body of the report (i.e., the introduction, method, results, and discussion) with a particular focus on the *research question, research hypothesis, participants, research method and design, major variables, instruments, statistical techniques, principal findings*, and *conclusions*?

The first half of the abstract does imply the study's research question, but it does not state it explicitly. Likewise, the research hypothesis is similarly implied, although we do not have a precise sense of the predicted comparison of the four levels of the manipulated IV relative to the four dependent variables.

We could, therefore, derive a sense of the research question that goes something like this: Is there a statistically significant difference among comprehensive massage therapy encompassing both soft tissue manipulation and remedial exercise with posture education, soft tissue manipulation only, remedial exercise with posture education only, and a placebo control of sham laser therapy, relative to function, pain, anxiety, and lumbar ROM experienced by participants suffering with subacute low-back pain?

The research hypothesis that we may, similarly, infer would read as follows: There is a statistically significant difference among comprehensive massage therapy encompassing both soft tissue manipulation and remedial exercise with posture education, soft tissue manipulation only, remedial exercise with posture education only, and a placebo control of sham laser therapy, relative to function, pain, anxiety, and lumbar ROM experienced by participants suffering with subacute low-back pain.

The abstract does acknowledge that 107 participants initially started the study and were baseline measured on the four outcome variables, but that only 98 and 91 of the original 107 completed the outcome measures after treatment and at one-month follow up, respectively. The abstract further indicates that of the 98 participants who remained in the study at least until the after treatment outcomes measures were recorded, the size of each

of the four comparison groups was 25, 25, 22, and 26, respectively.

The research method used in this study is true experimental/RCT and involved a randomized, comparative groups, pretest-posttest research design. The manipulated IV could be labeled as "nature of massage therapy intervention" and has four levels corresponding to the three experimental group interventions and one placebo control group cited earlier. The four DVs or outcome measures include function, pain, anxiety, and lumbar ROM.

The abstract further identifies by name the four instruments used to measure the four dependent variables. The actual statistical techniques used to analyze the study's data are not identified in the abstract. The major findings of the study, though, are summarized in the abstract in such a way as to indicate the effectiveness of the comprehensive massage therapy intervention over the other two treatments and the placebo on three of the four DVs to a statistically significant degree. Furthermore, both the comprehensive intervention and the soft tissue manipulation intervention demonstrated at least clinical significance on the remaining DV. An overarching conclusion is provided in the abstract in the form of an interpretation that massage therapy was shown to benefit patients with subacute low-back pain.

Introductory Section

3. Is the reader introduced to the *relevant professional literature* bearing on the study being reported by way of a *general overview of the research problem area* as well as a more *specific coverage of individual studies*?

This article's introductory literature review spans only the first paragraph and includes a total of nine citations from professional sources. A general overview of the problem area is provided; however, specific coverage of related studies is not provided in depth. Instead, the author chooses to characterize succinctly the available studies in terms of their demonstrating inconsistent findings, flawed methodologies, lack of compliance with a massage protocol by those providing treatment, and use of nonspecific massage as a control. This literature review does indicate the absence of studies that specifically investigated massage therapy as an intervention for low-back pain.

We need to recognize that although the majority of a research report's literature review typically appears in the introductory section, the three other sections constituting the report's main body will likely contain additional citations of literature sources. That is the case with this article, particularly regarding the literature citations appearing in the outcome measures part of the method section.

4. Is the purpose of the study identified by way of the *research question* being formulated at an *operational level*?

The second paragraph of the introductory section does indicate the study's purpose by stating what the study attempted. There is no operational formulation, however, of a research question per se. Instead, readers are required to identify the research question as it would presumably flow from the study's declarative purpose statement.

5. Is a *rationale or justification*, based on various features of the professional literature, presented as a context or framework for the study's *research hypothesis*?

6. Does the author state the study's *research hypothesis* in such a way that the predicted answer to the study's research question is clear and unambiguous?

These features are not provided at the outset of the article. We might assume, though, that the author's emphasis on correcting the methodological flaws and infidelity to established massage treatment protocols so pervasive in earlier studies may well represent a basis for anticipating some demonstrable effectiveness of massage therapy in treating low-back pain. Again, these are simply inferences we might make as readers in the absence of an explicitly stated rationale for an explicitly stated research hypothesis that is likewise missing.

Method Section

7. Are the study's *participants* clearly characterized along with the *inclusion and exclusion criteria* used for identifying them?

The first two paragraphs in the method section of the article do identify the professional setting for the study as well as the recruitment procedures and inclusion/exclusion criteria for identifying the initial sample of participants. Demographic characteristics of the participants, though, are not identified in detail until later in the results section.

8. Did the researchers justify the *number of participants* constituting the sample size by way of a *power analysis*?

Although positioned in a rather unusual location, the author does provide a documented power

analysis on which was based the decision to assign a minimum of 20 participants per comparison group. This reference to the power analysis appears in the last paragraph of the methods section and does justify the sample size on legitimate grounds.

9. Was an *accessible population* of potential participants acknowledged along with an indication of *how the sample was derived* from such a population, be it through random selection or some other procedure?

No, the article makes no mention whatever of an accessible population from which the sample was derived. Consequently, any possible discussion of selection methods for deriving the sample from a larger accessible population is moot.

10. Did the authors specify the manner in which the participants were *assigned* to the two or more comparison groups, be it through random assignment or some other means?

The third paragraph in the methods section does indicate that a table of random numbers was used to randomly assign participants to the four levels of the IV. This part of the report, though, does not mention the actual number of participants randomly assigned to each of the four comparison groups. Having already read the study's abstract, however, we do know that the comprehensive massage therapy, soft tissue manipulation only, remedial exercise with posture education only, and placebo of sham laser therapy groups had 25, 25, 22, and 26 participants, respectively, at the time of the posttreatment measurement of the four DVs.

11. Was any clarification provided as to how the *ethical aspects* of the study were governed, particularly in reference to the protection of the participants, the overall integrity of the research, and the earlier approval of the study by an IRB?

Yes, the initial paragraph of the methods section does acknowledge that approval was received from the Ethics Review Committee based at the university where the study was conducted. The author also states here that all participants gave informed consent prior to beginning their involvement in the study.

12. Was the nature of the research effort adequately characterized in terms of its position in the research continuum (i.e., its position regarding *research category, strategy, method, design, and defining procedures*)?

The title of the study, the abstract, and the third paragraph in the methods section do provide enough information to allow a reader to recognize that this investigation has the following characteristics: It is a study that belongs to the quantitative research category in that it employs a difference-oriented research strategy using a true experimental/RCT research method. Furthermore, this investigation represents a randomized, comparative groups, pretest-posttest research design in that it incorporates such research procedures as random assignment, pretesting, a manipulated IV, and posttesting.

13. Were the study's *variables operationalized* in a comprehensive fashion so that their manipulation or measurement could be replicated?

The treatment variable and outcome measures subsections of the article's methods section do provide considerable detail regarding the manipulation of the IV and the measurement of the four DVs at three different points in time.

Specifically, operational details are given that indicate precisely the type of treatment provided to each of the following four levels of the manipulated independent variable: Experimental Group 1, which received the comprehensive massage therapy encompassing soft tissue manipulation and remedial exercise with posture education; Experimental Group 2, which received soft tissue manipulation only; Experimental Group 3, which received remedial exercise with posture education only; and the Placebo Control Group, which received an inert treatment in the form of a sham low-level laser (infrared) therapy whereby the laser was set up to look as if it was functioning, but actually was not.

The two primary outcome measures or DVs are functionality and pain. These DVs are identified as being measured by the Roland Disability Questionnaire and the McGill Pain Questionnaire, respectively. Furthermore, the author provides for each of these two instruments descriptive information as well as documentation regarding their validity and reliability.

The two secondary outcome measures or DVs are anxiety and lumbar ROM. The author provides descriptive information as well as documented evidence for the validity and reliability of the two instruments that measured these secondary outcomes, namely, the State Anxiety Index and the Modified Schober Test.

14. Did the authors clearly specify the *equipment or instruments* used in the study for variable

manipulation or measurement purposes, along with a documentation of the technical characteristics of such including validity and reliability?

As discussed earlier, the author describes and justifies quite succinctly all instruments used in the study. The author also explains in detail the placebo control group that received the inert sham low-level laser (infrared) therapy. Furthermore, the study provides descriptive information regarding the four instruments used for measuring the four DVs as well as documentation of their validity and reliability.

Results Section

15. Were the *data analysis techniques* used in the study identified and justified?

Yes, though positioned at the end of the methods section, the author does cite the use of inferential techniques such as analysis of variance (ANOVA) and a subsequent Scheffe's post hoc multiple comparison test. Furthermore, in the results section it becomes apparent that descriptive statistics including the mean and standard deviation were used as well as another inferential technique of establishing 95% confidence intervals.

16. Were the results of the study communicated by an appeal to *descriptive and/or inferential statistics* consistent with the nature of the research question as well as the research method and measurement scales used?

Yes, the actual results communicated in the results section are consistent with the research question posed as well as the research method and measurement scales used. Specifically, descriptive statistics involving frequency counts are provided on the number of participants randomly assigned at the outset to the four comparison groups, the number of episodes of a given treatment either not started or not completed in its entirely, and the extent to which attrition occurred in each of the comparison groups. Extensive descriptive statistical results also appear on several baseline demographic characteristics of those 98 participants who received treatment.

Results based on the inferential techniques of ANOVA, the Scheffe test, and 95% confidence intervals–along with accompanying descriptive statistics of the mean and standard deviation–are indicated on all of the outcome measures.

17. Were the results of the data analysis related to an appropriate *decision* regarding the study's *null or statistical hypothesis*?

18. Was the decision regarding the null hypothesis acknowledged as a basis for inferring decisions concerning the *alternative and research hypotheses?*

These two questions/criteria are clustered together because the response in each case is essentially the same. The author does not explicitly state the null hypothesis or the alternative hypothesis in the results section, but instead apparently relies on the reader to make the necessary inferences. This is comparable to what the author does in the introductory section by not explicitly stating the research hypothesis but, instead, opting to assume that the prediction is clear to the reader. Even with the author implying each of these three hypotheses, there is no apparent attempt to relate explicitly the decision on the null hypothesis back to the alternative and research hypotheses. Perhaps this, too, is left to inference on the part of the reader.

As a final point, here, we must acknowledge in all fairness that the results presented by the author do provide the reader with all that is necessary to recognize those decisions that are functionally in place regarding the hypotheses. As summarized in the abstract, the results make it clear that massage therapy is significantly effective in treating subacute low-back pain where several important outcome measures are concerned.

19. If hypothesis testing was performed, were the analyses augmented with other statistical techniques such as *confidence interval estimation* or *effect size calculations?*

Yes, the results section does augment the hypothesis testing with calculations of 95% confidence interval estimations. No mention is made, though, of effect size being computed. If this had been provided, one option would have been for the author to demonstrate that proportion of the variability on each DV that can be attributed to, or explained by, the IV.

20. Were *tables and figures* appropriately used to make the data analyses more comprehensible?

The author makes excellent use of appropriate tables for displaying in a succinct way the results of the data analyses performed. This feature of the article allows the narrative to flow more easily and understandably because the reader has available a reference point in the form of the tables that provide an overview of the accumulated data. Figures were not necessary given the nature of the results presented.

Discussion Section

21. Did the researchers reflect on the manner in which the study was designed and conducted regarding any *limitations or delimitations* (i.e., intentional or unintentional boundaries)?

The fourth paragraph in the interpretation (i.e., discussion) section does acknowledge several limitations to the study. These deal with such concerns as the use of a single setting, a particular form of massage intervention provided by only two massage therapists, the failure to measure provider effects on the validity of the outcome measures, and the confines of the massage protocol that did not deviate in the number of sessions provided so as to accommodate varying degrees of severity or complexity of the problem treated.

The author also acknowledges that therapists with clinical experience and continuing education focusing on physiology provided the treatment. This latter point is perhaps more of a delimitation (i.e., boundary) of the study than an actual limitation (i.e., drawback). The same might be said about the reference earlier to the use of a single setting for the study, a fact that may speak more to the study's delimitations. In each instance we see a boundary of sorts rather than a limitation or drawback to the study.

22. Did the author *elaborate* on the *interpretation of the study's findings* beyond the interpretation that was begun in the results section?

Yes, the labeled section (i.e., interpretation) in this article that is equivalent to a standard discussion section does elaborate beyond the interpretation provided earlier. The presentation of the results in the previous section is couched somewhat in terms of an interpretation, yet this is followed with a more interpretive discussion later in the report.

23. Did the researcher address the *significance* of the study and its findings, particularly as they relate to earlier studies in the problem area investigated?

Yes, the author notes in the final paragraph of the article that this is the first randomized controlled trial of the effectiveness of massage therapy for subacute low-back pain. Furthermore, at several points throughout the results and interpretation sections, the researcher observes not only the occurrence of statistically significant findings, but also those results that are considered clinically significant.

These acknowledgments by the author take on considerably more meaning when we view them against the backdrop of the literature review that appears at the outset of the article. There the author cites various inconsistencies and flaws that permeate much of the available literature on the treatment of subacute low-back pain. The researcher also notes several methodological difficulties specifically with studies using massage therapy as an intervention. Furthermore, the final sentence of the article's literature review notes that no studies were found that specifically addressed massage therapy as an intervention for low-back pain. With this critical tone of the literature review in mind, the author does indeed succeed in highlighting the importance of this study's role in correcting several of the deficiencies found in earlier studies.

24. Did the discussion section address possible *intervening variables* in the study that might explain why the results obtained were indeed forthcoming?

This article does not speak to the issue of one or more intervening variables, or underlying mechanisms, that might explain why the results received were forthcoming.

25. Were *recommendations* suggested to the reader regarding needed follow-up studies that might replicate, fully or partially, the study?

Yes, the final two paragraphs of the article provide recommendations for further study needed in this area. These recommendations take the form of a call for both full and partial replications as well as a mention that varying types of low-back problems must be considered along with varying types of complicating factors in researching the potential of massage therapy as a viable intervention.

Concluding Section

26. Does the list of *references* accurately reflect each of the sources cited in the research report, with a consistent bibliographic citation style used?

Yes, the bibliographic information provided in the list of references does provide us with the full citation for each source acknowledged in the narrative. The formatting style, likewise, is consistent and should allow readers to pursue the cited sources for additional information.

27. Does the research report contain any *appendixes* that augment in greater detail information provided earlier in the article?

No appendixes are provided in this article.

28. Is there any information in the form of *author notes* providing insight regarding funding support for the study, contact directives for communicating with the author as a follow-up, or collegial assistance in completing the study?

Yes, the article does provide notes regarding funding support for the study, contact information for communicating with the author, and the acknowledgment of collegial assistance and support.

29. Are any *footnotes* provided that elaborate on one or more aspects of the study that would have been misplaced or distracting if they had been embedded in the main body of the report?

No footnotes appear in the article.

WHERE DO WE GO FROM HERE?

THE QUANTITATIVE RESEARCH CATEGORY (PART THREE): A MORE EXPANDED VIEW

Our attention in Chapters 3 and 4 was on the true experimental/randomized controlled trial research method. As we have seen, this method falls under the difference-oriented research strategy that is part of the broader quantitative research category. We have focused on this research approach from the outset for two valid reasons: (a) it is valued to a high degree in scientific inquiry because of the degree of refinement and control it exerts in investigating relationships between/among variables of interest and (b) it accommodates the intervention types of studies in which presumably most massage therapists and bodyworkers are interested and from which they would benefit the most. With this background in place, our next stop in the book is Part Three in which we cover the quantitative research category in a considerably broader and more expanded way.

THE DIFFERENCE-ORIENTED, ASSOCIATION-ORIENTED, AND DESCRIPTIVE-ORIENTED RESEARCH STRATEGIES

Chapter 5 will provide you with a more in-depth discussion of the *difference-oriented research strategy* family. In so doing we will see that there are three additional research methods beyond the true experimental/RCT method: the quasi-experimental, the single-case experimental, and the nonexperimental comparative groups research methods.

Chapter 6 then introduces you to the *association-oriented research strategy*. There we will examine the two major research methods that are part of the association-oriented research strategy: the correlational research method and the predictive research method.

In the final chapter of Part Three, Chapter 7, we will consider the *descriptive-oriented research strategy*.

This research strategy will give us the opportunity to learn about four additional research methods: the single-case quantitative analysis, the survey, the naturalistic/structural observational, and the case report methods.

REFERENCES

Chang, M. Y., Wang, S. Y., & Chen, C. H. (2002). Effects of massage on pain and anxiety during labour: A randomized controlled trial in Taiwan. *Journal of Advanced Nursing, 38*(1), 68–73.

Harris, S. (1992). *Chalk up another one: The best of Sidney Harris.* New Brunswick, NJ: Rutgers University Press.

Preyde, M. (2000). Effectiveness of massage therapy for subacute low-back pain: A randomized controlled trial. *Canadian Medical Association Journal, 162*(13), 1815–1820.

Van den Dolder, P. A., & Roberts, D. L. (2003). A trial into the effectiveness of soft tissue massage in the treatment of shoulder pain. *Australian Journal of Physiotherapy, 49*, 183–188.

ADDITIONAL RECOMMENDED RESOURCES

Cawley, N. (1997). A critique of the methodology of research studies evaluating massage. *European Journal of Cancer Care, 6,* 23–-31.

Hsieh, C-Y. J., Phillips, R. B., Adams, A. H., & Pope, M. H. (1992). Functional outcomes of low back pain: Comparison of four treatment groups in a randomized controlled trial. *Journal of Manipulative and Physiological Therapeutics, 15*(1), 4–9.

McMaster University Health Sciences Center, Department of Clinical Epidemiology & Biostatistics. (1981a). How to read clinical journals: IV. To determine etiology or causation. *Canadian Medical Association Journal, 124,* 985–990.

McMaster University Health Sciences Center, Department of Clinical Epidemiology & Biostatistics. (1981b). How to read clinical journals: V. To distinguish useful from useless or even harmful therapy. *Canadian Medical Association Journal, 124,* 1156–1162.

Westcombe, A. M., Gambles, M. A., Wilkinson, S. M., Barnes, K., & Fellowes, D. (2003). Learning the hard way! Setting up an RCT of aromatherapy massage for patients with advanced cancer. *Palliative Medicine, 17,* 300–307.

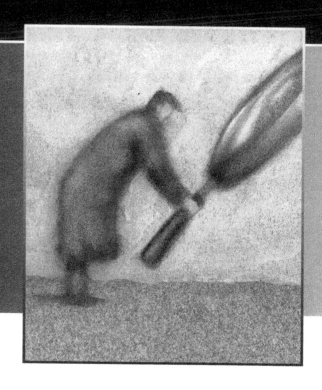

PART THREE

THE QUANTITATIVE RESEARCH CATEGORY

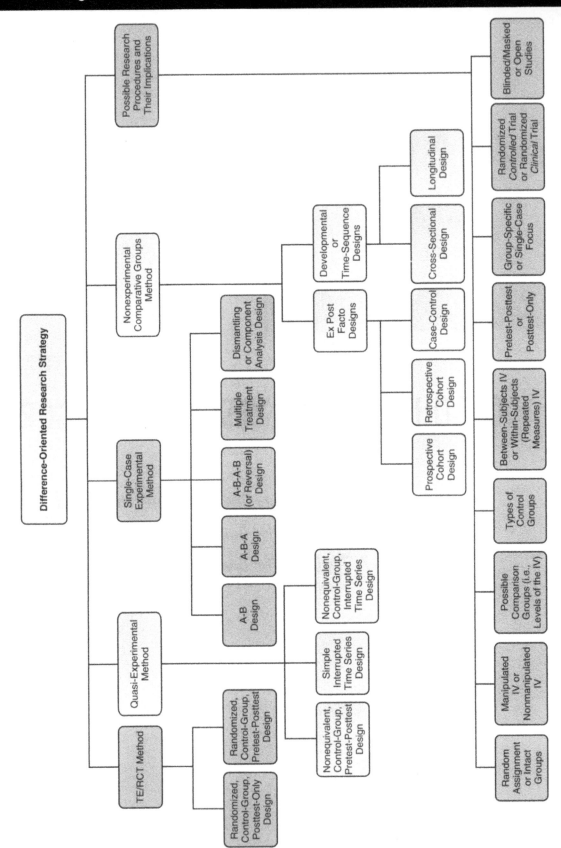

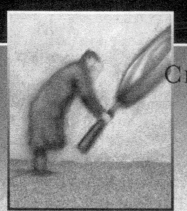

5

THE DIFFERENCE-ORIENTED RESEARCH STRATEGY

OUTLINE

OBJECTIVES

Upon completion of this chapter, the reader will have the information necessary to perform the following tasks:

1 List the four research methods that are included in the difference-oriented research strategy.

2 Identify and explain the two major research procedures that define the true experimental/randomized controlled trial research method.

3 List the two principal research designs that are included under the true experimental/randomized controlled trial research method, and address the following tasks for each:
    a. diagram and explain the research procedures that constitute the design;
    b. recognize, or be able to provide, an example of a study based on the design.

4 Identify and explain the two major research procedures that define the quasi-experimental research method.

5 List the three principal research designs that are included under the quasi-experimental research method, and address the following tasks for each:
    a. diagram and explain the research procedures that constitute the design;
    b. recognize, or be able to provide, an example of a study based on the design.

6 Identify and explain those major research procedures that define the single-case experimental research method.

7 List the five principal research designs that are included under the single-case experimental research method, and address the following tasks for each:
    a. diagram and explain the research procedures that constitute the design;
    b. recognize, or be able to provide, an example of a study based on the design.

KEY TERMS

A-B design
A-B-A design
A-B-A-B (or reversal) design
Between-subjects independent variable or
    design
Blinded/masked study
Cross-sectional design
Developmental or time-sequence designs
Difference-oriented research strategy
Dismantling or component-analysis
    design
Double-blind study
Evaluator-blinded trials
Ex post facto (or after the fact) designs
Intact groups
Level(s) of an independent variable
Longitudinal design
Manipulated independent variable

Multiple treatment design
No treatment (or "do nothing") control group
Nonequivalent, control-group, interrupted time
    series design
Nonequivalent, control-group, pretest-posttest
    design
Nonexperimental comparative groups
    method
Nonmanipulated independent variable
Open study
Placebo-attention control group
Placebo-sham treatment control group
Posttest-only design
Pretest-posttest
Previous/existing exposure and recent/
    present/future outcome focused
Prospective cohort design
Quantitative research category

Quasi-experimental method
Random assignment
Randomized, control-group, posttest-only
    design
Randomized, control-group, pretest-posttest
    design
Retrospective case-control design
Retrospective cohort design
Simple interrupted time series design
Single-blind study
Single-case experimental method
Standard treatment control group
Treatment/intervention focused
True experimental/randomized controlled trial
    research method
Waiting or wait-list control group
Within-subjects (or repeated measures)
    independent variable or design

8   Identify and explain the two major research procedures that
    define the nonexperimental comparative groups research
    method.

9   Identify and explain the two features, and implied research
    procedures, that define the three ex post facto (after-the-fact)
    designs included under the nonexperimental comparative
    groups research method.

10 List the three principal research designs that are considered ex
    post facto in nature, and address the following tasks for each:
    a. diagram and explain the research procedures that
        constitute the design;
    b. recognize, or be able to provide, an example of a study
        based on the design.

11 Identify and explain the two features, and implied
    research procedures, that define the two developmental or
    time-sequence designs included under the nonexperimental
    comparative groups research method.

12 List the two principal research designs that are considered
    developmental or time-sequence in nature, and address the
    following tasks for each:
    a. diagram and explain the research procedures that
        constitute the design;
    b. recognize, or be able to provide, an example of a study
        based on the design.

13 Distinguish between comparative groups that are formed by
    random assignment or as a result of being intact.

14 Distinguish between manipulated and nonmanipulated
    independent variables.

15 Explain the possible options that exist regarding comparative
    groups or levels of an independent variable.

16 Distinguish among the following five types of control groups:
    no treatment or "do nothing" control group, standard
    treatment control group, waiting-list control group,
    placebo-attention control group, and placebo-sham
    treatment control group.

17 Explain the distinction regarding a between-subjects
    independent variable and a within-subjects (repeated
    measures) independent variable.

18 Recognize the use of either a pretest-posttest, or
    posttest-only, set of measurement procedures in a
    hypothetical or actual research study, and explain the
    rationale behind each approach.

19 Regarding those research methods included in the
    difference-oriented research strategy, distinguish between
    a group-specific focus and a single-case focus.

20 Explain the subtle distinction between the expressions
    randomized controlled trial and randomized clinical trial.

21 Distinguish between a blinded/masked study and an
    open study.

WHERE HAVE WE BEEN AND WHERE ARE WE NOW? THE CONNECTION

The previous chapter provided in-depth coverage of the true experimental/randomized controlled trial (RCT) research method. Because of its highly respected position in scientific inquiry, we focused specifically on certain concepts, principles, and procedures that define this approach to doing research. We also considered the standard framework or structure that research reports follow as well as the functions served by such reports. We concluded Chapter 4 with an exhaustive critique of a published research article exemplifying the randomized controlled trial research method.

This chapter is the first of three chapters that constitute Part Three of this book and that focus on part of the quantitative research category. Specifically, we consider here the difference-oriented research strategy and its affiliated research methods and designs. The principal, though not exclusive, emphasis is on research methods and designs that accommodate treatment or intervention type studies. Consideration is also given, however, to those types of studies involving conditions or classifications that define certain research participants. Throughout the chapter we clarify the terminology used by researchers in the behavioral and health sciences that, although employing somewhat different terms and expressions, functionally means the same thing and serves the same purpose (Figure 5-1).

THE DIFFERENCE-ORIENTED RESEARCH STRATEGY: OVERVIEW OF ITS AFFILIATED RESEARCH METHODS AND DESIGNS

Four research methods constitute the **difference-oriented research strategy** addressed in this chapter. The first three of these methods focus on the type of research that involves some kind of treatment or intervention being introduced to participants in the study. These methods, which entail some type of treatment by way of a **manipulated independent variable**, are perhaps of most importance and relevance to massage therapists and related health science professionals. We can assume the vast majority of practitioners would have a particular interest in research that relates various interventions or modalities to certain client conditions. An example of any one of these first three research methods is when seated chair massage is contrasted with relaxation training in a corporate office setting for the purpose of determining which intervention is more effective in reducing workplace stress.

The fourth method involves studies in which a certain classification, status, or condition defines the two or more groups of research participants being compared on one or more factors. The two or more comparison groups of research participants, therefore, represent the two or more levels of a **nonmanipulated independent variable** (IV). An illustration of this fourth method could be the presence and absence of carpal tunnel syndrome (CTS) defining two groups of clerical workers who are

- Quantitative Research Category
  - • Difference-Oriented Research Strategy (Chapter 5)
    - • • True Experimental, or Randomized Controlled Trial, Method (treatment/intervention focused)
    - • • Quasi-Experimental Method (treatment/intervention focused)
    - • • Single-Case Experimental Method (treatment/intervention focused)
    - • • Nonexperimental Comparative Groups Method (focus on previous/existing exposure and recent/present/future outcome)
  - • Association-Oriented Research Strategy (Chapter 6)
    - • • Correlational Method
    - • • Predictive Method
  - • Descriptive-Oriented Research Strategy (Chapter 7)
    - • • Single-Case Quantitative Analysis Method
    - • • Survey Method
    - • • Observational Method
    - • • Case Report Method

FIGURE 5-1 ■ The quantitative research category: Its affiliated research strategies and their variable control-driven methods (bold emphasis designates coverage in Chapter 5).

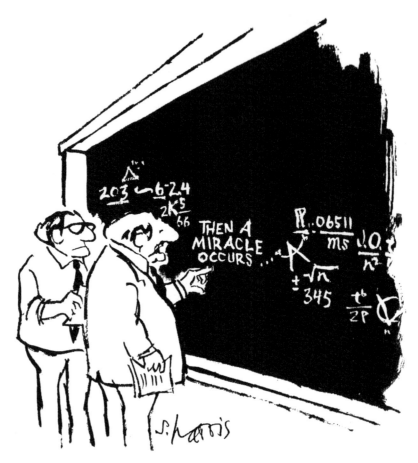

"I think you should be more explicit here in step two."

HUMOR BREAK ■ Hoping for a miracle at this stage in the book? A Humble Hymelian Observation: No, our continuing to make progress through what might seem like a "maze" of research concepts and terminology will not require a miracle, minor or major; just a lot of persistence and, we hope, "heaping servings" of intellectual delight along the way! (From Harris, S. [1977]. *What's so funny about science? Cartoons by Sidney Harris from* American Scientist. Los Altos, CA: W. Kaufman.)

being compared on the dependent variable (DV) of extent of appropriate workstation ergonomics in place.

Recall that each of these four research methods is considered difference-oriented because each investigates whether or not there is a significant difference between or among two or more levels of an IV relative to at least one DV. This should also serve as a reminder that the IV in each of these methods will always be manifested in at least two ways, as is the case, for example, when we are simply comparing an experimental group and a control group relative to some DV measure.

This chapter on the difference-oriented research strategy relates well to several excellent resources that include the following: Cassidy and Hart (2003); Christensen (2004); Dryden and Achilles (2003); Greenhalgh (2001); Hagino (2003); Hulley, Cummings, Browner, Grady, Hearst, and Newman (2001); Katz (2001); Kazdin (2003); Kendall, Butcher, and Holmbech (1999); Lewith, Jonas, and Walach (2002); Peat, Mellis, Williams, and Xuan (2002); Polit and Beck (2004); and Portney and Watkins (2000).

TRUE EXPERIMENTAL/RANDOMIZED CONTROLLED TRIAL METHOD: TREATMENT/INTERVENTION FOCUSED

Figure 5-2 provides a spotlight on the **true experimental/randomized controlled trial research method**, which is **treatment/intervention focused**, and its two affiliated research designs.

Two major research procedures define the true experimental/RCT research method: (a) the **random**

- Quantitative Research Category
  - • Difference-Oriented Research Strategy (Chapter 5)
    - • • **True Experimental, or Randomized Controlled Trial, Method (treatment/intervention focused)**
      - • • • **Randomized, Control-Group, Posttest-Only Design**
      - • • • **Randomized, Control-Group, Pretest-Posttest Design**
    - • • Quasi-Experimental Method (treatment/intervention focused)
    - • • Single-Case Experimental Method (treatment/intervention focused)
    - • • Nonexperimental Comparative Groups Method (focus on previous/existing exposure and recent/present/future outcome)

FIGURE 5-2 ■ Spotlight on the true experimental/randomized controlled trial research method and its affiliated research designs (bold emphasis designates coverage in this section).

assignment of participants to the two or more comparison groups, or **levels of an independent variable**, and (b) the use of a manipulated IV as the study's treatment or intervention. With these two essential research procedures in place, this method may assume any one of the following two research designs.

Randomized, Control-Group, Posttest-Only Design

Recall that Chapter 3 first introduced this design in the context of our effort to overview the true experimental/RCT method. The two essential features of the **randomized, control-group, posttest-only design**, random assignment and a manipulated IV, are followed by the participants being posttested on the study's one or more DVs. Box 5-1 displays in a succinct way the components and directional flow of this design's research procedures.

The earlier illustration of this design provided in Chapter 3 focused on the Chang, Wang, and Chen (2002) study. There the researchers contrasted massage intervention with its absence relative to pain and anxiety intensity experienced by the study's participants during childbirth. Although this study's abstract characterized the control group simply as not receiving the massage intervention, we can assume that the control group did receive

standard treatment in the maternity ward as opposed to its actually being a no-treatment control group. Additionally, this study involved two DVs that necessitated posttesting on each.

Randomized, Control-Group, Pretest-Posttest Design

Similar to the previous design, the critical features of the **randomized, control-group, pretest-posttest design** involve (a) the random assignment of participants to the experimental and control groups and (b) the use of a manipulated IV. What obviously distinguishes this design from the earlier one is the presence of pretesting of the participants before the levels of the IV are introduced. Once the two levels of the IV are introduced for the study's duration, the participants are then posttested on the one or more DVs. Box 5-2a shows these research procedures and their directional flow.

An illustration of this research design is a study by Field, Peck, Hernandez-Reif, Krugman, Burman, and Ozment-Schenck (2000) in which 20 burn victims were randomly assigned to a massage therapy or a standard treatment control group during the remodeling phase of wound healing. Pretest and posttest measures were taken not on one but on several DVs, such as postburn itching, pain, anxiety, and depression. This study demonstrated the overall effectiveness of the massage intervention.

Having introduced the randomized, control-group, pretest-posttest design, this is the most appropriate time to consider a slight variation of this design that still retains the essential features we just examined. The two comparison groups just discussed included an experimental group and a control group; hence, our display in Box 5-2a and the actual name of this design acknowledges these two groups as the basis for the difference-oriented comparison we are exploring. The same dynamics and logic apply if our research interest involves, for example, two experimental groups and a control group or three experimental groups and a control group.

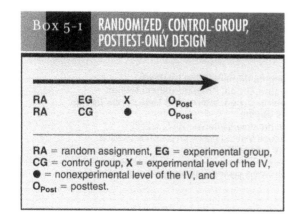

BOX 5-1   RANDOMIZED, CONTROL-GROUP, POSTTEST-ONLY DESIGN

RA   EG   X O_{Post}
RA   CG   ● O_{Post}

RA = random assignment, **EG** = experimental group, **CG** = control group, **X** = experimental level of the IV, ● = nonexperimental level of the IV, and O_{Post} = posttest.

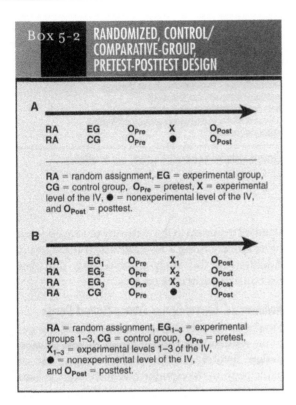

Box 5-2 RANDOMIZED, CONTROL/COMPARATIVE-GROUP, PRETEST-POSTTEST DESIGN

A

| RA | EG | O_{Pre} | X | O_{Post} |
| RA | CG | O_{Pre} | ● | O_{Post} |

RA = random assignment, EG = experimental group, CG = control group, O_{Pre} = pretest, X = experimental level of the IV, ● = nonexperimental level of the IV, and O_{Post} = posttest.

B

RA	EG_1	O_{Pre}	X_1	O_{Post}
RA	EG_2	O_{Pre}	X_2	O_{Post}
RA	EG_3	O_{Pre}	X_3	O_{Post}
RA	CG	O_{Pre}	●	O_{Post}

RA = random assignment, EG_{1-3} = experimental groups 1-3, CG = control group, O_{Pre} = pretest, X_{1-3} = experimental levels 1-3 of the IV, ● = nonexperimental level of the IV, and O_{Post} = posttest.

following: Experimental Group 1, which received the comprehensive massage therapy encompassing soft tissue manipulation and remedial exercise with posture education; Experimental Group 2, which received soft tissue manipulation only; Experimental Group 3, which received remedial exercise with posture education only; and the Placebo-Sham Treatment Control Group, which received an inert treatment in the form of a sham low-level laser (infrared) therapy whereby the laser was set up to look as if it was functioning but actually was not. Preyde, in effect, was investigating whether or not there was a statistically significant difference among these four levels of the IV relative to two primary DVs and two secondary DVs. The primary DVs, once again, were functionality and pain; the secondary DVs were anxiety and lumbar range of motion (ROM). The participants in this study were pretested as well as posttested on these four DVs.

The Preyde study, therefore, is labeled as a *randomized, comparative (or comparison) groups, pretest-posttest design*. Furthermore, its research procedures and directional flow are illustrated in Box 5-2b as follows and, accordingly, represent a variation of what we saw in Box 5-2a.

Regardless of how the two or more levels of our manipulated variables are operationalized and named, we are still investigating whether or not there is a significant difference between two levels or among three or more levels of our manipulated IV.

To appeal to a study that we considered in Chapter 4, the Preyde (2000) investigation provides an excellent example of a possible research design variation mentioned in the preceding paragraph. You may recall that in the Preyde study, the manipulated IV was designated as the nature/extent of massage therapy in treating subacute low-back pain. This manipulated IV was manifested by way of four levels, with each level constituting one of the four groups compared. They included the

QUASI-EXPERIMENTAL METHOD: TREATMENT/INTERVENTION FOCUSED

Figure 5-3 highlights the quasi-experimental research method and its three affiliated research designs.

The **quasi-experimental method** is the second of four research methods included in the difference-oriented research strategy family. The following two research procedures determine this method: (a) the use of "intact" groups of participants—that is, two or more participant groups already formed or in place—for comparison purposes, rather than randomly assigning the study's participants to the comparison groups as is done in the true experimental/RCT method; and (b) the use of a manipulated IV as the study's treatment or intervention.

- Quantitative Research Category
  - • Difference-Oriented Research Strategy (Chapter 5)
    - • • True Experimental, or Randomized Controlled Trial, Method (treatment/intervention focused)
    - • • **Quasi-Experimental Method (treatment/intervention focused)**
      - • • • **Nonequivalent, Control-Group, Pretest-Posttest Design**
      - • • • **Nonequivalent, Control-Group, Interrupted Time Series Design**
      - • • • **Simple Time Series Design**
    - • • Single-Case Experimental Method (treatment/intervention focused)
    - • • Nonexperimental Comparative Groups Method (focus on previous/existing exposure and recent/present/future outcome)

FIGURE 5-3 ■ Spotlight on the quasi-experimental research method and its affiliated research designs (bold emphasis designates coverage in this section).

It should be apparent, then, that the only distinction between the true experimental and quasi-experimental methods is the use of random assignment in the former and its absence in the latter, where comparison group formation is concerned. Both true experimental and quasi-experimental methods, however, do involve a manipulated IV. With these two defining features of the quasi-experimental method understood, let us now consider the three research designs available for implementing this method.

Nonequivalent, Control-Group, Pretest-Posttest Design

Because the comparison groups are not formed as a result of random assignment, we cannot assume that the groups are equivalent at the outset on the various extraneous variables present in the study. In other words, we cannot assume that the extraneous variables are being controlled and do not run the risk of functioning as confounding variables. This is the basis for the word *nonequivalent* in the design's name, the **nonequivalent, control-group, pretest-posttest design**.

In an attempt to establish some basis for determining if indeed the comparison groups are functionally equivalent on one or more of the most potentially threatening extraneous variables, the researcher administers a pretest on one or more of these variables. Based on the pretest results, the researcher is able to judge whether or not the comparison groups are essentially the same at the outset of the study prior to the IV being introduced.

In its most basic form, the manipulated IV is introduced at this point, thereby establishing the experimental and control groups. These groups are then compared in terms of the study's DV, which is assessed by way of the posttest. Box 5-3 shows the directional flow of these research procedures.

A hypothetical illustration of this research design might be the two intact sections of a university-level

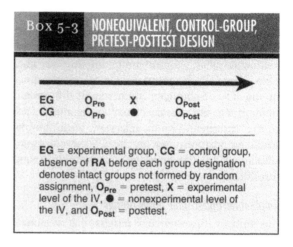

BOX 5-3   NONEQUIVALENT, CONTROL-GROUP, PRETEST-POSTTEST DESIGN

EG O_{Pre} X O_{Post}
CG O_{Pre} ● O_{Post}

EG = experimental group, **CG** = control group, absence of **RA** before each group designation denotes intact groups not formed by random assignment, O_{Pre} = pretest, **X** = experimental level of the IV, ● = nonexperimental level of the IV, and O_{Post} = posttest.

dance course in which students from one section receive massage therapy and students from the other section are on a waiting list to receive the massage intervention subsequent to the study being concluded (cf. Leivadi et al., 1999). Essentially, we would be comparing the massage treatment experimental group with a waiting list control group on one possible outcome measure, such as shoulder abduction ROM.

Nonequivalent, Control-Group, Interrupted Time Series Design

The second of three possible designs available for the quasi-experimental method, the **nonequivalent, control-group, interrupted time series design**, is almost identical to the previously discussed design, except for the presence here of multiple pretest and multiple posttest measures. Part of the rationale for the multiple pre- and posttest measures appearing in both comparison groups is to foster a somewhat greater reliability or consistency of measurement before and after the introduction of the manipulated IV. The layout of this design, then, appears as shown in Box 5-4.

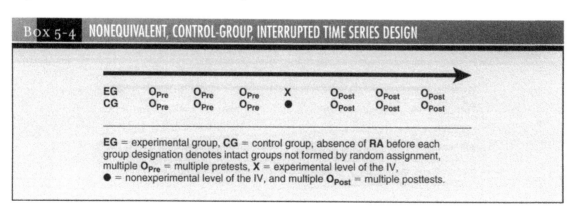

BOX 5-4   NONEQUIVALENT, CONTROL-GROUP, INTERRUPTED TIME SERIES DESIGN

EG O_{Pre} O_{Pre} O_{Pre} X O_{Post} O_{Post} O_{Post}
CG O_{Pre} O_{Pre} O_{Pre} ● O_{Post} O_{Post} O_{Post}

EG = experimental group, **CG** = control group, absence of **RA** before each group designation denotes intact groups not formed by random assignment, multiple O_{Pre} = multiple pretests, **X** = experimental level of the IV, ● = nonexperimental level of the IV, and multiple O_{Post} = multiple posttests.

An example of this research design could be a slight extension of the hypothetical university-level dance course study cited earlier. In this instance of a nonequivalent, control-group, interrupted time series design, both groups would be premeasured on the DV of shoulder abduction ROM several times prior to the massage therapy being introduced to the treatment group. Likewise, both groups would be postmeasured on the DV several times subsequent to the massage intervention being introduced.

Simple Interrupted Time Series Design

The third of three research designs that we might use in implementing a quasi-experimental method, the **simple interrupted time series design**, is actually a variation of the previous design. It is designated as a "simple" interrupted time series design because only one group is involved in the study, with multiple pretest measures being recorded prior to the treatment's introduction and multiple posttest measures afterward. The basis for comparison here is limited to the aggregate of pretest measures contrasted with the aggregate of posttest measures of the DV. This is the only comparative basis available given the fact that there is no second group against which to compare the first. Box 5-5 displays the sequence of these procedures.

An example of this research design could be a scaling back of the hypothetical study just discussed, wherein only one section of the university-level dance course is investigated. In this instance, the participants in this one section would be premeasured on the DV several times prior to the massage intervention being introduced, and then they would be postmeasured several times subsequent to the treatment being introduced. The obvious drawback to this design is the fact that although we would have a pretest versus posttest basis for

comparison, there is no control group available for between-group comparisons.

SINGLE-CASE EXPERIMENTAL METHOD: TREATMENT/INTERVENTION FOCUSED

Figure 5-4 overviews the single-case experimental research method and its five research designs.

The **single-case experimental method** is the third of four research methods found in the difference-oriented research strategy. Helpful resources available for placing this method in proper context are those by Graziano and Raulin (2004), Hilliard (1993), and Kiene and von Schon-Angerer (1998). As the name indicates, this method focuses on one participant in a study who has been exposed to a manipulated IV. The single-case aspect of this method refers to the one specific participant, rather than a group of participants, who is the focus of the study. It is included here as an experimental method primarily because of the presence of a given treatment or intervention–a manipulated IV–to which the single participant is being exposed. For these reasons, this research method is of particular relevance to massage therapists as well as other manual therapists.

The attention to an individual client presenting certain signs and symptoms of a condition in need of treatment, and the therapist's decision to intervene with an appropriate treatment modality, obviously sets the stage for documenting the impact of that intervention across the various phases that span this research method. The term *phase* refers to a series of observations/measurements across time of the same individual under the same condition. It is precisely the options available regarding phases prior to, during, and subsequent to treatment that define the several research designs constituting this method. Boxes 5-6 through 5-10 display those options.

Box 5-5   SIMPLE INTERRUPTED TIME SERIES DESIGN

| EG | O_{Pre} | O_{Pre} | O_{Pre} | X | O_{Post} | O_{Post} | O_{Post} |

EG = experimental group, multiple O_{Pre} = multiple pretest measures of the DV prior to the treatment being introduced, **X** = experimental "level" of the IV representing the treatment, multiple O_{Post} = multiple posttest measures of the DV subsequent to the treatment being introduced.

- Quantitative Research Category
  - • Difference-Oriented Research Strategy (Chapter 5)
    - • • True Experimental, or Randomized Controlled Trial, Method (treatment/intervention focused)
    - • • Quasi-Experimental Method (treatment/intervention focused)
    - • • **Single-Case Experimental Method (treatment/intervention focused)**
      - • • • **A - B Design**
      - • • • **A - B - A Design**
      - • • • **A - B - A - B Design (or Reversal Design)**
      - • • • **Multiple Treatment Design**
      - • • • **Dismantling or Component-Analysis Design**
    - • • Nonexperimental Comparative Groups Method (focus on previous/existing exposure and recent/present/future outcome)

FIGURE 5-4 ■ Spotlight on the single-case experimental research method and its affiliated research designs (bold emphasis designates coverage in this section).

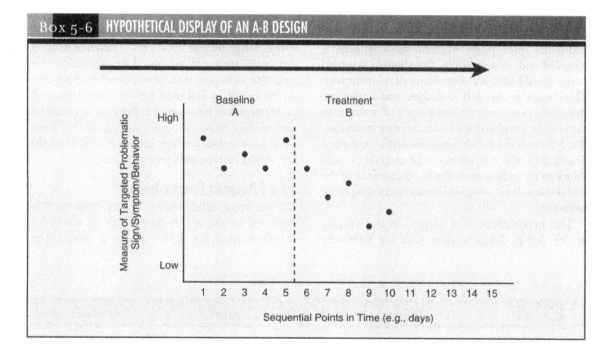

Box 5-6   HYPOTHETICAL DISPLAY OF AN A-B DESIGN

A-B Design

The simplest scenario for explaining the **A-B design** is documenting over a period of time—several days or weeks, for example—the signs/symptoms/behavior presented by a client who (a) is initially in need of treatment not yet provided and (b) is then provided with the treatment. The initial phase, during which the client is not receiving any intervention, is labeled the *baseline phase* and designated by the letter "A." During this baseline phase, the targeted signs/symptoms/behaviors of the client are measured at each of several points in time spanning, perhaps, a certain number of days or weeks. These measurements or observations are termed the baseline observations. Once the treatment begins, the study is then said to

be in the treatment phase and is designated by the letter "B." During the treatment phase, measurements or observations of the client's presenting problematic signs/symptoms/behaviors are again recorded at each of several points in time and are labeled *treatment observations*. Box 5-6 illustrates the A-B design in that hypothetical case of the treatment having the desired effect of reducing the targeted problematic condition originally presented by the client.

An illustrative example of the A-B design could be an individual case of cervicobrachial pain syndrome for which a massage therapy protocol is used during a treatment phase B following an initial baseline phase A. Measures of range of shoulder abduction at several points during each of these two phases would quantify this dependent variable. An extension (A-B-C) of the design we are now considering was actually used in a study by Cowell and Phillips (2002) in which a baseline phase A was followed sequentially by treatment phases B and C. During treatment phase B, manipulative physiotherapy was used; this was then followed in treatment phase C by a home exercise regimen. At several points during each of these three phases the researchers measured such DVs as pain intensity, functional disability, and cervical and shoulder mobility, and they subsequently documented the beneficial effects of the two interventions.

A-B-A Design

A slight extension of the A-B design involves an additional third phase wherein the treatment is removed and, consequently, the client is returned to the initial baseline circumstance of no treatment. This design is the **A-B-A design,** and it demonstrates the outcome or consequence of a return to the client's initial status of not receiving treatment. Box 5-7 shows the A-B-A design for that hypothetical situation in which a return to the original circumstance of no treatment results in a recurrence of the initial high level of problematic sign/symptom/behavior.

The hypothetical data shown in this display of the A-B-A design suggest that the treatment provided during phase B was apparently effective because not only did the client's presenting problem subside during the treatment phase, but the initiating high levels of the problem returned when the treatment was discontinued. We can visually inspect the pattern of changes in the targeted problem as we move from the initial baseline phase to the treatment phase and then back to the baseline phase. We could also quantitatively calculate, and then visually display on the figure, the actual mean level of the targeted problem during each phase as well as the change in mean level of the targeted problem as the study progressed across the three phases.

The earlier hypothetical illustration of the A-B design could easily be extended to exemplify this A-B-A design. In this instance, the baseline phase A involving measures of shoulder abduction for someone suffering with cervicobrachial pain syndrome might be followed by a treatment phase B of massage intervention, followed by a return to the baseline phase A. Again, during each of these three phases—two baseline and one treatment—the DV would be measured several times.

A-B-A-B Design (or Reversal Design)

The apparent effectiveness of the treatment as displayed in the A-B-A design can be somewhat corroborated if the A-B-A design is extended to

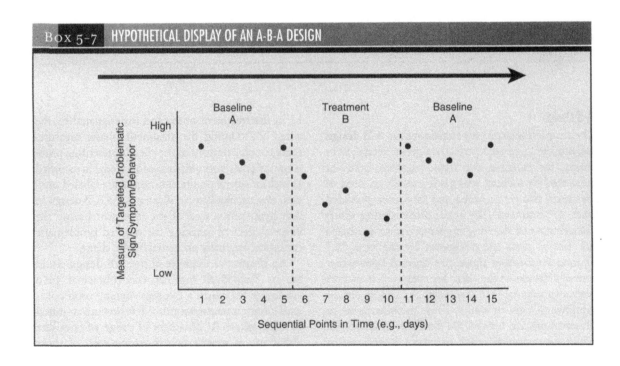

BOX 5-7   HYPOTHETICAL DISPLAY OF AN A-B-A DESIGN

include a return to the treatment during a fourth phase. This would constitute what is known as an **A-B-A-B (or reversal) design** and could provide further evidence of the treatment's role in reducing the level of the client's initial presenting problem. Box 5-8 displays this A-B-A-B reversal design for hypothetical data consistent with this pattern.

An example of this design is a study conducted by Lovas, Craig, Segal, Raison, Weston, and Markus (2002) that investigated the effects of massage therapy on the human immune response in healthy adults. The design was applied separately to two participants for whom the baseline phase A was followed on two occasions by a treatment phase B involving relaxing massage as an intervention. Several DVs involving biochemistry and anxiety measures were considered in conjunction with each of the two baseline phases and two treatment phases.

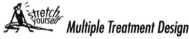

Multiple Treatment Design

Our discussion so far of the single-case experimental method has been founded on the idea of a baseline phase defined by the absence of any type of treatment and followed by a treatment phase during which some type of intervention is implemented. This is, in a sense, the single-case counterpart to our earlier discussions of a true experimental or quasi-experimental research method wherein a control group is contrasted with an experimental group

relative to a DV. The control condition, of sorts, in our present discussion is represented by the baseline phase, and the experimental condition is obviously the treatment phase. Under both conditions–control and experimental–our single participant (or subject or case) is being monitored over a designated time period on the target problem that drew our attention in the first place (i.e., the study's DV).

Just as a true experimental or quasi-experimental research method can investigate two or more treatment interventions in a given study, so too can a single-case experimental method focus on two or more treatments along with the baseline or control condition. Such is the case with the **multiple treatment design**, wherein the study contrasts a baseline phase with two or more treatment phases involving two or more types of intervention. Box 5-9 shows the hypothetical sequence and resulting observations of a multiple treatment design with two treatments designated as "B" and "C."

As a hypothetical example of this multiple treatment design, a client may be presenting evidence of CTS as a consequence of extensive computer keyboarding. The initial intervention (B) used by the therapist might be to prescribe a massage protocol, with a subsequent treatment plan (C) that relies on hydrotherapy. A baseline phase A would immediately precede each of the two treatment phases B and C as displayed earlier, with measures

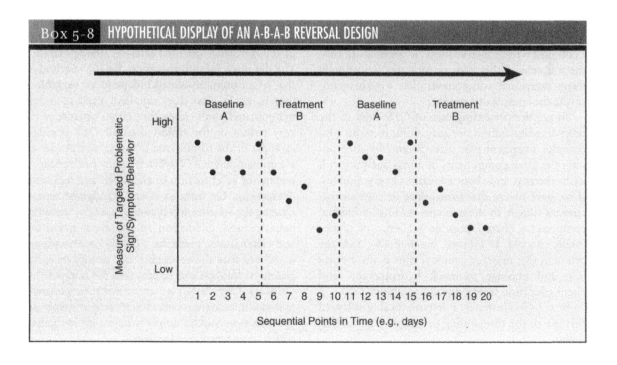

BOX 5-8   HYPOTHETICAL DISPLAY OF AN A-B-A-B REVERSAL DESIGN

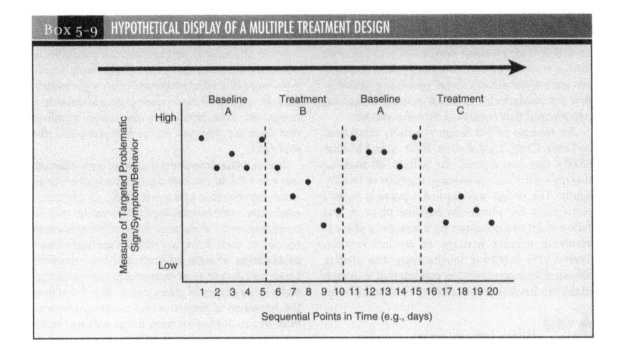

BOX 5-9   HYPOTHETICAL DISPLAY OF A MULTIPLE TREATMENT DESIGN

of pain reduction occurring several times during each of the four phases.

Dismantling or Component-Analysis Design

Our discussion regarding the multiple treatment design probably has caused you to anticipate this final design in our coverage of the single-case experimental method. The **dismantling or component-analysis design** allows the researcher to use a series of treatment phases for the purpose of investigating a complex type of intervention. To accomplish this, the researcher either adds or subtracts sequentially those individual components that together constitute the complex treatment.

To use the presenting case of CTS cited in the preceding illustration, we may think in terms of a complex treatment plan that potentially incorporates the three components of a massage protocol, hydrotherapy, and client education in ergonomics. If we were to use the dismantling or component-analysis design by sequentially adding individual components, then a possible sequence of phases might proceed as follows: baseline (A); massage protocol (B); massage protocol plus hydrotherapy (C); and massage protocol, hydrotherapy, and client education in ergonomics combined (D).

Box 5-10 illustrates a hypothetical display of this use of the dismantling or component-analysis design.

NONEXPERIMENTAL COMPARATIVE GROUPS METHOD: FOCUS ON PREVIOUS/EXISTING EXPOSURE AND RECENT/PRESENT/FUTURE OUTCOME

Figure 5-5 highlights the nonexperimental comparative groups research method, its two major subdivisions, and the several affiliated research designs.

The **nonexperimental comparative groups method** is the last of four research methods included in the difference-oriented research strategy family. The defining research procedure for this method is that of a **nonmanipulated independent variable**—that is, an IV that does not lend itself to being manipulated by the researcher, either because of its very nature or for ethical reasons. One possible example of the former case is that of sex/gender as a nonmanipulated IV whereby pain perception is researched as a function of masculine and feminine distinctions. Or, from an ethical standpoint, investigating the relationship between extent of smoking behavior and inclination to use complementary and alternative medicine (CAM) interventions mandates that the researcher use already existing groups of smokers and nonsmokers for comparison purposes. Obviously, one would not even consider cultivating smoking behavior among a group of previous nonsmokers simply to have a group against which to compare nonsmokers.

- Quantitative Research Category
  - • Difference-Oriented Research Strategy (Chapter 5)
    - • • True Experimental, or Randomized Controlled Trial, Method (treatment/intervention focused)
    - • • Quasi-Experimental Method (treatment/iIntervention focused)
    - • • Single-Case Experimental Method (treatment/intervention focused)
    - • • **Nonexperimental Comparative Groups Method (focus on previous/existing exposure and recent/present/future outcome)**
      - • • • **Ex Post Facto ("after the fact") Designs**
        - • • • • **Prospective Cohort Design**
        - • • • • **Retrospective Cohort Design**
        - • • • • **Retrospective Case-Control Design**
      - • • • **Developmental or Time-Sequence Designs**
        - • • • • **Cross-Sectional Design**
        - • • • • **Longitudinal Design**

FIGURE 5-5 ■ Spotlight on the nonexperimental comparative groups research method and its affiliated research designs (bold emphasis designates coverage in this section).

A second research procedure that defines the nonexperimental comparative groups method involves the manner in which the two or more comparison groups are formed. There is a certain degree of latitude in that the comparison groups may be formed in one of two possible means. In the first instance, the comparison groups may represent **intact groups** of participants who are already formed or in place, and not randomly assigned. The earlier example of comparing already established smokers and nonsmokers in an available sample illustrates this scenario. In the second case, random selection results in the formation of the two or more comparison groups based on some factor of interest that becomes the nonmanipulated IV. An illustration might be that of randomly selecting from an accessible population male and female participants for whom comparisons may be made regarding pain perception.

The critical features, then, of the nonexperimental comparative groups method are (a) a nonmanipulated IV and (b) the designation of comparative groups based on a trait, characteristic, or previous treatment/condition exposure of the participants that already exists rather than a new treatment to which the participants are now being subjected. In this latter case, the group membership of the participants is a matter of already being in place or intact as members, or being randomly selected from two or more strata in the accessible population. Appropriate resources that elaborate on the nonexperimental comparative groups method are

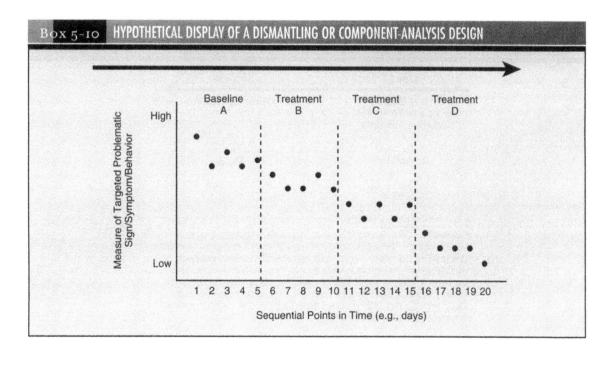

BOX 5-10 **HYPOTHETICAL DISPLAY OF A DISMANTLING OR COMPONENT-ANALYSIS DESIGN**

the following: Christensen (2004), Katz (2001), Peat (2002), and Portney and Watkins (2000).

At an even more specific level, the nonexperimental comparative groups method involves two possible types of research designs: the ex post facto (after the fact) designs and the developmental (or time sequence) designs.

Ex Post Facto (After the Fact) Designs

In the **ex post facto (or after the fact) designs**, the participants selected have (a) *already* been exposed to a particular treatment/condition or (b) *already* exhibit a particular trait, characteristic, or outcome. The *italic* emphasis on the word *already* is critical in that it conveys the "afterward" theme of these "after the fact" designs regarding either a treatment/condition previously exposed to or a trait, characteristic, or outcome previously exhibited. These designs involve the following three: prospective cohort design, retrospective cohort design, and retrospective case-control design.

Prospective Cohort Design: Focus on Existing Exposure and Future Outcome.

In the **prospective cohort design**, the two or more comparative groups are formed in the present based on an already existing exposure to treatment/condition variations, and then they are followed into the future with a view toward one or more outcomes being measured.

For instance, a researcher may designate the nonmanipulated IV as duration (in hours) of a typical workweek with the following two levels: comparative group 1 of ≤ 30 hours and comparative group 2 of ≥ 50 hours. The DV or outcome of interest here might be that of frequency of episodes of tension headaches. In schematic form, this design appears as indicated in Box 5-11.

Retrospective Cohort Design: Focus on Previous Exposure and More Recent Outcome.

In the **retrospective cohort design**, the two or more comparative groups were formed in the more distant past based on a previous exposure to treatment/condition variations, and then they were followed forward to the more recent past with a view toward one or more outcomes having been measured.

To continue with a variation of our earlier example, a researcher may define the nonmanipulated IV as duration of a typical workweek with the same two levels as designated before (i.e., ≤ 30 hours and ≥ 50 hours of work per week). Again, the DV or outcome of interest may be the frequency of tension headache episodes. The major consideration in this retrospective cohort design—as contrasted with the previous design—is that here the treatment/condition variations occurred previously in the more distant past while the outcome of interest occurred in the more recent past. Box 5-12 displays this design.

Retrospective Case-Control Design: Focus on Present Outcome and Previous Exposure.

In the **retrospective case-control design**, the two comparative groups are

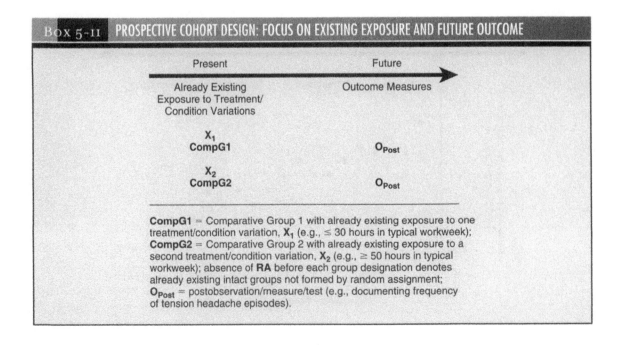

Box 5-11   PROSPECTIVE COHORT DESIGN: FOCUS ON EXISTING EXPOSURE AND FUTURE OUTCOME

Present   Future

Already Existing   Outcome Measures
Exposure to Treatment/
Condition Variations

X_1
CompG1 O_{Post}

X_2
CompG2 O_{Post}

CompG1 = Comparative Group 1 with already existing exposure to one treatment/condition variation, X_1 (e.g., ≤ 30 hours in typical workweek); **CompG2** = Comparative Group 2 with already existing exposure to a second treatment/condition variation, X_2 (e.g., ≥ 50 hours in typical workweek); absence of **RA** before each group designation denotes already existing intact groups not formed by random assignment; O_{Post} = postobservation/measure/test (e.g., documenting frequency of tension headache episodes).

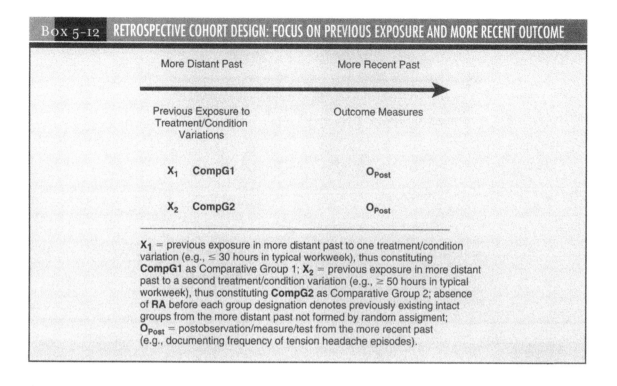

BOX 5-12 RETROSPECTIVE COHORT DESIGN: FOCUS ON PREVIOUS EXPOSURE AND MORE RECENT OUTCOME

X_1 = previous exposure in more distant past to one treatment/condition variation (e.g., $\leq$ 30 hours in typical workweek), thus constituting **CompG1** as Comparative Group 1; X_2 = previous exposure in more distant past to a second treatment/condition variation (e.g., $\geq$ 50 hours in typical workweek), thus constituting **CompG2** as Comparative Group 2; absence of **RA** before each group designation denotes previously existing intact groups from the more distant past not formed by random assigment; O_{Post} = postobservation/measure/test from the more recent past (e.g., documenting frequency of tension headache episodes).

formed in the present based on the presence of an outcome (i.e., the case) and the absence of the same outcome (i.e., the control), and then they are traced backward in time with a view toward past exposure to a treatment/condition.

Building on our earlier illustration, a researcher may designate the nonmanipulated IV as the extent of tension headache episodes presently occurring, with the following two levels: comparative group 1, comprised of individuals for whom tension headaches are present, and comparative group 2, consisting of individuals for whom tension headaches are absent. The researcher then traces backward in time with a focus on the duration in hours of a typical workweek for the participants, thereby defining the study's DV. In effect, a present outcome measure—resulting in a case of interest and its absence—is traced retrospectively to a previous exposure to a presumed precipitating treatment/condition. The dynamics of this design are shown in Box 5-13.

Developmental or Time-Sequence Designs

Developmental or time-sequence designs investigate human development changes and/or the sequencing of behaviors/conditions over time. The nonmanipulated IV here is either age specific or time interval specific.

In the first instance of age specificity, a researcher may be interested in the relationship between age during adolescence and knowledge of healthy dietary habits. In the second instance, one may investigate the relationship between length of time engaged in a keyboarding-intensive occupation and the development of CTS. In both instances, a distinction can be made between a cross-sectional study and a longitudinal study based on the way in which the investigated changes are documented.

Cross-Sectional Design. In the **cross-sectional design**, the researcher identifies representative samples of individuals at the specific age or time interval levels of interest and then measures them on the DV at only one point in time. For example, representative samples of 13-, 15-, and 17-year-olds might be measured at the same point in time on their knowledge of healthy dietary habits. Or, in the case of the second previous example, representative samples of data processors with one, three, and five years of ongoing keyboarding experience could be assessed concurrently for symptoms of CTS. Box 5-14 displays the layout of a cross-sectional design appropriate to these two examples.

The advantage with a cross-sectional design is the efficiency with which a DV might be measured across two or more age levels or time intervals.

BOX 5-13 RETROSPECTIVE CASE-CONTROL DESIGN: FOCUS ON PRESENT OUTCOME AND PREVIOUS EXPOSURE

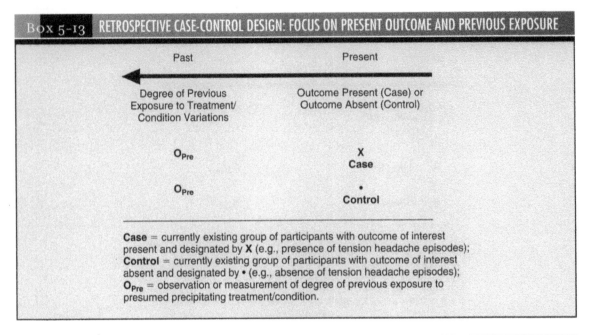

Case = currently existing group of participants with outcome of interest present and designated by **X** (e.g., presence of tension headache episodes); **Control** = currently existing group of participants with outcome of interest absent and designated by • (e.g., absence of tension headache episodes); O_{Pre} = observation or measurement of degree of previous exposure to presumed precipitating treatment/condition.

BOX 5-14 CROSS-SECTIONAL DESIGN

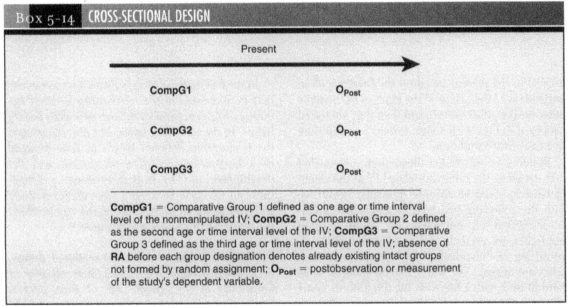

CompG1 = Comparative Group 1 defined as one age or time interval level of the nonmanipulated IV; **CompG2** = Comparative Group 2 defined as the second age or time interval level of the IV; **CompG3** = Comparative Group 3 defined as the third age or time interval level of the IV; absence of **RA** before each group designation denotes already existing intact groups not formed by random assignment; O_{Post} = postobservation or measurement of the study's dependent variable.

The principal drawback, however, is that even with the random selection of representative samples, the fact remains that one is comparing two or more groups of participants with no guarantee that all extraneous variables are controlled, particularly those that pertain to individual differences.

Longitudinal Design. In the **longitudinal design**, the investigator selects a single group of participants and then measures them on the DV of interest at each of several points across time corresponding to

the age levels or time intervals defining the IV. In the first example suggested earlier, the researcher would measure a select group of 13-year-olds on knowledge of dietary health habits and then would repeat the measurement of the DV two and four years later when the original participants are 15 and 17 years old, respectively. In a comparable fashion, the other suggested study would assess a select group of data processors with one year of experience keyboarding for the presence of CTS and then would repeat the assessment on the identical

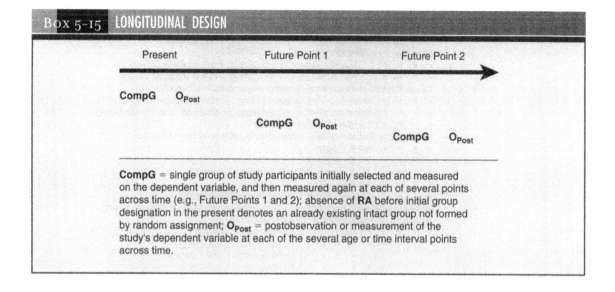

BOX 5-15 LONGITUDINAL DESIGN

CompG = single group of study participants initially selected and measured on the dependent variable, and then measured again at each of several points across time (e.g., Future Points 1 and 2); absence of **RA** before initial group designation in the present denotes an already existing intact group not formed by random assignment; O_{Post} = postobservation or measurement of the study's dependent variable at each of the several age or time interval points across time.

participants two and four years later. Box 5-15 shows the basic form of a longitudinal design appropriate to these two examples.

The principal advantage of a longitudinal design is that the same individuals constitute the study's participants across each of the two or more levels of the IV. This is an optimal way to control those extraneous variables related to the individual differences of the participants because the same individuals are present across the levels of the IV. The glaring drawback to the longitudinal design, though, is the time commitment necessitated by all involved due to the protracted duration of the study. This frequently results in attrition on the part of study participants with no viable recourse in terms of replacements.

DETAILED SUMMARY

Figure 5-6 provides a detailed summary of the difference-oriented research strategy as well as the affiliated research methods and research designs that have been covered in this chapter.

POSSIBLE RESEARCH PROCEDURE OPTIONS AND THEIR IMPLICATIONS

Our journey so far in Chapter 5 has covered a variety of research methods, research designs, and research procedures that are rather basic to the difference-oriented research strategy. At every step along the way, we have made decisions regarding research procedures that really involved options that were available and that we acknowledged.

In some cases, though, other research procedure options were not identified and discussed because of a need to lay out the basics before exploring possible variations. Now we must identify and explain those variations and provide even more of an explanation of what we have already covered.

RANDOM ASSIGNMENT OR INTACT GROUPS

As a reminder, the essential distinction between the true experimental/randomized control trial method and the quasi-experimental method involves the random assignment of participants to the two or more levels of the IV. In the former case, the participants are indeed randomly assigned to the comparative groups. In the latter instance, though, the comparative groups are formed not as a result of random assignment but rather as a function of the groups already being intact or in place.

The presence of random assignment in the true experimental/randomized control trial method is one of two critical procedures necessary to derive cause-and-effect conclusions. The other critical procedure involves the IV being manipulated or governed by the researcher. This issue brings us to the next option that requires a decision on the part of researchers.

MANIPULATED INDEPENDENT VARIABLE OR NONMANIPULATED INDEPENDENT VARIABLE

You may recall from our earlier discussions that the IV in a difference-oriented study is also known as a stimulus variable, input variable, or possibly as a causal variable. Certain research questions require that the researcher manipulate or actually govern the

- Quantitative Research Category
  - • Difference-Oriented Research Strategy (Chapter 5)
    - • • True Experimental, or Randomized Controlled Trial, Method (treatment/intervention focused)
      - • • • Randomized, Control-Group, Posttest-Only Design
      - • • • Randomized, Control-Group, Pretest-Posttest Design
    - • • Quasi-Experimental Method (treatment/intervention focused)
      - • • • Nonequivalent, Control-Group, Pretest-Posttest Design
      - • • • Nonequivalent, Control-Group, Interrupted Time Series Design
      - • • • Simple Time Series Design
    - • • Single-Case Experimental Method (treatment/intervention focused)
      - • • • A - B Design
      - • • • A - B - A Design
      - • • • A - B - A - B Design (or Reversal Design)
      - • • • Multiple Treatment Design
      - • • • Dismantling or Component-Analysis Design
    - • • Nonexperimental Comparative Groups Method (focus on previous/existing exposure and recent/present/future outcome)
      - • • • Ex Post Facto ("after the fact") Designs
        - • • • • Prospective Cohort Design
        - • • • • Retrospective Cohort Design
        - • • • • Retrospective Case-Control Design
      - • • • Developmental or Time-Sequence Designs
        - • • • • Cross-Sectional Design
        - • • • • Longitudinal Design

FIGURE 5-6 ■ Detailed summary of the difference-oriented research strategy and its affiliated research methods and designs covered in Chapter 5.

dynamics associated with the IV. This is certainly the case in any study involving a treatment or intervention being delivered in the present to the study's participants. This is also the type of IV that is the focal point in those research efforts that are perhaps of most interest to massage therapists and other health science professionals who are curious about various treatment modalities and their impact on certain client outcomes.

Equally important among our research procedure options regarding the IV are those circumstances wherein the research question is not addressing a treatment or intervention in the present, but rather concerns itself with traits, characteristics, or conditions that do not (or should not) lend themselves to being actually manipulated or governed by the researcher. In those instances, we are dealing with the nonmanipulated IV. Our earlier discussion of the nonexperimental comparative groups method and its affiliated research designs provided several illustrations of this type of IV.

In the context of a difference-oriented research strategy, the IV being addressed is always manifested in two or more ways regardless of whether or not it is being manipulated. This issue—not coincidentally—leads us to yet another option that must be addressed by researchers.

POSSIBLE COMPARATIVE GROUPS OR LEVELS OF THE INDEPENDENT VARIABLE

Any IV in a difference-oriented study, whether it is manipulated or not, always involves two or more ways in which it is shown or manifested. As we have seen before, another name for these ways in which the IV presents itself is the levels of the IV. A true experimental design, for example, may in its simplest form investigate the difference between an experimental group and a control group relative to the study's DV. In a more extended manner, the same type of design may investigate the differences among three groups—two experimental groups and a control group—regarding a DV.

The nature of a study's research question is what leads eventually to the determination of how many comparative groups or levels of the IV will be explored for differences regarding the DV. Accordingly, any researcher involved in a difference-oriented study has basically two decisions to make as a reflection of the research question that is prompting the study in the first place: (a) whether the IV is manipulated or nonmanipulated and (b) whether the IV entails two or more comparative groups or levels that reflect the manner in which the IV is made manifest.

TYPES OF CONTROL GROUPS

As we have seen, a control group is one of the possible comparative groups or levels of an IV investigated in a difference-oriented research strategy. Several types of control groups may appear in a study, with each variety serving a particular and unique purpose. The possible versions of a control group include the following: (a) the no treatment or "do nothing" control group, (b) the standard treatment control group, (c) the waiting-list control group, (d) the placebo-attention control group, and (e) the placebo-sham treatment control group.

The **no treatment (or do nothing) control group** entails precisely what its name implies. Although this type of control group is appearing considerably less frequently in research studies, its use does occur when the researcher is interested in comparing one or more treatment groups to a comparable group of participants for whom no treatment or involvement is planned.

The **standard treatment control group** simply involves study participants who are receiving whatever health care treatment or intervention is recognized as standard or typical for their presenting condition. This standard treatment of care is contrasted with the one or more experimental versions or levels of the IV to ascertain if indeed any differences exist between or among the interventions relative to one or more outcome measures of interest (i.e., DVs). The study by Chang, Wang, and Chen (2002) that was excerpted and discussed initially in Chapter 3 illustrates a control group wherein the 30 participants undergoing childbirth obviously received standard medical treatment, but without the massage intervention as was the case in the experimental group.

The **waiting or wait-list control group** is that group of participants who are initially not receiving the investigative treatment or intervention during the actual conduct of the study but are instead literally on a waiting list of people who are scheduled to receive the treatment once the study is completed. This approach to constituting a control group for purposes of comparison to an experimental or treatment group is one way to ensure participant welfare when (a) those initially in the control group have a noncritical/nonemergency condition that potentially can benefit from the treatment and (b) the investigative treatment is of relatively brief duration so that the waiting period is not too protracted. As a reminder, the van den Dolder and Roberts (2003) study addressed earlier in Chapter 4 included a waiting-list control group.

The fourth of five possible types of control groups is the **placebo-attention control group**. In this situation, a group of study participants not receiving the experimental treatment is exposed to a stimulus experience that is inert with respect to any direct anticipated impact on the outcome being investigated. Although inert as just described, the stimulus experience is typically in the form of interpersonal contact and support that provides those participants with a sense of being attended to and involved. This essentially creates in both the experimental group and the placebo-attention control group a common experience of being engaged. Consequently, this allows any outcome differences between the groups to be attributed to the one *un*common feature across the two groups, namely, the presumed dynamic nature of the experimental treatment. As an illustration, a childbirth labor study reported by Field, Hernandez-Reif, Taylor, Quintino, and Burman (1997) compared partners massaging women in labor against partners simply being present and reacting spontaneously during labor, usually in terms of the breathing exercise coaching learned earlier in prenatal classes.

The fifth possible variety of control groups is known as the **placebo-sham treatment control group**. In this instance, study participants being contrasted with the experimental treatment group are exposed to a simulated treatment that *feigns* the intervention of a viable treatment. In reality, though, the *presumed* dynamic or viable treatment provided to the control group is actually a pretended or impostor-type intervention with no actual dynamic potential to influence the outcome measure(s). The Preyde (2000) study referenced in Chapter 4 included among the four levels of its manipulated IV a sham laser (infrared) therapy intervention positioned to appear as if it were functioning when in actuality it was not operative.

BETWEEN-SUBJECTS INDEPENDENT VARIABLE OR WITHIN-SUBJECTS (REPEATED MEASURES) INDEPENDENT VARIABLE

The distinction involving a *between-subjects* IV and a *within-subjects* (*repeated measures*) IV is one that we have not made thus far. This distinction, however, is critical with respect to two important considerations: (a) the way in which study's participants become affiliated with the IV's comparative groups and (b) the type of statistical technique eventually used to analyze the acquired data on the DV.

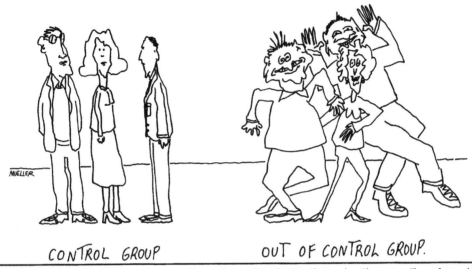

CONTROL GROUP   OUT OF CONTROL GROUP.

HUMOR BREAK ■ Yet another type of control group? Another Humble Hymelian Observation: The professional literature seems to be silent on the actual existence of this type of control group distinction; therefore, please exercise caution if and when an author refers to an alleged "out of control" group! (From Mueller, P. S. [nd]. *P. S. Mueller cartoons*. © 1984, 2004 P. S. Mueller. www.psmueller.com.)

In the case of how participants become affiliated with the two or more comparative groups in a study, the **between-subjects independent variable or design** (variously known as a between-subjects design) simply implies that each level of the IV involves a separate and distinct group of individuals affiliated with it. If, for example, the IV has three levels that are being contrasted regarding the study's DV, then three separate and distinct groups of participants will constitute those three levels of the IV.

The advantage to a between-subjects IV is that the experiences of a given group in a given level of the IV remain there and entail no other participation with any of the other levels of the IV. An important consequence of this is that the participants' measures on the DV are specific to what they experienced within that one particular group or IV level.

The disadvantage to a between-subjects IV, however, is that even with the random assignment of a distinct group of participants to a specific level of the IV, there is no definitive guarantee that the two or more comparative groups are actually equivalent in terms of, for example, those individual differences that we are trying to control. Researchers in this circumstance often act on the assumption that the comparative groups are indeed equivalent on those extraneous variables that take the form of individual differences; however, this is still in the realm of an assumption.

In the instance of the **within-subjects (or repeated measures) independent variable or design** (likewise variously known as a within-subjects design), a specific group of participants actually experiences each and every one of the IV's levels. If the IV has three levels, for example, that are being compared regarding the study's DV, then one and the same group of participants will experience what each of the three levels of the IV has to offer.

The advantage to the within-subjects design is that it represents an optimal way to control extraneous variables that are rooted in individual differences across participants. This is the case simply because the same participants—along with the same individual differences that they represent—are present within each of the IV's levels. By implication, also, this same group of participants is repeatedly measured on the DV within each of the IV's levels. Accordingly, the within-subjects IV or design is also referred to as a *repeated measures* IV or design.

The disadvantage to a *within-subjects* or *repeated measures* IV is that the participants' experience of a given level of the IV runs the risk of carrying over to their experience of the one or more other levels of the IV. When we consider that the participants are being repeatedly measured on the DV in the context of each level, then the possibility certainly exists that their responses to the DV under the conditions of one level may be influenced by their earlier experience of a preceding level of the IV. This problem of carryover effect can and should be counteracted by a procedure known as counterbalancing. Ideally, counterbalancing calls for the participants to experience each level of the IV in every sequential position in which the IVs two or more levels can be positioned. The participants' repeated measures on the DV are then aggregated for analysis purposes across all of the possible sequential positions in which any given level might have appeared. The ultimate intent, therefore, is for counterbalancing to counteract the carryover effects.

At the outset of this section we mentioned that a second important consideration that depends on an IV being either between subjects or within subjects has to do with the statistical technique selected to analyze the data collected on the DV. Although this fact is addressed in Appendix D, we can acknowledge now that the distinction involving between-subjects and within-subjects IVs is one of several criteria that researchers must use in difference-oriented studies to ensure the selection of the most appropriate statistical technique. As an illustration, the independent group's t-test would be a *possible* selection for data analysis purposes in a difference-oriented study wherein the IV is between subjects and involves only two levels. In a similar circumstance involving a between-subjects IV with three or more levels, the one-way between-subjects analysis of variance might be a possible selection. The word *possible* is emphasized in both of these illustrations because more criteria must come into play before a final selection of either statistical technique could be justified. More on these statistical matters awaits you in Appendix D.

PRETEST-POSTTEST OR POSTTEST-ONLY

Some of the designs encountered earlier in this chapter specified a pretest or preobservation procedure relatively early in the design's sequence and, specifically, prior to the introduction of the IV. In some cases, the pretest is for the purpose of establishing a baseline record of the participants' reactions to the DV under consideration prior to any type of intervention being introduced. In other cases, the pretesting may be for the purpose of collecting data that become the basis for identifying the two or more levels of the IV.

Virtually all of the designs examined thus far in this chapter entailed a posttest of the participants on the study's DV. In some instances, this is for the purpose of examining the contrast between pretest and posttest performances. In those cases wherein only a posttest is administered, the intent is to rely exclusively on the contrast between or among the two or more levels of the IV relative to the posttest measures only.

Although this section speaks in terms of a single measure of a DV, it is actually more typical to encounter studies in which two or more DVs are examined. Furthermore, pretesting that occurs in a study is often—though not exclusively—focused on the accumulation of demographic and other types of participant characterizing data that inform the researcher of the broader context in which and about whom the study is being undertaken.

GROUP-SPECIFIC OR SINGLE-CASE FOCUS

Three of the four research methods included under the difference-oriented research strategy involve manipulated and nonmanipulated IVs whose levels take the form of *groups* of participants that are being contrasted with respect to the study's DV. These three methods are the following: true experimental/randomized controlled trial, quasi-experimental, and nonexperimental comparative groups. Because each of these methods entails the comparison of groups per se, the previously discussed issue of between-subjects versus within-subjects IVs is always present and an important consideration.

One of the four research methods in the difference-oriented research strategy does not rely on groups of participants, but instead involves individual participants. This is the *single-case* experimental method, wherein the focus is on a *single participant* who may be exposed to baseline measures, treatment variations, and postmeasures somewhat comparable to those experienced in the group-specific methods. This single-case experimental method holds a great deal of potential for practitioners in therapeutic massage who have an interest in research that may be integrated in the context of their individual practice. Different clients presenting varying signs and symptoms of conditions that call for the informed use of appropriate interventions and modalities all represent a possible scenario wherein practitioners may contribute to the scientific advancement of our profession. Of course, it is critical to emphasize here that standard prerequisites would have to be in place regarding such issues as the practitioner's research literacy and capacity, membership on a viable research team, mentor-collegial supervision, client/participant protection, and the overall ethical integrity of the research effort.

RANDOMIZED CONTROLLED *TRIAL OR* RANDOMIZED CLINICAL *TRIAL*

This chapter started with a discussion of the first of four research methods included under the difference-oriented research strategy. True experimental or randomized controlled trial was the name identified with that method. Our explanation of this method involved a comparison between an experimental or treatment group and a control group. It is precisely in this context that the expression randomized controlled trial is used, namely, when the group being compared to the experimental group is a no treatment or "do nothing" control group or, possibly, a waiting-list control group. As Hagino (2003) pointed out, however, the expression *randomized clinical trial* is preferred when the comparison to the experimental group involves a comparison treatment control group. In this case, three other options for control groups become a possibility and include the following: standard treatment control group, placebo-attention control group, and placebo-sham treatment control group.

BLINDED/MASKED OR OPEN STUDIES

A **blinded/masked study** refers to the research procedure whereby one or more parties in a study are unaware of the level of the IV to which a participant belongs. In a **single-blind study**, participants are unaware of their group membership. A **double-blind study**, however, involves neither the investigator nor the participant being aware of the participant's affiliated level of the IV. As noted by Ernst (2002, p.17), "blinding patients in trials of massage therapy is probably not achievable. The same obviously applies to the therapist. In essence this means that in clinical massage research only the **evaluator-blinded trials** are feasible." By virtue of the distinctions just made, the complete absence of any form of blinding or masking defines an **open study**.

WHERE DO WE GO FROM HERE?

THE DIFFERENCE-ORIENTED RESEARCH STRATEGY: FIRST OF THREE "SERVINGS" IN OUR "INTELLECTUAL FEAST" KNOWN AS THE QUANTITATIVE RESEARCH CATEGORY

We have concluded our introductory survey of those several research methods that define the difference-oriented research strategy. Our earlier chapters indicated that the broad-based **quantitative research category** encompasses three research strategies: difference-oriented, association-oriented, and descriptive-oriented. We are now set to delve into the second of these three.

NEXT "SERVING": THE ASSOCIATION-ORIENTED RESEARCH STRATEGY

Chapter 6 addresses the association-oriented research strategy. In so doing, we will examine the two principal research methods that define this approach to doing quantitative research: the correlational research method and the predictive research method. Trusting that the "food," "meal," "serving," and "feast" metaphors have not presented too much of a distraction to you (as in possibly putting the book aside to engage in some "gustatory delights"), let us now continue the intellectual feast to see precisely what the association-oriented research strategy part of the menu has to offer.

REFERENCES

Cassidy, C. M., & Hart, J. A. (2003). Methodological issues in investigations of massage/bodywork therapy: Part IV–Experimental research design. *Journal of Bodywork and Movement Therapies, 7*(4), 240–250.

Chang, M. Y., Wang, S. Y., & Chen, C. H. (2002). Effects of massage on pain and anxiety during labour: A randomized controlled trial in Taiwan. *Journal of Advanced Nursing, 38*(1), 68–73.

Christensen, L. B. (2004). *Experimental psychology* (9th ed.). Boston: Pearson/Allyn & Bacon.

Cowell, I. M., & Phillips, D. R. (2002). Effectiveness of manipulative physiotherapy for the treatment of a neurogenic cervicobrachial pain syndrome: A single case study–experimental design. *Manual Therapy, 7*(1), 31–38.

Dryden, T., & Achilles, R. (2003). *Massage therapy research curriculum kit.* Evanston, IL: AMTA Foundation.

Ernst, E. (2002). Evidence-based massage therapy: A contradiction in terms? In G. J. Rich (Ed.), *Massage therapy: The evidence for practice* (pp. 1–25). New York: Mosby.

Field, T., Hernandez-Reif, M., Taylor, S., Quintino, O., & Burman, I. (1997). Labor pain is reduced by massage therapy. *Journal of Psychosomatic Obstetrics & Gynaecology, 18*(4), 286–291.

Field, T., Peck, M., Hernandez-Reif, M., Krugman, S., Burman, I., & Ozment-Schenck, L. (2000). Postburn itching, pain, and psychological symptoms are reduced with massage therapy. *Journal of Burn Care and Rehabilitation, 21,* 189–193.

Graziano, A. M., & Raulin, M. L. (2004). *Research methods: A process of inquiry (with student CD-ROM)* (5th ed.). Boston: Pearson/Allyn & Bacon.

Greenhalgh, T. (2001). *How to read a paper: The basics of evidence based medicine* (2nd ed.). London: BMJ Books.

Hagino, C. (2003). *How to appraise research: A guide for chiropractic students and practitioners.* New York: Churchill Livingstone.

Harris, S. (1977). *What's so funny about science? Cartoons by Sidney Harris from* American Scientist. Los altos, CA: Wm. Kaufman.

Hilliard, R. B. (1993). Single-case methodology in psychotherapy process and outcome research. *Journal of Consulting and Clinical Psychology, 61*(3), 373–380.

Hulley, S. B., Cummings, S. R., Browner, W. S., Grady, D., Hearst, N., & Newman, T. B. (2001). *Designing clinical research: An epidemiologic approach* (2nd ed.). Philadelphia: Lippincott Williams & Wilkins.

Katz, D. L. (2001). *Clinical epidemiology & evidence-based medicine: Fundamental principles of clinical reasoning & research.* Thousand Oaks, CA: Sage.

Kazdin, A. E. (Ed.). (2003). *Methodological issues & strategies in clinical research* (3rd ed.).Washington, DC: American Psychological Association.

Kendall, P. C., Butcher, J. N., & Holmbeck, G. N. (1999). *Handbook of research methods in clinical psychology* (2nd ed.). New York: John Wiley & Sons.

Kiene, H., & von Schon-Angerer, T. (1998). Single-case causality assessment as a basis for clinical judgment. *Alternative Therapies, 4*(1), 41–47.

Leivadi, S., Hernandez-Reif, M., Field, T., O'Rourke, M., D'Arienzo, S., Lewis, D., et al. (1999). Massage therapy and relaxation effects on university dance students. *Journal of Dance Medicine & Science, 3*(3), 108–112.

Lewith, G., Jonas, W. B., & Walach, H. (Eds.). (2002). *Clinical research in complementary therapies: Principles, problems, and solutions.* New York: Churchill Livingstone.

Lovas, J. M., Craig, A. R., Segal, Y. D., Raison, R. L., Weston, K. M., & Markus, M. R. (2002). The effects of massage therapy on the human immune response in healthy adults. *Journal of Bodywork and Movement Therapies, 6*(3), 143–150.

Mueller, P. S. (nd). *P. S. Mueller cartoons.* www.psmueller. com.

Peat, J. K., Mellis, C., Williams, K., & Xuan, W. (2002). *Health science research: A handbook of quantitative methods.* Thousand Oaks, CA: Sage.

Polit, D. F., & Beck, C. T. (2004). *Nursing research: Principles and methods* (7th ed.). Philadelphia, PA: Lippincott Williams & Wilkins.

Portney, L. G., & Watkins, M. P. (2000). *Foundations of clinical research: Applications to practice* (2nd ed.). Upper Saddle River, NJ: Prentice Hall Health.

Preyde, M. (2000). Effectiveness of massage therapy for subacute low-back pain: A randomized controlled trial. *Canadian Medical Association Journal, 162*(13), 1815–1820.

Van den Dolder, P. A., & Roberts, D. L. (2003). A trial into the effectiveness of soft tissue massage in the treatment of shoulder pain. *Australian Journal of Physiotherapy, 49,* 183–188.

ADDITIONAL RECOMMENDED RESOURCES

Bailey, D. M. (1997). *Research for the health professional: A practical guide* (2nd ed.). Philadelphia: F. A. Davis.

Batavia, M. (2001). *Clinical research for health professionals: A user-friendly guide.* Boston: Butterworth-Heinemann.

Burns, N., & Grove, S. K. (2003). *Understanding nursing research* (3rd ed.). Philadelphia: W. B. Saunders.

Domholdt, E. (2000). *Physical therapy research: Principles and applications* (2nd ed.). Philadelphia: W. B. Saunders.

Field, A., & Hole, G. (2003). *How to design and report experiments.* Thousand Oaks, CA: Sage.

Gillis, A., & Jackson, W. (2002). *Research for nurses: Methods and interpretation.* Philadelphia: F. A. Davis.

Goodwin, C. J. (2005). *Research in psychology: Methods and design* (4th ed.). Hoboken, NJ: John Wiley & Sons.

Gravetter, F. J., & Forzano, L. B. (2003). *Research methods for the behavioral sciences.* Belmont, CA: Thomson Wadsworth.

Hicks, C. M. (1999). *Research methods for clinical therapists: Applied project design and analysis* (3rd ed.). New York: Churchill Livingstone.

Menard, M. B. (2002). Methodological issues in the design and conduct of massage therapy research. In G. J. Rich (Ed.), *Massage therapy: The evidence for practice* (pp. 27–41). New York: Mosby.

Menard, M. B. (2003). *Making sense of research: A guide to research literacy for complementary practitioners.* Toronto: Curties-Overzet.

Moher, D., Jadad, A. R., & Tugwell, P. (1996). Assessing the quality of randomized controlled trials: Current issues and future directions. *International Journal of Technology Assessment in Health Care, 12*(2), 195–208.

Sackett, D. L, Haynes, R. B., Guyatt, G. H., & Tugwell, P. (1991). *Clinical epidemiology—A basic science for clinical medicine.* London: Little, Brown.

Sackett, D. L., Straus, S. E., Richardson, W. S., Rosenberg, W., & Haynes, R. B. (2000). *Evidence-based medicine: How to practice and teach EBM* (2nd ed.). New York: Churchill Livingstone.

Stommel, M., & Wills, C. E. (2004). *Clinical research: Concepts and principles for advanced practice nurses.* Philadelphia: Lippincott Williams & Wilkins.

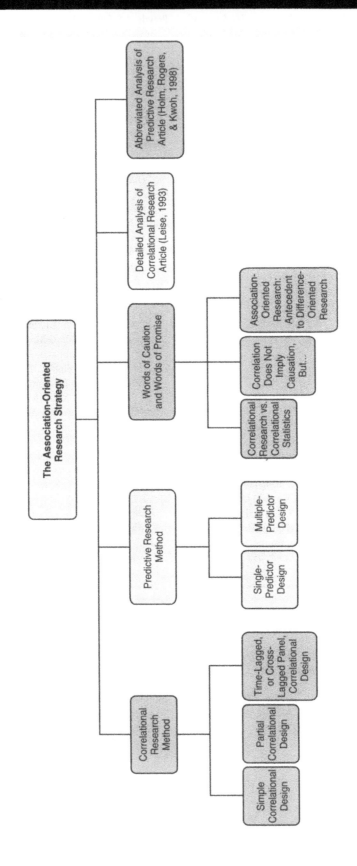

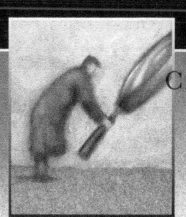

CHAPTER 6

THE ASSOCIATION-ORIENTED RESEARCH STRATEGY

OUTLINE

OBJECTIVES

Upon completion of this chapter, the reader will have the information necessary to perform the following tasks:

1　List the two research methods that are included in the association-oriented research strategy.

2　Identify and explain the three major research procedures that define the correlational research method.

3　List the three principal research designs that are included under the correlational research method, and address the following tasks for each:
　a. diagram and explain the research procedures that constitute the design;
　b. recognize, or be able to provide, an example of a study based on the design.

4　Identify and explain the six research procedures that define the predictive research method.

5　List the two principal research designs that are included under the predictive research method, and address the following tasks for each:
　a. diagram and explain the research procedures that constitute the design;
　b. recognize, or be able to provide, an example of a study based on the design.

6　Distinguish between correlational research and correlational statistics.

7　Explain the relationship between correlation and causation.

8　Explain how association-oriented research may function as a precursor to difference-oriented research.

9　Read and critique published research reports that exemplify the correlational research method and the predictive research method.

Association-oriented research strategy
Coefficient of determination
Correlational research method
Correlational statistics
Correlation-causation relationship
Criterion variable (or Y variable)
Cross-lagged correlation
Directionality problem
Multiple coefficient of determination value

Multiple correlation coefficient
Multiple linear regression
Multiple-predictor design
Partial correlation coefficient
Partial correlational design
Pearson correlation coefficient
Predictive research method
Predictor variable (or X variable)
Quantitative research category

Simple correlational design
Simple linear regression
Single-predictor design
Synchronous correlation
Test-retest correlation
Time-lagged, or cross-lagged panel, correlational design

WHERE HAVE WE BEEN AND WHERE ARE WE NOW? THE CONNECTION

The previous chapter provided an introduction to the first of three research strategies constituting the **quantitative research category**, namely, the difference-oriented research strategy. We considered those designs affiliated with the following four research methods: (a) the true experimental/randomized controlled trial method, (b) the quasi-experimental method, (c) the single-case experimental method, and (d) the non-experimental comparative groups method.

The emphasis in Chapter 5 spoke to those types of research studies that attract most extensively the attention and interest of massage therapists and related health science professionals. This is the case because the difference-oriented research encompasses those methods and designs used for investigating various treatments or interventions that perhaps hold some potential for affecting desired outcomes among clients with various presenting conditions.

In this second of three chapters that constitute Part Three, we focus on the quantitative research category by considering the association-oriented research strategy and its affiliated research methods and designs (Figure 6-1). As the expression implies, this research strategy investigates how two or more variables are related in an associational fashion. For example, in one of the most basic research methods included under the association-oriented research strategy, we consider how two dependent variables (DVs) might be related—associated—in terms of how one co-relates, or correlates, with the other. Accordingly, we may research the correlation between two DVs in an effort to determine if they are directly related, inversely related, or unrelated.

Throughout this chapter, keep in mind that research studies of an associational nature are frequently the ones that initially attract the attention of researchers, and only afterward does a research problem area sometimes necessitate an

- **Quantitative Research Category**
  - • Difference-Oriented Research Strategy (Chapter 5)
    - • • True Experimental, or Randomized Controlled Trial, Method (treatment/intervention focused)
    - • • Quasi-Experimental Method (treatment/intervention focused)
    - • • Single-Case Experimental Method (treatment/intervention focused)
    - • • Nonexperimental Comparative Groups Method (focus on previous/existing exposure and recent/present/future outcome)
  - • **Association-Oriented Research Strategy (Chapter 6)**
    - • • **Correlational Method**
    - • • **Predictive Method**
  - • Descriptive-Oriented Research Strategy (Chapter 7)
    - • • Single-Case Quantitative Analysis Method
    - • • Survey Method
    - • • Naturalistic/Structured Observational Method
    - • • Case Report Method

FIGURE 6-1 ■ The quantitative research category: Its affiliated research strategies and their variable control-driven methods (bold emphasis designates coverage in Chapter 6).

appeal to the difference-oriented research strategy. Also, some research problems are of such a nature that an association-oriented research strategy is precisely what is needed, even in the absence of any potential follow-up that would invoke the difference-oriented option. Examples of these two possibilities will follow as the specifics of this chapter unfold.

THE ASSOCIATION-ORIENTED RESEARCH STRATEGY: OVERVIEW OF ITS AFFILIATED RESEARCH METHODS AND DESIGNS

Two research methods constitute the **association-oriented research strategy** covered in this chapter. As already mentioned, this research strategy focuses on investigating a relationship between or among variables with an initial focus on the possible existence of an association between or among them. This possible association may take the form, for example, of a co-relationship, or correlation, between two DVs such as pain intensity and anxiety level experienced by a client suffering from chronic low-back pain.

The first method we examine in this chapter is the **correlational research method**. Although we will be exploring three research designs included under this method, the most basic feature of this method is that in its simplest form we investigate the correlation between two DVs (again, for example, pain intensity and anxiety level).

The second method under the association-oriented research strategy is the **predictive research method**. Our coverage of this method will span two research designs. In each there is a reliance on research data available from an earlier correlational study that allows one to explore in greater detail the identical variables. For example, with a correlational study of pain intensity and anxiety level already in place, one could rely on that earlier data set and be able to predict an anticipated anxiety level for a client experiencing a measured degree of pain intensity due to a chronic condition.

Recommended resources that might serve to elaborate on the content of this chapter include the following: Cozby (2004); Goodwin (2005); Gravetter and Forzano (2003); Healey (2005); Holm, Rogers, and Kwoh (1998); Jaccard and Becker (2002); Leise (1993); Portney and Watkins (2000); and Rosnow and Rosenthal (2005).

CORRELATIONAL RESEARCH METHOD

Figure 6-2 spotlights the correlational research method and its three affiliated research designs.

Three major research procedures define the correlational research method: (a) the existence of a sample or group of participants that may or may not have been formed by random selection, (b) the measurement of each participant in the sample on two or more DVs, and (c) the application of correlational statistical techniques to analyze the data set generated by the measures of the DVs. With these three essential research procedures acknowledged, this method may be implemented by any one of the three research designs discussed in the next three subsections.

Before proceeding to those three designs, though, this is an appropriate point to discuss the way in which we will deal with the statistics underlying the association-oriented research strategy. Basically, the content covered in this chapter focuses on those concepts and procedures that allow us to conduct both correlational and predictive studies. Our discussion of those concepts and procedures does, out of necessity, make reference to related statistical techniques. We do not, however, attempt to delve into the actual computational aspects of those techniques. Part of Appendix D provides an overview of statistical techniques inclusive of the correlation-based statistical methods referred to in this chapter.

Simple Correlational Design

The **simple correlational design** allows us to investigate the relationship between two DVs, DV_1 and DV_2. We are basically exploring whether or not there is an association between these two variables

---

- Quantitative Research Category
  - • Association-Oriented Research Strategy (Chapter 6)
    - • • **Correlational Method**
      - • • • **Simple Correlational Design**
      - • • • **Partial Correlational Design**
      - • • • **Time-Lagged, or Cross-Lagged Panel, Correlational Design**
    - • • Predictive Method
      - • • • Single-Predictor Design
      - • • • Multiple-Predictor Design

FIGURE 6-2 ■ Spotlight on the correlational research method and its affiliated research designs (bold emphasis designates coverage in this section).

or, stated another way, whether or not they co-relate, or are correlated, with each other.

Depending on the two DVs being investigated, a researcher may determine that the two DVs are directly related or, perhaps, inversely related. A third possibility is that the two DVs are simply not related at all in a straight line or linear fashion. Box 6-1 shows how we might visualize a simple correlational design, along with graphic displays of the first two of three possibilities just mentioned.

The third possibility of the two DVs not being related at all in a linear manner would simply be displayed by a collection of points on the graph that do not approximate a straight line either ascending or descending from left to right. An illustration of a simple correlational design could be a study wherein the researchers investigate the association, or correlation, between client progress regarding trunk flexion range of motion (ROM) (i.e., the DV_1) and therapist verbal acknowledgment/approval of the progress (i.e., DV_2) across a sample of 25 client-therapist pairs (or dyads). The graphical results could easily resemble those of the first possibility shown in Box 6-1 in that there is a *direct* relationship between the two DVs as displayed by the accumulation of points on the graph that approximates a straight line ascending from left to right. More specifically, what this shows is that as the extent of client progress increases, so does the extent of therapist approval and vice versa, thus suggesting a moderately strong direct relationship.

Additionally, the graph (also called a scatterplot) could be accompanied by what is known as a **Pearson correlation coefficient** designated by lowercase letter r. In this example, one could encounter, say, an $r = .40$, indicating a moderately strong positive correlation between the two DVs. Because r can range from a -1.0 (perfect negative correlation, implying a perfect inverse relationship) to a $+1.0$ (perfect positive correlation, implying a perfect direct relationship), the hypothetical $r = .40$ being used here would indicate a moderately strong positive correlation that gives quantifiable evidence to what we already know from our graph (scatterplot) to be a moderately strong direct relationship.

Building on the insights provided by the scatterplot and the Pearson correlation coefficient, r, we could further calculate quite easily what is known as the **coefficient of determination** that is designated by the symbol r^2. In this instance, with $r = .40$, r^2 (or r times itself, $.40 \times .40$) would equal $.16$. At this value of $r^2 = .16$, the meaning or interpretation is that 16% of the variations that we notice on one DV (e.g., the measures of client progress, DV_1) are explained by the variations that exist on the other DV (e.g., the measures of therapist approval, DV_2).

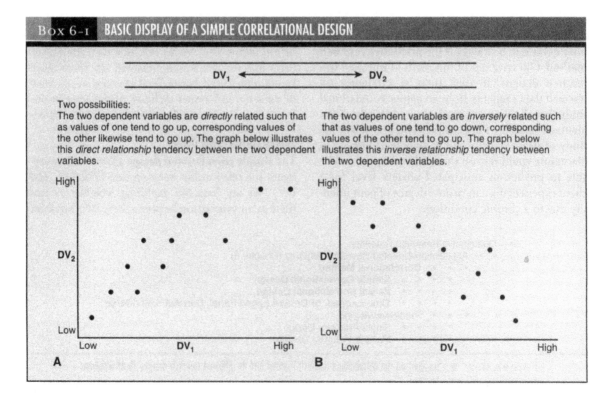

BOX 6-1   BASIC DISPLAY OF A SIMPLE CORRELATIONAL DESIGN

$DV_1 \longleftrightarrow DV_2$

Two possibilities:
The two dependent variables are *directly* related such that as values of one tend to go up, corresponding values of the other likewise tend to go up. The graph below illustrates this *direct relationship* tendency between the two dependent variables.

The two dependent variables are *inversely* related such that as values of one tend to go down, corresponding values of the other tend to go up. The graph below illustrates this *inverse relationship* tendency between the two dependent variables.

A

B

Also, the r^2 just cited, the coefficient of determination, is an example of an *effect size* statistic first introduced in Chapter 3. In this instance, it is an effect size calculation appropriate to the simple correlational design we are discussing.

Partial Correlational Design

The illustration just used to demonstrate a possible simple correlational study focused on only two DVs. In the vast majority of similar research studies, however, one seldom encounters an actual situation wherein the two DVs are exclusively related one to the other with no additional influence from one or more other variables. Quite often there is at least a third variable that can be identified as potentially influencing the relationship between the first two DVs. When this occurs, it is referred to as a "third variable problem" because the third variable's influence on the first two DVs is confusing, or confounding, our interpretation of what the true relationship is between DV_1 and DV_2.

One possible solution to this third variable problem is what is known as a **partial correlational design**. In this type of design, the researchers investigate the correlation between the two DVs of principal interest (i.e., DV_1 and DV_2), but with an adjustment made so that the influence of the third DV (DV_3), is cancelled or "partialed" out. This procedure, then, allows us to obtain a more accurate reading on the correlation between the first two DVs in that the unwanted influence of the third DV is mathematically eliminated. Otherwise, the correlation between the two principal DVs—without adjustments made for the third DV—would be termed spurious. The symbolization for the partial correlation between DV_1 and DV_2, but with DV_3 partialed

out, is $r_{12.3}$. Box 6-2 shows how a partial correlational design might be visualized.

In the earlier example of an interest in the correlation between extent of client progress regarding trunk flexion ROM (DV_1) and extent of therapist verbal acknowledgment/approval of the progress (DV_2), a possible confounding third DV might be the degree of known client compliance with a between-session stretching regimen assigned by the therapist (DV_3). Given that known client compliance with the stretching regimen is most likely correlated with client progress as well as therapist approval, it would be crucial to partial out those measures of client compliance so as to remove at least that one confounding variable.

Time-Lagged, or Cross-Lagged Panel, Correlational Design

The use of a partial correlational design to address the so-called third variable problem helps to counteract the unwanted influence of a third DV, thereby aiding researchers in avoiding a misleading spurious correlation. Although such a design is indeed beneficial, there still exists another potential difficulty in the correlational research method that investigates the association between two DVs, the *directionality problem*. Let us return to our original simple correlational study focusing on client progress and therapist approval in an effort to understand this directionality problem.

You will recall that in our earlier example we discussed the trend of points constituting a scatterplot that suggested a moderately strong direct relationship between client progress (DV_1) and therapist approval (DV_2). This was the case because the points on the graph approximated a straight line ascending from

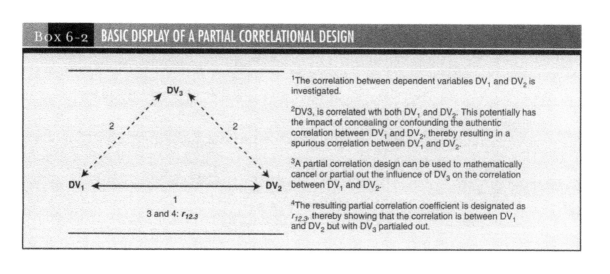

BOX 6-2 BASIC DISPLAY OF A PARTIAL CORRELATIONAL DESIGN

[1]The correlation between dependent variables DV_1 and DV_2 is investigated.

[2]DV3, is correlated wth both DV_1 and DV_2. This potentially has the impact of concealing or confounding the authentic correlation between DV_1 and DV_2, thereby resulting in a spurious correlation between DV_1 and DV_2.

[3]A partial correlation design can be used to mathematically cancel or partial out the influence of DV_3 on the correlation between DV_1 and DV_2.

[4]The resulting partial correlation coefficient is designated as $r_{12.3}$, thereby showing that the correlation is between DV_1 and DV_2 but with DV_3 partialed out.

DV_3

2   2

DV_1 ⟷ DV_2

1

3 and 4: $r_{12.3}$

left to right. We also discussed quantifying this relationship by calculating the Pearson correlation coefficient with a value of $r = .40$, thus suggesting a moderately strong positive correlation. The fact still remains, however, that in a correlational study one cannot infer a cause-and-effect relationship between the two DVs. In other words, correlation does not imply causation. As discussed earlier in the book, researchers have the potential to infer cause-and-effect relationships only in the context of a true experimental/randomized controlled trial study.

Having made that disclaimer regarding correlation not implying causation, we must acknowledge that researchers might still wonder in a correlational study if indeed one of the DVs is the antecedent, or precursor, to the other DV. For example, in our earlier illustration, is it a matter of client progress being antecedent to or preceding therapist approval, or is it more the case that therapist approval is antecedent to or precedes client progress? Although we are not talking in terms of cause and effect, the issue of which DV is antecedent to or precedes the other DV is a legitimate and practical concern. This issue, essentially, is the **directionality problem** in that we are asking if the direction of influence or dynamics is from client progress to therapist approval, or vice versa. It is precisely to this directionality problem that the **time-lagged**, or **cross-lagged panel**, **correlational design** speaks.

To address the directionality problem, a time-lagged correlational design measures the study's participants on the two DVs at two different points across time. Once this is done, the researchers then calculate the Pearson r for the two DVs at both time point 1 and time point 2. This allows one to then examine further the correlation coefficients for several pairs of DVs at different points in time. This explanation is aided greatly by Box 6-3 in that it displays the several possible correlation coefficients that can be examined as well as the implied insights that may be gathered regarding directionality (cf. Rosnow & Rosenthal, 2005).

As displayed previously, the two **synchronous correlations** are essentially the same. Such is the case, likewise, for the two **test-retest correlations**. The two **cross-lagged correlations**, however, are substantially different in that the correlation coefficient for DV_1 at time point 1 and DV_2 at time point 2 is .67, whereas the correlation coefficient for DV_2 at time point 1 and DV_1 at time point 2 is only .36. These cross-lagged correlational patterns, therefore, suggest a directionality influence moving from client progress to therapist approval whereby client progress may be thought of as the antecedent, or precursor, to therapist approval.

PREDICTIVE RESEARCH METHOD

Figure 6-3 spotlights the predictive research method and its two affiliated research designs.

Six principal research procedures constitute the predictive research method: (a) the presence of a

---

Box 6-3   DISPLAY OF TIME-LAGGED CORRELATIONAL DESIGN FOR HYPOTHETICAL CLIENT PROGRESS–THERAPIST APPROVAL STUDY

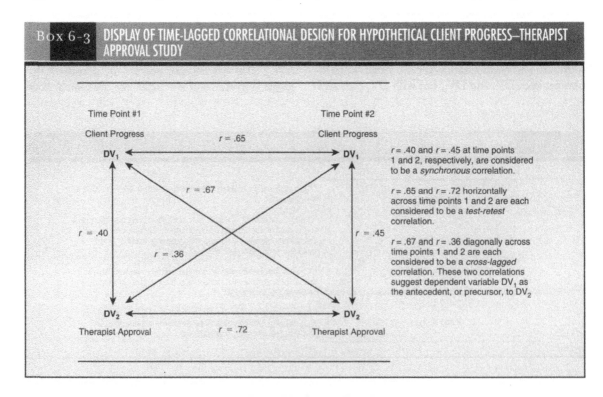

- Quantitative Research Category
  - • Association-Oriented Research Strategy (Chapter 6)
    - • • Correlational Method
      - • • • Simple Correlational Design
      - • • • Partial Correlational Design
      - • • • Time-Lagged, or Cross-Lagged Panel, Correlational Design
    - • • **Predictive Method**
      - • • • **Single-Predictor Design**
      - • • • **Multiple-Predictor Design**

FIGURE 6-3 ■ Spotlight on the predictive research method and its affiliated research designs (bold emphasis designates coverage in this section).

sample of participants or pairs of participants that may or may not have been formed by random selection, (b) the availability of a correlational data set reflecting two or more original DVs, (c) the measurement of each participant in the sample on one or more of the original DVs, (d) the designation of one of the original DVs as a criterion variable (CV), (e) the designation of one or more of the original DVs as one or more predictor variables (PV), and (f) the application of correlation-based statistical techniques that reflect an earlier data set of two or more DVs and that allow predictions.

The preceding paragraph may have come across as somewhat confusing. Cutting across all of the bases that needed to be touched, the bottom line is that the predictive research method reflects and builds on the correlational research method discussed earlier. In one respect, we are simply extending and expanding what we learned in the previous section on correlational methods so as to make possible the prediction of values on a DV of interest. Now let us proceed to the wonders to be found in the predictive research method.

Single-Predictor Design

Let us continue with the hypothetical study and data we introduced earlier that investigated the relationship between client progress regarding trunk flexion ROM (DV$_1$) and therapist acknowledgment/approval of the progress (DV$_2$) for a sample of 25 client-therapist dyads. Recall that each of the 25 clients was measured on DV$_1$ just as each of the 25 therapists was measured on DV$_2$. We also projected for our hypothetical data set the following: (a) a scatterplot of points on a graph that approximates a straight line ascending from left to right, (b) a Pearson correlation coefficient of $r = .40$, and (c) a coefficient of determination value of $r^2 = .16$.

With these correlational data and statistics in place, a researcher could conduct a predictive study using the **single-predictor design** that would allow

the prediction of one of our original DVs based on knowledge of the other original DV. For example, working with a hypothetical 26th client-therapist pair, if we measure the client on his or her progress regarding trunk flexion ROM (DV$_1$), we could use that information to predict the extent of the therapist's approval (DV$_2$).

The single-predictor design, then, uses a *known* value on one of the original DVs (say, client progress, DV$_1$) to predict a *currently unknown* value on the other original DV (say, therapist approval, DV$_2$). When this is done in the context of a predictive study, the known variable used for the prediction is called the **predictor variable** (PV), while the currently unknown but soon-to-be predicted variable is called the **criterion variable** (CV). Also, the DV$_1$ or PV may be designated as the **X variable**; correspondingly, the DV$_2$ or CV may be designated as the **Y variable**.

The extension of the Pearson correlation coefficient technique that makes this type of prediction possible involves another statistical technique known as **simple linear regression**. The word *simple* in the expression indicates that only one PV is being used to predict the CV. A detailed discussion of this statistical technique is beyond the intent and scope of this book; however, Box 6-4 displays the concept of a single-predictor design as well as the generic formula used for simple linear regression. Also, Appendix D provides more detailed coverage of the measurement and statistical considerations addressed in the book.

Multiple-Predictor Design

As the expression implies, the **multiple-predictor design** actually builds on the single-predictor design in that two or more PVs are used to predict a single CV. Just as the single-predictor design requires a correlational data set already in place that gives values to a DV$_1$ (or X) and a DV$_2$ (or Y), in a similar but extended fashion the multiple-predictor design has certain correlational data set prerequisites.

More specifically, to conduct a multiple-predictor study, a researcher would first need to have access to a data set that contains values for three or more original DVs. For example, the hypothetical study we have been using with values available on extent of both client progress (DV$_1$) and therapist approval (DV$_2$) could be enhanced by also obtaining measures on a third DV, namely, the degree of client compliance with a between-session stretching regimen assigned by the therapist (DV$_3$).

Box 6-4   DISPLAY OF A SINGLE-PREDICTOR DESIGN, USING SIMPLE LINEAR REGRESSION, TO PREDICT ONE CRITERION VARIABLE FROM ONE KNOWN PREDICTOR VARIABLE

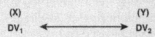

(X)   (Y)

DV_1 ⟷ DV_2

Measured values of DV_1 and DV_2 are already in place for a sample of participants (or pairs of participants).

Scatterplot showing the graph of the relationship between DV_1 and DV_2 is available as well as the value of the Pearson r.

For a *new* participant (or pair of participants) not part of the original sample, a measure of DV_1 or X can be made (e.g., extent of client progress), becomes known, and is labeled as the *predictor variable (PV)*. This value of the PV then can be used to predict DV_2 or Y, which is currently unknown yet is being predicted and labeled as the *criterion variable (CV)*. The following illustrates this progression:

DV_1 or X = PV ⟶ DV_2 or Y = CV
(Measured and known)   (Unknown but predicted)

The basic form of the *simple linear regression equation* that drives the prediction of Y based on X is $\hat{Y} = a + bX$, where $\hat{Y}$ is the predicted value of Y or the CV; X is the known value of the PV; a is a numerical constant representing the y-intercept of the regression line through the original scatterplot of data points; and b is a weighted factor based on the slope of the regression line, that is multiplied by X.

If indeed data were available on all three of these DVs for, say, a sample of 25 participants or pairs of participants, then a *multiple linear regression equation* could be formulated. This would, in turn, allow a researcher to use known values on two of the three original DVs for a given participant to predict a value for a currently unknown third DV. Or, in the terminology developed in the previous section, two known PVs could be used to predict a currently unknown CV. To accomplish this multiple-predictor task, one would have to rely on yet another correlation-based statistical technique known as **multiple linear regression**. In this instance, the word *multiple* implies that two or more PVs are used to predict one CV. Box 6-5 continues our reliance on displaying the concept underlying a multiple-predictor design as well as a generic formula used for multiple linear regression.

One final point deserves mention before leaving the topic of a multiple-predictor design.

Box 6-5   DISPLAY OF A MULTIPLE-PREDICTOR DESIGN, USING MULTIPLE LINEAR REGRESSION, TO PREDICT ONE CRITERION VARIABLE FROM TWO (OR MORE) KNOWN PREDICTOR VARIABLES

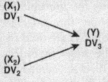

(X_1)
DV_1

(Y)
DV_3

(X_2)
DV_2

Measured values of dependent variables DV_1, DV_2, and DV_3 are already in place for a sample of participants (or pairs of participants).

A correlation matrix and Pearson *r*s quantifying the correlations across the three dependent variables are available. Also, a *multiple correlation coefficient* designated by upper-case *R* is available to indicate the correlation between a combined set of two or more dependent variables (e.g., DV_1 and DV_2 used as predictor variable [PVs]) and one remaining dependent variable (e.g., DV_3 used as the criterion variable [CV]).

For a *new* participant (or pair of participants) not part of the original sample, measures can be taken of DV_1 or X_1 (e.g., extent of client progress) and DV_2 or X_2 (e.g., extent of therapist approval). These variables become known and are labeled as PV_1 and PV_2. These values on the PVs can then be used to predict DV_3 or Y, which is currently unknown yet is being predicted and labeled as the *CV*. The following illustrates this progression:

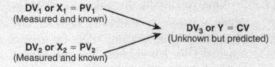

DV_1 or X_1 = PV_1
(Measured and known)

DV_3 or Y = CV
(Unknown but predicted)

DV_2 or X_2 = PV_2
(Measured and known)

The basic form of the *multiple linear regression equation* that drives the prediction of Y based on X_1 and X_2 is $Y = a + b_1X_1 + b_2X_2$, where Y is the predicted value of Y or the criterion variable, CV; X_1 and X_2 are the known values for the predictor variables PV_1 and PV_2; a is a numerical constant; and b_1 and b_2 are weighted factors multiplied by the values for X_1 and X_2, respectively.

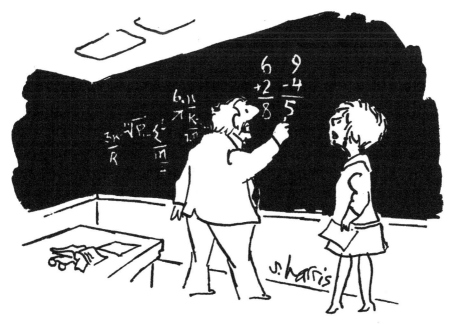

"Every once in a while I just like to unwind with a little addition and subtraction."

HUMOR BREAK ■ Are we starting to feel like the guy at the chalkboard? (From Harris, S. [1992]. *Chalk up another one: The best of Sidney Harris.* New Brunswick, NJ: Rutgers University Press.)

The **multiple correlation coefficient, R,** as cited in Box 6-5, is typically reported in prediction studies and represents the correlation between a combined set of two or more PVs and the one predicted CV. Also, reports of prediction studies usually indicate a **multiple coefficient of determination value,** or **R^2,** which designates the proportion of variability on the CV that can be explained by the combined set of two or more PVs. Further elaboration on these concepts, as well as the implications of the so-called beta weights (e.g., b_1 and b_2 introduced earlier), can be found in Jaccard and Becker (2002).

DETAILED SUMMARY

Figure 6-4 provides a detailed summary of the association-oriented research strategy as well as its

- Quantitative Research Category
  - • Association-Oriented Research Strategy (Chapter 6)
    - • • Correlational Method
      - • • • Simple Correlational Design
      - • • • Partial Correlational Design
      - • • • Time-Lagged, or Cross-Lagged Panel, Correlational Design
    - • • Predictive Method
      - • • • Single-Predictor Design
      - • • • Multiple-Predictor Design

FIGURE 6-4 ■ Detailed summary of the association-oriented research strategy and its affiliated research methods and designs covered in Chapter 6.

affiliated research methods and research designs that have been covered in this chapter.

FURTHER OBSERVATIONS ON THE ASSOCIATION-ORIENTED RESEARCH STRATEGY: WORDS OF CAUTION AND WORDS OF PROMISE

CORRELATIONAL RESEARCH VERSUS CORRELATIONAL STATISTICS: BEWARE OF THE DISTINCTION

It is important to keep in mind that a distinction exists between correlational research on one hand and techniques using **correlational statistics** on the other. Correlational research that investigates the relationship between or among two or more DVs will of necessity bring into play correlation-based statistical techniques. The same can be said for predictive studies that are founded on correlational data, for they too will of necessity employ statistical analyses that are rooted in correlation-based concepts and techniques.

On the other hand, the use of correlation-based statistics in a research study does not necessarily imply that the study itself is correlational in nature. For example, a researcher could be conducting a true experimental/randomized controlled trial study wherein one of the study's outcomes involves exploring the correlation between two variables of interest. The study itself is difference-oriented in nature rather than association-oriented, yet a Pearson correlation coefficient may be calculated to quantify the outcome of interest. A particularly valuable resource on this issue is the research textbook by Goodwin (2005).

CORRELATION DOES NOT IMPLY CAUSATION, BUT . . .

As discussed earlier in this chapter, correlation does not necessarily imply causation. Two DVs may be strongly correlated in either a positive or negative direction, thus implying a strong direct or inverse relationship, respectively. This does not, however, necessarily imply that one is the cause of the other. For example, the hypothetical correlation of an $r = .40$ between client progress and therapist approval does not necessarily imply that either DV is the cause of the other. Association-oriented research simply does not involve the degree of control that is essential to arriving at research findings that hold out the possibility of cause-and-effect conclusions. Such a potential for possibly arriving at cause-and-effect research conclusions remains in the exclusive domain of only a true experimental/ randomized controlled trial type of difference-oriented study.

It can be said, though, that causation does imply correlation. If, for instance, a true experimental study leads to findings that suggest a causal linkage between the independent variables (IVs) and DVs, then it can be concluded likewise that the two variables are obviously correlated.

To summarize this brief section, it might be helpful to think along the following lines about the **correlation-causation relationship**: (a) correlation does not necessarily imply causation; (b) causation, however, does indeed imply causation; and finally, (c) correlation is a necessary but insufficient condition for causation.

ASSOCIATION-ORIENTED RESEARCH AS AN ANTECEDENT, OR PRECURSOR, TO DIFFERENCE-ORIENTED RESEARCH

Precisely because correlation is a necessary but insufficient condition for causation, it follows that studies of an association-oriented nature, be they in terms of the correlational or predictive method, hold the potential for leading to difference-oriented studies. This chapter's example of investigating the correlation between the extent of client progress regarding a certain condition and the extent of

therapist feedback of approval could easily give rise to a related difference-oriented study.

Perhaps, for example, a cross-lagged correlational study of client progress and therapist approval might prompt a follow-up nonexperimental comparative groups study. In this case, for instance, the extent of client progress might be designated as the nonmanipulated IV with low, moderate, and high levels of progress; the DV, in turn, might be the extent of therapist approval. Although this type of difference-oriented study would still not have the potential for demonstrating cause and effect, the results could, nonetheless, inform to an even greater extent the conclusions reached in the earlier cross-lagged study.

It is not uncommon, then, in many areas of health science and behavioral science research to witness a historical progression from association-oriented to difference-oriented studies. Furthermore, the catalyst for starting this progression logically has its roots in descriptive-oriented studies. An example of this three-step progression could be a descriptive-oriented study on the prevalence of complementary and alternative medicine (CAM) use in North America giving rise to an association-oriented study on demographic and health condition factors that predict the likelihood to use CAM. In turn, this predictive study may lead a difference-oriented investigation of the relationship between frequency of chair massage intervention and stress reduction among clerical workers in a corporate setting.

ILLUSTRATION OF THE CORRELATIONAL RESEARCH METHOD USING A SIMPLE CORRELATIONAL DESIGN: A DETAILED ANALYSIS OF A COMPLETE RESEARCH ARTICLE

Box 6-6 provides, in its entirety, a research article by Leise (1993) that represents a correlational research study using a simple correlational research design. As the title and abstract indicate, the researcher investigated the correlation between chronic pain in individuals with rheumatoid arthritis and a healthy sense of humor.

Based on your careful reading of the Leise (1993) study, let us now critique the research article. In so doing, we will rely on the 29 critique questions that appeared in Chapter 4 and that represent the various criteria that should be helpful as we work our way through this report of a correlational study.

Catherine McMullen Leise, M.S.N., R.N.

Thiel College

The purpose of this study was to examine the relationship between chronic pain and a healthy sense of humor in individuals with rheumatoid arthritis. It was hypothesized that women with a diagnosis of rheumatoid arthritis who scored higher on the sense of humor scales would have a lower score on the pain scale. Likewise, if a lower score was obtained on the humor scales, it was expected that the subject would have a higher pain score. The sample population consisted of thirty women from the Northeast section of the United States, randomly chosen, between the ages of 33 and 66 years, diagnosed with rheumatoid arthritis. The results of this study showed a significant positive correlation ($r = .31$, $p < .01$) between humor and pain, which was contrary to the stated hypothesis. Findings also showed that, except for age, there were no significant relationships between the demographic data and the subjects' perception of pain or humor. It was found that age was negatively correlated with both humor and pain. Possible reasons for the findings are discussed, and nurses are encouraged to consider all the functions of humor in working with patients.

Pain is a very common experience. At one time or another, almost everyone has experienced pain, yet it is at times difficult to describe (Melzack, 1973). Pain is the chief cause of physical disability in the United States today, making it a major problem of this century (Ball, 1984; Brena, 1978). Health care professionals dedicate much time and energy to pain relief (Eland, 1988; Hedlin & Dostrovsky, 1979). Also pain stimulates a person to seek professional health care more often than does any other symptom (Allerton & Exley, 1982; McCaffery, 1980). Every day, health care professionals care for millions of people in chronic pain. Approximately 21 million of these people in chronic pain are arthritis sufferers, disabled not only by the degenerative process of arthritis but also by the pain (Arthritis Foundation, 1989; Brena, 1978).

Rheumatoid arthritis is the most common form of this disorder, affecting more than 7 million Americans. It is a chronic disease, usually with pain as the first and major symptom (Arthritis Foundation, 1989). In this study, chronic pain was studied by questioning women diagnosed with rheumatoid arthritis.

In the past, the relief of chronic pain focused on physical factors such as pharmacological manipulation, physiological stimulation, and surgical intervention. These methods remain important components of pain therapy today. Also, various psychological treatments of chronic pain have become known. Biofeedback, distraction, and relaxation have been used (Broome & Khorshidian 1982; Whipple, 1987). Yet to be added to this list of methods used in controlling pain is the therapeutic use of humor.

Although a common experience in daily living, humor is not a component of health education, nor is it widely used in health care settings (Ellis, 1978). Today, humor and its beneficial effects are widely studied (Metcalf, 1987; Ruxton, 1988; Schunior, 1989; Sullivan & Deane, 1988); however, it is seldom used in the health care setting (Ruxton, 1988).

The purpose of this study was to examine the relationship between chronic pain and a healthy sense of humor in individuals with rheumatoid arthritis. It was hypothesized that women diagnosed with rheumatoid arthritis who possess a healthy sense of humor would experience less pain than would those individuals without a healthy sense of humor. It was expected that subjects who scored higher on the sense of humor scale would score lower on the pain scale, and conversely. The major objective was to demonstrate to health professionals that well-placed humor can be an effective tool in caring for clients; humor can be therapeutic.

Humor as reported by the individual is the ability to perceive absurdity in serious situations. A healthy sense of humor is an expression of humor that is constructive, not destructive; it is the ability to make the best of a bad situation. It is measured in this study using the Situational Humor Response Questionnaire (SHRQ) and the Coping Humor Scale (CHS; Martin & Lefcourt, 1983).

Pain is a perception of an event; it is "whatever the experiencing person says it is, existing whenever he says it does" (McCaffery, 1980, p. 26). Chronic pain is a perpetual sensation of hurting lasting longer than 6 months. It may be cyclic in nature with exacerbations and remissions. It is measured in this study using the McGill-Melzack Pain Questionnaire (Melzack, 1975).

Review of the Literature

Humor and pain have been studied since ancient history, although both remain indefinable. As Robinson (1977) stated, humor cannot be defined with one all-inclusive definition. There remain many unanswered questions and much controversy concerning humor. Humor cannot be placed in one discipline, for it can be used in all disciplines (Robinson, 1978).

Humor and Health

Research on humor is endless; however, research pertaining to humor and health is limited (Van Zandt & La Font, 1985). Historically, the belief is that humor has a positive effect on one's health and well-being (Moody, 1978). Proverbs 17:22 states, "A merry heart doeth good like a medicine; but a broken spirit drieth the bones."

Continued

Box 6-6   THE CORRELATION BETWEEN HUMOR AND THE CHRONIC PAIN OF ARTHRITIS — CONT'D

In 1923, McDougall made known his belief that laughter and humor evolved, just as did humans, as a necessary correction of the effects of sympathy. Without humor, McDougall believed that humans could not have survived, because it is nature's antidote to the depressing and sad events around humanity. McDougall felt that humor was a response to pain rather than to pleasure.

Freud, considered to be the primary theorist of humor, suggested that in humor the ego takes on the viewpoint of the superego. From this vantage point, one can view the anxieties with a certain detachment. Humor turns an otherwise negative event into a less significant one, thus saving "psychic energy" (Freud, 1928).

Van Zandt and La Font (1985), like many previous researchers, believed humor to be therapeutic. In the Lincoln General Hospital humor study, Van Zandt and La Font studied nurses in acute care settings and their use of humor. The purpose of the study was to examine the therapeutic value of humor. In a questionnaire, the nurses simply reported their use of humor with patients. All but one subject reported humor as having a positive outcome.

In his study of humor, Fry (1971) found that laughter increased heart rate and blood pressure, thus exercising the heart. Fry contended that humor is a potential life saver, for humor is directly opposite to emotions such as fear and rage. Fry felt that humor relieves fear and acts as a buffer against rage, thus decreasing ill effects such as heart attacks. Humor is also antagonistic to stress both in its psychological and physical aspects. The stress caused by emotional tension is decreased by means of the "cathartic" effects of humor (Fry, 1971, 1979, 1980).

Williams (1986) also studied the effects of humor on health. Like Fry (1971), Williams (1986) found that humor decreases anxiety, increases heart and respiratory rates, and improves muscle tone. He also found that humor enhances an individual's tolerance to pain.

Dossey, Keegan, Guzzetta, and Kolkmeier (1988) go one step further in their description of humor as having a body-mind connection. They surmise that play and laughter makes a person feel better emotionally as well as physically. They also feel that humor is used as a coping mechanism and helps keep individuals whole. In using humor therapeutically with patients, Dossey et al. (1988) also describe the nursing process.

Today, studies document humor's positive effect on patients diagnosed with cancer and on the elderly (Ruxton, 1988; Schunior, 1989; Simon, 1988; Sullivan & Deane, 1988). Sullivan and Deane (1988) found that humor benefited elderly patients with the opportunity for better communication. Patients were more willing to communicate their concerns through the use of humor. Simon (1988) states that the elderly also use humor as a coping mechanism.

Martin and Lefcourt (1983) investigated the historical belief that a sense of humor is therapeutic. They believed that humor could be used as a coping mechanism in times of stress. They hypothesized that a sense of humor "reduces the deleterious impact of stressful experiences" (p. 1313).

In their study of humor, Martin and Lefcourt (1983) provided evidence for the hypothesis of this study. After they developed the SHRQ, a self-report measure of humor production, Martin and Lefcourt (1983, 1984) tested their questionnaire using three studies dealing with the effects of humor on stress. The findings of these studies showed an inverse relationship between humor production and life stressors and between humor production and negative moods. They also reported that subjects who experienced high stress levels also produced more humor (Martin and Lefcourt, 1983). These findings supported their hypothesis that humor is therapeutic in that it reduces the impact of stress. These studies also validated the SHRQ as a valid measure of humor production (Martin & Lefcourt, 1983, 1984).

Like humor, pain is a perception which influences a person's emotions. Meinhart and McCaffery (1983) remind us that mind and body are inseparable; one cannot feel pain physiologically without emotionally feelings the effects of pain. Therefore, pain can be described as being both a physiologic and psychologic event (Meinhart & McCaffery, 1983; Allerton & Exley, 1982). Evidence has also shown that pain is changeable and variable. Different people perceive pain differently depending on their past experience with pain, cultural learning, what the situation means to them, expectations of a painful experience, and stress (Melzack, 1973).

Pain research has chiefly been done to examine the relationship of pain to demographic data such as age and sex, or to psychological aspects, such as anxiety (Kim, 1980). Most of these studies, however, have been conducted in the laboratory setting, where pain was measured by pain tolerance or pain threshold, not actual clinical pain.

Clinically, Jacox and Stewart (1973) studied the relationship between sex of subject and pain. They found that the diagnosis, not sex, affected the pain. In two separate studies, Barber and Cooper (1972) and Blitz and Dinnerstein (1971), distraction was found to reduce the patient's perception of pain.

In his studies of pain, Melzack (1975) devised a self-report method to measure pain: The McGill-Melzack Pain Questionnaire. To test his questionnaire, Melzack (1975) used 297 patients diagnosed with pain due to 12 different disease entities, including arthritis. Results of the study showed high intercorrelations ($r > 0.9$, $p < 0.01$ in all cases) among all categories of the questionnaire, which confirmed the McGill-Melzack Pain Questionnaire as a valid measure of pain. Extensive testing by Melzack (1975) during the development of this questionnaire demonstrated interval consistency reliability.

In the research for this article, chronic pain, the perpetual sensation of hurting, was studied through rheumatoid arthritis. Rheumatoid arthritis is a chronic disease resulting in progressive physical debilitation and chronic pain. It affects women more often than men, and there is a higher prevalence in the northeast section of the country. Rheumatiod arthritis has also been associated with stress and depression (Luckman & Sorenson, 1974; O'Dell, 1977; Spitz, 1984).

Box 6-6 THE CORRELATION BETWEEN HUMOR AND THE CHRONIC PAIN OF ARTHRITIS — CONT'D

Methodology

This research was conducted in a major city in northeastern Ohio. The sample population consisted of 30 women between the ages of 33 and 66 years of age with a diagnosis of rheumatoid arthritis and no other chronic health problem, and who lived in the areas of northeastern Ohio and northwestern Pennsylvania. Subjects were randomly selected from the three available arthritis clinics. Permission was obtained from human subjects, the clinic administration, and the physicians who treated the women. Clinic physicians supplied names of subjects who met the criteria ($N = 81$). All of these potential subjects were given an explanation of the study and asked to participate. Of the 81 names given, 51 agreed to participate in the study. To ensure confidentiality, all participants were given identification numbers. Of these numbers, 30 were then chosen randomly using a random number table. The same information and instructions were given to all participants, and informed consent was obtained from each subject.

Chronic pain was measured using the McGill-Melzack pain Questionnaire (Melzack, 1975), a self-report questionnaire that measures pain quantitatively. Three types of date were obtained from this questionnaire: The Pain Rating Index (PRI), the number of words chosen (NWC), and the present pain intensity (PPI). The PRI, which describes pain quality, was obtained from a list of 20 groups of words ranked in order that describe pain. Subjects were asked to circle the words that described their pain. The score could range from 0 (for the subject who chose none of the words) to the highest score of 78. It must be noted that in this study subjects were asked to describe their usual pain, not the pain they felt at the time, which is what the questionnaire originally intended. The NWC was simply the number of words that the subject chose to describe her pain. The range for the NWC is from 0 to 20. The PPI, which describes pain intensity, was obtained from the number-word combination of the overall pain intensity, which is numbered from 1 to 5 (Melzack, 1975). Subjects chose one word from a list of five words with a number from 1 to 5 — mild (1) to excruciating (5) — that best described the pain that they experienced at the time. The lowest score for this measure is 1 and the highest possible score is 5.

Humor was measured using the SHRQ, which measures humor production, and the CHS, which measures the use of humor as a coping mechanism (Martin & Lefcourt, 1984). The SHRQ consisted of 18 items where common situations were described. Each item was followed by a 5-point Guttman-type scale that ranges from I would have not been amused (1) to I would have laughed heartily (5). Subjects were asked to put themselves in each situation and answer accordingly. Three additional nonsituational self-descriptive items were presented. In these times, the subjects are essentially asked to rate their sense of humor; the lowest and highest possible scores for the SHRQ are 21 and 104, respectively (Martin and Lefcourt, 1984).

Reliability was measured by administering the SHRQ to 497 subjects. An interval consistency reliability of .70 to .79 was obtained for this measure (Martin & Lefcourt, 1984). Three studies of validity were reported (Martin & Lefcourt, 1983). All three studies supported the validity of the SHRQ as a quantitative measure of humor.

The CHS, also developed by Martin and Lefcourt (1983), consists of seven statements that subjects responded to. The statements are answered on a 4-point scale ranging from strongly disagree (1) to strongly agree (4). Analysis based on data from 56 subjects produced an internal consistency reliability of .61. The lowest possible score for the CHS was 7 and the highest was 28 (Martin & Lefcourt, 1983).

The three questionnaires were administered to each subject privately in her home. Demographic data, which included age, educational level, marital status, employment status, arthritis data, and medication regime, was collected first. The pain questionnaire was then given. This was to rule out any bias of the humor tests affecting the subjects' pain. Immediately following the pain questionnaire, the SHRQ and the CH were given in that order. Instructions were given, and each questionnaire was read aloud to each subject by the researcher so that no instructions were missed or misunderstood. All tests combined took no more than 40 minutes for each subject to complete.

Quantitative analysis of the data was completed. The mean and the standard deviation were computed for each score obtained in the three instruments used. Correlations between these scores were measured using the Pearson product-moment correlation coefficient. Intercorrelations and correlations among these questionnaires were measured using this statistic. Length of illness and its effect on humor were also examined. In other words, did the length of illness have a negative effect on a person's sense of humor? This question was answered using the Pearson product-moment correlation coefficient.

Results

Analysis of the data did not support the hypothesis for this study. The findings of this study showed that the demographic data that were collected , except for age, were not related to the subjects' perception of pain and humor. Age showed a negative correlation between both humor and pain ($r = -.26$, $p < .17$; $r = -.44$, $p < .01$, respectively). It was found that with increased age, subjects reported less pain as well as less humor. Demographic data is presented in Table 1. As seen in this table, the educational level of the subjects was rather high. Most of these subjects were married, and all but one were either working outside of the home or as a housewife or both. All subjects had been diagnosed with rheumatoid arthritis between 1 and 10 years prior to this study. The number of years the subject was diagnosed also had no effect on their perception of humor or pain. The arthritis data that were collected, such as time of day pain was experienced, how long the pain lasted, medication regime, and alterations in physical ability had no significant effect on their reporting of pain or humor.

The three measures derived from the pain questionnaire as described previously are the PRI, NWC, and the PPI. The PRI describes pain quality. The lowest reported score for the PRI was 6 and the highest score was 20 with a mode of 10. Only two subjects reported a score of 20.

Continued

Box 6-6   THE CORRELATION BETWEEN HUMOR AND THE CHRONIC PAIN OF ARTHRITIS — CONT'D

The PPI describes present pain intensity. One subject did report a score of 0 stating that she was not experiencing pain at that time. No one reported a score higher than 2. Half of the subjects reported this score, and the other 14 reported a score of 1.

For the humor indices, the lowest score of the SHRQ reported by the subjects was 34 and the highest was 73. For the CHS, subjects reported a low score of 15 and a high score of 27. Scores were negatively skewed. Table 2 illustrates the mean and standard deviation of each measure.

Intercorrelations between two of the pain scales (PRI and NWC) and between the two humor indices were significantly positive; however, it was much lower for the humor indices than for the pain scales (.92 and .48, respectively). There were no significant correlations between the PRI and NWC and the third pain scale, the PPI. This was expected, because the PRI and the NWC measured overall pain and the PPI measured pain presently experienced.

The results of the correlations between the humor and pain scales were somewhat surprising. These correlations showed a significant positive correlation at the .01 alpha level. Using two of the pain indices and one humor scale (between the PRI and the SHRQ and between the NWC and the SHRQ), correlation coefficients were .31 and .33, respectively. In other words, subjects who reported a high index of pain also reported a high index of humor. However, when using the PRI, a significant negative correlation between this pain index and the SHRQ was found. When using the second humor scale, the CHS, no significant correlation could be found between it and any of the pain indices. Table 3 shows the correlations among the humor and pain indices.

TABLE 1   DEMOGRAPHIC DATA OF SUBJECTS, WITH MEAN SCORES AND STANDARD DEVIATIONS

VARIABLE	N	PERCENTAGE
Age (in years)		
30-40	5	17
41-50	5	17
51-60	14	47
61-66	6	19
Mean	52.5	
SD	9.3	
Marital Status		
Divorced	3	10
Married	24	80
Widowed	3	10
Education (in years)		
10-11	4	13
12	17	57
13+	9	30
Mean	12.55	
SD	1.6	
Employment Status		
Management	2	7
Professional	4	13
Housewife	16	53
Labor	2	7
Unemployed	1	3
Other	5	17
Year Diagnosed		
1978-1982	11	37
1983-1987	19	63
Mean	(19)	82.6
SD	4.8	

TABLE 2   DESCRIPTIVE DATA OF THE HUMOR AND PAIN INDICES

VARIABLE	MEAN	SD	RANGE
PRI	25.8	10.2	12-48
NWC	11.9	4.0	6-20
PPI	1.5	0.6	0-02
SHRQ	54.6	8.6	35-73
CHS	21.4	3.4	15-27

Note: PRI = Pain Rating Index; NWC = number of words chosen; PPI = present pain intensity; SHRQ = Situational Humor Response Questionnaire; CHS = Coping Humor Scale.

TABLE 3   ZERO-ORDER CORRELATION MATRIX OF THE HUMOR (SHRQ AND CHS) AND PAIN (PRI, NWC, AND PPI) INDICES

		PRI	NWC	PPI	SHRQ
NWC	R	0.92			
	P	0.00			
PPI	R	0.21	0.15		
	P	0.27	0.44		
SHRQ	R	0.31	0.33	0.04	
	P	0.10	0.07	0.82	
CHS	R	0.09	0.05	−0.30	0.48
	P	0.63	0.80	0.11	0.01

Note: PRI = Pain Rating Index; NWC = number of words chosen; PPI = present pain intensity; SHRQ = Situational Humor Response Questionnaire; CHS = Coping Humor Scale

Discussion

The hypothesis for this study was not substantiated. A negative correlation was expected between pain and humor; instead a positive correlation was found between two of the pain indices and humor (between the PRI and SHRQ and the NWC and SHRQ). Also, an inverse relationship was found between the PPI and humor.

One reason for the outcome may be that people who report high overall pain perception need more humor in their lives to cope with pain. McDougall (1923) believed humor to be a response to pain not to pleasure. He also believed that for people to live through the ages humor was used as a buffer against depression and pain. When one experienced a negative event, humor was used to combat this (McDougall, 1923). These people who must face a life time of pain need humor to be able to live with the pain and survive. Consequently, people in pain need humor, hence the positive correlation between humor and pain. These findings also correlate well with the study done by Martin and Lefcourt (1983) cited earlier. In their study, they found that subjects produced more humor when experiencing high levels of stress. Pain is a known stressor; the positive correlation between overall pain and humor found in this study substantiates the findings of Martin and Lefcourt (1983). Martin and Lefcourt (1983, 1984) also found an inverse relationship between humor production and life stressors and between humor production and negative moods. This parallels the inverse relationship between present pain and humor found in this study.

This correlation, which, is in direct contrast to the positive correlation between the other pain indices (PRI and NWDC) and the SHRQ seems to substantiate the hypothesis for this study. The first difference is that although all of the pain indices do measure pain, two different types of pain are being measured. The PPI measures present pain, whereas the PRI and the NWC measure the overall pain that a person usually experiences. This may explain the differences in the correlations among the humor and pain indices. People may use humor to decrease the pain they experience at the present, hence the inverse relationship between the SHRQ and the PPPI. At the same time, people who experience chronic pain have a greater need to use humor. This would explain why the subjects who reported experiencing more "usual" pain. Moreover, one cannot overlook the fact that the PPI is scored with only one item and the range of the scores were reported was restricted.

The third area to be addressed is the reason that the CHS did not correlate with any of the pain indices, whereas the other humor index (SHRQ) did. First, it must be noted that although there was a positive correlation between these two scales, it was low. Also, the CHS is only a 7-item questionnaire, whereas the SHRQ is a 21-item questionnaire, leading one to question the reliability of the CHS. Another reason is that although both questionnaires are designed to measure humor, they measure two different aspects of humor. The CHS measures how much people used humor as a coping mechanism, and the SHRQ measures overall humor production. All of these reasons may have contributed to the nonsignificant correlations that were computed.

Because the research did not substantiate the hypothesis and the findings were inconclusive, this subject needs further study. There are many applications for further study. Replication and expansion of this study using a larger population or use of a different pain population would be useful. Also, research concerning if and how humor is used in different health care settings by nurses would be profitable. A comparison of the use of humor between males and females may also be useful. It may be said that humor has a positive effect on health; however, it cannot be concluded that humor has a direct positive impact on the disease process itself. Before this conclusion can be made, more research is needed in the body-mind connection to increase the knowledge of the total body's response to life.

Implications

If a negative relationship exists between a healthy sense of humor and chronic pain, then nursing practices and nursing education can be modified to include humor therapy. Humor can then be implemented by the nurse as an intervention in the nurse-client relationship, thus being incorporated in the client's care plan. The effects of humor therapy can then be evaluated and may provide evidence of behavioral changes. An increased awareness amount health professionals about the effects of humor could lead to the use of humor as a creative professional and therapeutic tool.

Humor offers many benefits and is viewed as a valuable asset by many individuals. Humor must not be seen as a panacea but must be used in connection with other treatment modalities. Nurses need to consider all of the functions of humor in working with patients. Nurses can potentially use humor as a therapeutic intervention in many situations with any age group in health care settings.

References

Allerton, B. & Exley, E. (1982, October). Pain: What do we really know about it? *Critical Care Update*, pp. 28-31.

Arthritis Foundation. (1989). *Overcoming rheumatoid arthritis*. Atlanta, GA: Author.

Ball, R. (1984). Chronic pain. *Jefferson Journal of Psychiatry*, 2, 11-24.

Barber, T. & Cooper, B. (1972). Effects on pain of experimentally induced and spontaneous distraction. *Psychological Reports*, 31, 647-651.

Blitz, B. & Dinnerstein, A. (1971). Role of attentional focus is pain perception manipulation of response to noxious stimulation by instructions. *Journal of Abnormal Psychology*, 77(1), 42-45.

Brena, S. (1978). The staggering cost of chronic pain. In S. F. Brena (Ed.), *Chronic pain: America's hidden epidemic* (pp. 3-11). New York: Artheneum.

Broome, A. & Khorshidian, C. (1982). Psychological treatments of chronic pain. *Nursing Times*, 4, 1305-1306.

Continued

| BOX 6-6 | THE CORRELATION BETWEEN HUMOR AND THE CHRONIC PAIN OF ARTHRITIS — CONT'D |

Dossey, B., Keegan, L., Guzzetta, C., & Kolkmeier, L. (1988). *Holistic nursing: A handbook for practice.* Rockville, MD: Aspen.

Eland, J. (1988). Pain management and control. *Journal of Gerontological Nursing, 14*(4), 10-15.

Ellis, S. (1978). Humor the wonder drug. *Nursing Times, 74,* 1792-1793.

Freud, A. (1928). Humor. *International Journal of Psychoanalysis, 9,* 1-6.

Fry, W. (1971). Laughter: Is it the best medicine? *Stanford M.D., 10*(1), 16-20.

Fry, W. (1979, April). *Using humor to save lives.* Paper presented at the meeting of the American Orthopsychiatric Association, Washington, DC.

Fry, W. (1980, January). *Humor and healing.* Paper presented at the University of California, San Francisco.

Hedlin, A., & Dostrovsky, J. (1979). Understanding the physiology of pain. *Canadian Nurse, 75,* 28-30.

Jacox, A., & Stewart, M. (1973). *Psychosocial contingencies of the pain experience.* Iowa City: University of Iowa.

Kim, S. (1980). Pain: Theory, research and nursing practice. *Advances in Nursing Science, 2,* 43-59.

Luckman, J., & Sorenson, K. (1974). *Medical surgical nursing: A psychophysiologic approach* (pp. 1220-1228), Philadelphia: W.B. Saunders.

Martin, R.A., & Lefcourt, H. (1983). Sense of humor as a moderator of the relation between stressors and moods. *Journal of Personality and Social Pyschology, 45*(6), 1313-1324.

Martin, R.A., & Lefcourt, H. (1984). Situational humor response questionnaire: Quantitative measure of sense of humor. *Journal of Personality and Social Psychology, 47*(1), 145-155.

McCaffery, M. (1980). Understanding your patient's pain. *Nursing, 10,* 26-31.

McDougall, M. (1923). *An outline of psychology.* London: Metheum.

Meinhart, N., & McCaffery, M. (1983). *Pain: A nursing approach to assessment and analysis.* CT: Appleton-Century-Croft.

Melzack, R. (1973). *The puzzle of pain.* London: Penguin.

Melzack, R. (1975). The McGill Pain Questionnaire: major properties and scoring methods. *Pain, 1,* 277-279.

Metcalf, C. (1987). Humor, life, and death. *Oncology Nursing Forum, 14*(4), 19-21.

Moody, R. (1978). *Laugh after laugh: The healing power of humor.* Clearwater, FL: Headwater Press.

O'Dell, A. (1977). Pain associated with arthritis and other rheumatic disorders. In A. Jacox (Ed.), *Pain: A source book for nurses and other health professionals* (pp. 349-515). Boston: Little, Brown.

Robinson, V. (1977). *Humor and health professions.* Thorofare, NJ: Charles B. Slack.

Robinson, V. (1978). Humor in nursing. In C. Carlson & B. Blackwell, (Eds.), *Behavioral concepts and nursing interventions* (pp. 191-210). Philadelphia: J.B. Lippincott.

Ruxton, J. (1988). Humor intervention deserves our attention. *Holistic Nursing Practice, 2*(3), 54-62.

Schunior, C. (1989). Nursing and the comic mask. *Holistic Nursing Practice, 3*(3), 7-17.

Simon, J. (1988). The therapeutic value of humor in aging adults. *Journal of Gerontological Nursing, 14*(8), 9-13.

Spitz, P. (1984). The medical, personal and social costs of rheumatoid arthritis. *Nursing Clinics of North America, 19,* 575-582.

Sullivan, J. & Deane, D. (1988). Humor and health. *Journal of Gerontological Nursing, 14*(1), 20-24.

Van Zandt, S. & La Font, C. (1985). Can a laugh a day keep the doctor away? *Journal of Practical Nursing, 35*(3), 33-35.

Whipple. B., (1987). Methods of pain control: review of research and literature. *Image: Journal of Nursing Scholarship, 19*(3), 142-146.

Williams, H. (1986). Humor and healing: Therapeutic effects in geriatrics. *Gerontion, 1*(3), 14-17.

Catherine McMullen Leise, M.S.N., R.N., is a graduate of Pennsylvania State University and an instructor of community health nursing at Thiel College in Greenville, Pennsylvania.

From Leise, C.M. (1993). The correlation between humor and the chronic pain of arthritis. *Journal of Holistic Nursing, 11*(1), 82–95.

PRELIMINARY SECTION

1. Does the *title* of the study provide a basis for identifying the *type of study*, *major variables*, and *participants*?

The title does indicate that the study is correlational in nature and, by implication, belongs to the association-oriented research strategy. Also, the title identifies the two major variables investigated in the study as being those of humor and chronic arthritic pain. The participants are obviously individuals suffering from arthritis, although the title does not clarify the actual nature of the arthritic condition.

2. Does the *abstract* synthesize the main body of the report (i.e., the introduction, method, results, and discussion) with a particular focus on the *research question, research hypothesis, participants, research method and design, major variables, instruments, statistical techniques, principal findings*, and *conclusions*?

The abstract does appropriately summarize many of the principal themes that a reader would expect to encounter in greater detail in the main body of the report. The research question is implied by virtue of the abstract's first sentence, which states the study's purpose. Also, the research hypothesis, participants, research method and design, and major variables are addressed. Although the abstract is silent on the instruments used to measure the study's variables, it does acknowledge the correlational statistical technique used along with the study's findings. The conclusions, for the most part, are delayed until the article's actual discussion section.

INTRODUCTORY SECTION

3. Is the reader introduced to the *relevant professional literature* bearing on the study being reported by way of a *general overview of the research problem area* as well as a more *specific coverage of individual studies*?

The author provides a comprehensive review of the literature pertaining to the study's two principal variables of humor and the chronic pain of arthritis. The progression in this literature review is from a fairly general overview to a more detailed consideration of relevant studies and concepts. Somewhat misleading, though, is the manner in which the untitled introduction is followed by the sections labeled "Review of the Literature" and "Humor and Health." In fact, the literature review is actually provided prior to, within, and subsequent to the section designated as "Review of the Literature." It should be noted that the section titled "Humor and Health" does cover relevant literature, not only on humor and health in general but also as these two areas relate specifically to the experience of pain. It appears that the professional literature review provided does succeed in establishing an appropriate context within which the author's study can be considered.

4. Is the purpose of the study identified by the *research question* being formulated at an *operational level*?

The fifth paragraph of the introductory section does provide an explicit statement of the study's purpose along with an acknowledgment of its overall major objective where health professionals are concerned. The detailed statement of the research hypothesis in this same paragraph does operationalize somewhat how the study's purpose is to be addressed. Although there is no formal statement of the study's research question per se, it is certainly implied by virtue of the information provided in the introductory section, particularly the paragraph just referenced.

5. Is the *rationale or justification*, based on various features of the professional literature, presented

as a context or framework for the study's *research hypothesis*?

Although distributed throughout the first three parts of the article leading up to the "Methodology" section, the professional literature reviewed does indeed establish a context within which the study's research hypothesis is justified. A reader should easily recognize—based on the literature reviewed—precisely why the investigator is predicting the types of outcomes that are hypothesized. The rationale for the study's hypothesis, though, might have been enhanced if the author had delayed until the latter part of the introductory section the actual statement of the hypothesis.

6. Does the author state the study's *research hypothesis* in such a way that the predicted answer to the study's research question is clear and unambiguous?

Yes, the introductory section does contain an explicit statement of the research hypothesis. The prediction is that participants diagnosed with rheumatoid arthritis who possess a healthy sense of humor would experience less pain than would those individuals without a healthy sense of humor. This is followed by an indication of the pattern of scores expected on the measures of both humor and pain.

METHOD SECTION

7. Are the study's *participants* clearly characterized along with the *inclusion and exclusion criteria* used for identifying them?

The first paragraph in the "Methodology" section identifies certain demographics of the sample of 30 participants. An inclusion criterion of having been diagnosed with rheumatoid arthritis is cited, along with an implied exclusion criterion of any other chronic health problems.

8. Did the researchers justify the number of participants constituting the sample size by way of a *power analysis*?

No, the method section of this article is silent on any type of power analysis justifying the decision to include 30 participants in the sample. A fairly clear indication is given, however, of the steps actually taken to derive the sample of 30.

9. Was an *accessible population* of potential participants acknowledged along with an indication of *how the sample was derived* from such a population, be it through random selection or some other procedure?

The accessible population of potential participants was based at three available arthritis clinics; however, the size of the accessible population is not identified. Random selection was used to arrive at the sample size of 30. The first paragraph in the method section also characterizes the information provided to the potential participants prior to the selection process actually being conducted.

10. Did the author specify the manner in which the participants were *assigned* to the two or more comparison groups, be it through random assignment or some other means? (Please note that this critique question remained in our listing of 29 for the expressed purpose of emphasizing that the issue of assigning participants to comparison groups is nonexistent where a correlational study is concerned.)

A correlational study of this type simply involves a single sample of participants on whom measures a re recorded for at least two DVs. There is no assignment of participants to two or more comparison groups as is the case in certain difference-oriented studies. Consequently, the critique question posed here is irrelevant to a correlational study.

11. Was any clarification provided as to how the *ethical aspects* of the study were governed, particularly in reference to the protection of the participants, the overall integrity of the research, and the earlier approval of the study by an institutional review board?

The first paragraph of the "Methodology" section acknowledges that permission for possible involvement in the study was sought from the potential participants, arthritis clinic administrators, and attending physicians. Potential participants meeting the inclusion/exclusion criteria were given an explanation of the study and invited to participate. Of those who agreed to take part in the study, identification numbers were assigned so as to ensure confidentiality. Informed consent was also obtained from the study's participants. No mention is made, however, of the study's proposal being submitted to and approved by an institutional review board.

12. Was the nature of the research effort adequately characterized in terms of its position in the research continuum (i.e., its position regarding *research category, strategy, method, design,* and *defining procedures*)?

The article's "Methodology" section did adequately characterize the reported study as reflecting a correlational research method using a simple correlational design. This is apparent in that procedures were used to measure the two DVs and correlate them by way of an appeal to the Pearson product-moment correlation coefficient. The study's method, design, and procedures suggest an association-oriented research strategy that is one of several options available in the quantitative research category.

13. Were the study's *variables operationalized* in a comprehensive fashion so that their manipulation or measurement could be replicated?

Yes, the study's two DVs were operationalized very well in that chronic pain was measured by three indices and humor was measured by two indices. This made possible a correlation matrix whereby the correlation between any two of the five indices could be examined. Anyone reading this research report would indeed be able to replicate the manner in which the two DVs were operationalized and measured. Additional information was also provided regarding the collection of data on several relevant demographic variables.

The issue of one or more variables being manipulated in this study is actually irrelevant in that the principal focus is only on DVs. There are no IVs to be manipulated as would possibly be the case in certain difference-oriented studies.

14. Did the author(s) clearly specify the *equipment or instruments* used in the study for variable manipulation or measurement purposes, along with a documentation of the technical characteristics of such including validity and reliability?

The only relevant issue here is the three instruments used to measure chronic pain and humor among the 30 participants. The one instrument used for measuring chronic pain generated three types of data or indices. The two instruments employed for measuring humor resulted in two types of data or indices on this variable. For all three instruments, technical characteristics were reported in terms of instrument description, scores generated, validity, and reliability. Demographic data of a standard nature were collected at the outset of the study prior to the measures being taken on pain and humor.

RESULTS SECTION

15. Were the *data analysis techniques* used in the study identified and justified?

Yes, the article reports appropriate data analysis techniques used as well as their justification given the purposes of this study and the nature of the data collected. Descriptive statistics, Pearson correlation coefficients, and the results of null hypothesis significance tests are reported clearly and justified, thereby leading to the results being quite understandable.

16. Were the results of the study communicated by an appeal to *descriptive and/or inferential*

statistics consistent with the nature of the research question as well as the research method and measurement scales used?

As alluded to in the previous statement, the article does indeed report appropriate descriptive and inferential statistics. The reported means, standard deviations, ranges, and Pearson *r*s are all appropriate descriptive statistics in this study. Furthermore, the Pearson *r*s were also used in an inferential sense in that the statistical significance or nonsignificance of each correlation coefficient was determined for the purpose of null hypothesis testing.

17. Were the results of the data analysis related to an appropriate *decision* regarding the study's *null or statistical hypothesis or hypotheses?*

Yes, the results section does report appropriate decisions regarding the null hypothesis significance tests. An important ethical point illustrated in this study is the fact that a researcher is obligated to report accurately the results of a study even when some of the study outcomes are contrary to what was hypothesized at the outset. This author does precisely this in a forthright manner.

18. Was the decision regarding the null hypothesis acknowledged as a basis for inferring decisions concerning the *alternative and research hypotheses?*

The decision regarding the study's null hypothesis actually manifested itself several ways in that three indices for chronic pain are used along with two indices for humor. Consequently, the study speaks in terms of several decisions based on the null hypothesis significance test results. For each of these several results, regardless of whether the decision was in terms of statistical significance or nonsignificance, the implications are identified explicitly for the variations of the research hypothesis and implicitly for the alternative hypothesis.

19. If hypothesis testing was performed, were the analyses augmented with other statistical techniques such as *confidence interval estimation* or *effect size calculations?*

This study does not report any other statistical analyses that would augment the hypothesis testing that occurred.

20. Were *tables and figures* appropriately used to make the data analyses more comprehensible?

The author did use three tables very effectively to display in a succinct manner the results of the data analyses. No figures were used, perhaps because the tables seemed sufficient to the tasks at hand.

DISCUSSION SECTION

21. Did the researchers reflect on the manner in which the study was designed and conducted regarding any *limitations or delimitations* (i.e., intentional or unintentional boundaries)?

The researcher did acknowledge that it would be useful in replicating and expanding this study if a larger population (actually sample) were used as well as possibly a different pain population. Also, rather than using only female participants, the author proposes possibly looking at gender differences in the use of humor.

22. Did the author *elaborate* on the *interpretation of the study's findings* beyond the interpretation that was begun in the results section?

The author does an exemplary job of discussing at length those results that are both consistent and inconsistent with the study's original predictions. The author appeals extensively to the professional literature—both historical and current—on both humor and pain in an effort to interpret the seemingly contradictory and unanticipated outcomes of the study. This feature of the article may indeed represent its greatest strength in that the researcher displays an impressive degree of intellectual honesty and rigor in an appeal to concepts, principles, and past research relevant to humor, pain, and their interrelationship.

23. Did the researcher address the *significance* of the study and its findings, particularly as they relate to earlier studies in the problem area investigated?

As indicated in the response to the previous question, the author did indeed address at length the significance of the study in the context of both the anticipated and unanticipated results. Again, this discussion appealed extensively to earlier conceptual and empirical studies in the areas of humor and pain. In so doing, the author succeeded in identifying different perspectives from which humor, pain, and their interconnectedness might be considered. The researcher also built into the significance of the study an extrapolation or extension of sorts in that the discussion of the study's implications delves into such areas as the body-mind connection, nursing practice and education, humor as a complementary therapeutic tool, and humor's role among health professionals in general.

24. Did the discussion section address possible *intervening variables* in the study that might explain why the results obtained were indeed forthcoming?

Although not identified by the expression intervening variable per se, this is another area in which the author does an exemplary job in discussing the study's findings. Specifically, the researcher goes to great lengths to explain plausible reasons why the study's findings are what they are, and this is precisely what a discussion of a study's intervening variable(s) should concern.

More to the point, the author relies on a historical source to speculate that humor may well be a response more attuned to pain than to pleasure in order to "buffer against" depression and pain itself. The author also speculates that, consistent with more recent research, because humor production has been associated with high stress levels and pain is indeed a stressor, it would follow that humor would be directly related to pain level as uncovered in this study. Other plausible reasons cited for why the results of the study are what they are relate to the following themes: (a) the pain indices used in the study actually reflect two types of pain (i.e., present pain and overall chronic pain usually experienced), thereby possibly engaging the use of humor in different ways; and (b) likewise, the humor indices used in the study reflect two aspects of humor (i.e., humor as a coping mechanism and overall humor production), thereby complicating the effort to correlate "humor" with the varieties of "pain" just cited.

25. Were *recommendations* suggested to the reader regarding needed follow-up studies that might replicate, fully or partially, the current study?

Yes, as indicated in the responses to questions 21 and 23, the author does make valuable recommendations regarding needed follow-up studies. These essentially appeal to possible replicated studies that would alter somewhat the nature of the pain population studied, the size of the sample, the gender of the participants, and the overall broadening of research into humor's role among health care professionals.

CONCLUDING SECTION

26. Does the list of *references* accurately reflect each of the sources cited in the research report, with a consistent bibliographic citation style used?

It appears that the list of references accomplishes what it is intended to do. Presumably a reader would be able to follow up the various citations if interested in exploring in greater detail the author's use of any given source.

27. Does the research report contain any *appendixes* that augment in greater detail information provided earlier in the article?

No appendixes are provided in this article.

28. Is there any information in the form of *author notes* that provide insight regarding funding support for the study, contact directives for communicating with the author as a follow-up, or collegial assistance in completing the study?

The only information of this type is the author's institutional affiliation as identified immediately after the list of references.

29. Are any *footnotes* provided that elaborate on one or more aspects of the study that would have been misplaced or distracting if they had been embedded in the main body of the report?

No footnotes appear in the article.

ILLUSTRATION OF THE PREDICTIVE RESEARCH METHOD USING A MULTIPLE-PREDICTOR DESIGN: AN ABBREVIATED ("QUICKIE") ANALYSIS OF A COMPLETE RESEARCH ARTICLE

Box 6-7 displays the complete research article by Holm, Rogers, and Kwoh (1998) that illustrates the predictive research method using a multiple-predictor research design. As reflected in the title and abstract of this study, the researchers investigated the impact of several PVs on the functional disability of a rheumatoid arthritis sample of participants.

After carefully reading the Holm et al. (1998) study, we are now in a position to do an abbreviated or "quickie" critique of this research article. A detailed analysis of this study using our usual listing of 29 critique questions would perhaps be an instance of overkill given that we just completed such an exercise in the previous section on the correlational research method. We can, however, briefly overview this study by highlighting those features of the study that most define it as an example of a multiple-predictor design. So, with that game plan in mind, let us proceed!

At first glance, this study may seem intimidating. Rest assured, though, that it is quite comprehensible if examined in a systematic way that takes into account what we have already covered in this chapter on a multiple-predictor design.

Text continued on p. 118

BOX 6-7 PREDICTORS OF FUNCTIONAL DISABILITY IN PATIENTS WITH RHEUMATOID ARTHRITIS

Margo B. Holm, Joan C. Rogers, and C. Kent Kwoh

Objective. Using the World Health Organization's classification system of the consequences of disease, this study sought to examine the impact of physical and psychological impairment variables, beyond that contributed by social, demographic, and disease variables, on the functional disability of a rheumatoid arthritis (RA) sample. Data collected during an acute episode were used to predict concurrent and future disability status.

Method. A secondary data analysis of 85 adults hospitalized for exacerbations in arthritis was undertaken. Disability was assessed with the Health Assessment Questionnaire. Physical impairment was measured with the Keitel Function Test and Pain Analog Scales, and psychological impairment was measured with the center for Epidemiologic Studies Depression Scales and the Perceived Self-Efficacy Scales for People with Arthritis.

Results. Our findings indicated that physical impairment, demographic, and disease variables accounted for 64% of the explained variance in disability during the concurrent episode. Psychological impairment as well as demographic and disease variables accounted for 49% of the explained variance in future disability status.

Conclusion. The combined influence of demographic characteristics and the consequences of the pathology of RA experienced as physical and psychological impairments contributed differentially to disability during concurrent and future time periods.

Key words. Rheumatoid arthritis; Disability; Impairment.

Introduction

The World Health Organization (WHO) classifies the consequences of pathology at 3 levels, i.e., impairment, disability, and handicap (1). WHO defines impairment as the loss or abnormality of an anatomic, physiologic, cognitive, or emotional structure or function. For the person with rheumatoid arthritis (RA), impairments can include restricted joint mobility, pain with movement, depression, and low self-efficacy for function. According to WHO, disability is concerned with the activities of a person that are required to carry out daily life tasks. Examples of disabilities are problems in everyday tasks such as eating, dressing, bathing, and shopping. Everyday tasks, when coalesced in different combinations, form the basis of social roles (e.g., mechanic, homemaker, student). If task disabilities are severe, social role performance can become dysfunctional and the person will no longer be able to enact roles satisfactorily. The experience of pathology at this level is referred to as handicap. Handicap involves a social disadvantage such that the individual is limited or prevented from fulfilling a social role that is regarded as appropriate based on age, sex, and social and cultural norms.

The development of self-report instruments, such as the Health Assessment Questionnaire (HAQ; 2) and the Arthritis Impact Measurement Scales (3), has facilitated the assessment of health and disability status in persons with arthritis (4). The ability to perform activities of daily living (ADL) is one component of health status, and disability, or task performance dysfunction, reflects the cumulative impact of disease on daily life tasks. Numerous studies have sought to elucidate the nature of disability in persons with arthritis by examining the relationship between the ability to perform ADL and impairment expressed in factors such as impaired mobility (5-7), pain (8-11), depression (8, 10, 12-14), and self-efficacy beliefs (15).

Restricted joint mobility and joint pain are salient impairments of arthritis that are commonly cited by patients as limiting ADL. Although significant correlations have been found between impaired upper and lower extremity mobility restrictions and disability (6,7), the magnitude of these correlations have been low to moderate (e.g., $r = 0.36–0.57$). The ADL categories of arising, walking, and hygiene seem to be particularly sensitive to impairment expressed as joint mobility restrictions in both the upper and lower extremities. By grouping ADL into units emphasizing impairment of restricted joint mobility, such as bending down, Badley et al (5) found slightly stronger relationships (e.g., $r = 0.42–0.78$) between joint motion and ADL. Likewise, Hakala et al (16) found moderately strong relationships ($r = 0.75$) between the impairment of restricted joint mobility assessed on the Keitel Function Test and the ADL of the HAQ. Patients' perceptions of pain have also been found to be significantly correlated with disability (8-11), with higher levels of pain related to greater disability.

In terms of psychological impairment, the relationship between depressive affect and disability has received the most attention, but the findings are inconsistent and the extent to which a depression — disability linkage is exaggerated by the somatic content of depression instruments remains an open question (10, 17-19). Using instruments with known sensitivity to the somatic aspects of RA (17), an association between depression and disability was found by Peck et al (10) but not by Serbo and Jajic (8). Using a scale with little somatic content, Katz and Yelin (14) demonstrated that subjects exhibiting depressive symptoms had poorer function than those without depressive symptoms. Anderson et al (12) found that depression was related to physicians' ratings of disability but not to patients' self-assessments. Hawley and Wolfe (13) ascertained that disability contributed to the variance in depression and that changes over 3 years in disability were related to changes in depression. More recently, perceived self-efficacy has emerged as an important psychological construct in disability management (20). Self-efficacy refers to individuals' beliefs in their competence to perform a particular behavior or task in the future (21). Schiaffino et al (15) found that patients who expressed greater self-efficacy had lower levels of functional disability, regardless of level of pain experienced.

Continued

Box 6-7   PREDICTORS OF FUNCTIONAL DISABILITY IN PATIENTS WITH RHEUMATOID ARTHRITIS—CONT'D

Previous research, as well as the WHO model, suggests that impairments such as restricted joint mobility, joint pain, depression, and low perceived self-efficacy are related or may lead to task disability. In the present study, we sought to examine the impact of these physical and psychological impairment variables, beyond that contributed by social, demographic, and disease variables, on the functional disability of a RA sample at two points in time (11, 15, 22). Concurrent disability was predicted from the measures taken at admission to the hospital for arthritis-related reasons (concurrent episode/time1), and disability one year after discharge (future status/time 2) was predicted using the same measures.

Patients and Methods

Subjects. Subjects included in this secondary data analysis were patients from the inpatient rheumatology service of St. Margaret Memorial Hospital, Pittsburgh, Pennsylvania, between 1989 and 1992, who had agreed to participate in a prospective longitudinal study on the use and adequacy of assistive devices, a study reported elsewhere (23-25). All subjects had a definitive diagnosis of RA made by a rheumatologist. The sample of the current study, 85 subjects with RA, had a mean age of 61.5 years (SD 12.6). The majority were female (82%), Caucasian (95%), and married (58%). Seventy-three percent of the subjects lived with a spouse, friend, or family member, and 27% lived alone. Thirty-eight percent of the subjects had not completed high school, 40 % had a high school diploma, and 22% had more than a high school education. The annual family income level of those subjects who reported their incomes (53%) was $15,000 to $19,999.

All subjects were admitted to the hospital due to exacerbations of their RA. Subjects reported being diagnosed with RA for a mean of 16.4 years (SD 14.5). All subjects met the 1987 American College of Rheumatology (ACR; formerly the American Rheumatism Association) revised criteria for RA (26). The mean number of ACR criteria per subject was 5.3 (SD 1.0). Ninety percent of the patients had documentation of morning stiffness lasting greater than 30 minutes, 46% included radiographic confirmation of erosion of one or more joints, and 85% had a rheumatoid factor (RF) latex titer >1.60. Twenty-one subjects (25%) were lost to attrition at the 1-year followup, but only 9 were unaccounted for: 4 were deceased; 3 had moved to long-term care settings; 5 subjects refused to participate in the interview or were too confused to provide reliable information; and 9 had disconnected telephones or were not traceable.

Procedures. Subjects were referred to the original study within three days of hospitalization. After informed consent was obtained, demographic and social variables were determined using a structured interview, disease variables were obtained during the structured interview and from chart review, and the time 1 impairment measures were administered in the patient's room and adjoining hallway following the standardized procedures for each instrument. Time 2 measures were collected via telephone interview one year following discharge from the hospital. Patients were sent a copy of the HAQ in the mail, as well as a card summarizing possible responses that would facilitate response by telephone.

Measures. The social and demographic predictor variables of age, gender, living situation, marital status, and educational level were gathered by the research therapists during the structured interview at time 1. One disease predictor variable, the number of tender joints, was gathered from the patient using a checklist of 14 bilateral joint regions, which, in addition to the cervical spine and lumbar spine, made a total of 30 possible tender joint regions. All other disease variables (i.e., duration of RA, ACR criteria, and RF latex titer) were obtained from chart review.

The impairment predictor variables were derived from instruments used to measure physical and psychological status. The Keitel Function Test (KFT) consists of 24 performance test items that evaluate active range of motion in the upper and lower extremities and the vertebral column (27). Total scores range from 4 to 100; the higher the score, the more restricted the joint mobility. The KFT is sensitive to change (28, 29) and has been used as both a predictor variable (30) and an outcome measure (31). For the purposes of the current study, the KFT was adapted in 3 ways; 1) items 6 and 7 on wrist flexion and extension were expanded to include a scale item for less than 45 degrees of flexion and extension; 2) item 22 on walking 30 meters was expanded to include a scale item for accomplishing the 30 meters, although exceeding the 40 seconds inherent in the KFT; and 3) items 23 and 24 on stair climbing were eliminated due to safety concerns. In the current study, then, the KFT scores for items 6 and 7 ranged from 1 to 4 and from item 22 ranged from 0 to 7, and thus, with the elimination of items 23 and 24 (i.e., 6 points) and the expansion of items 6, 7, and 22 (i.e., an additional 5 points), the range on the KFT was 4 to 99 points. Interrater reliability among 5 dyads of raters, evaluating 10 patients, ranged from 0.94% to 0.97% agreement. The total KFT score was used as a physical impairment predictor variable. Pain perception was examined by adding task-specific visual pain analog scales to 7 of the major ADL assessed on the HAQ (2): dressing, arising from a bed or chair, eating, walking, bathing, toileting, and shopping. This was done to establish the pain level associated with specific activities. Interrater reliability with the task-specific pain scales was established at 0.95% agreement among 4 raters while testing 15 subjects. Pain perception, the overall summed score of the 7 adapted pain visual analog scales, was the second physical impairment predictor variable.

The Center for Epidemiologic Studies Depression Scale (CES-D; 32) consists of 20 statements that reflect depressive symptoms such as crying and loss of appetite. Scores on the CES-D have been found to correlate with scores on the Beck (r = 0.81) and Zung (r = 0.90) depression scales (33, 34). Items are scored on a 4-point scale indicating how often these symptoms were experienced during the past week (i.e., less than

Box 6-7   PREDICTORS OF FUNCTIONAL DISABILITY IN PATIENTS WITH RHEUMATOID ARTHRITIS—CONT'D

1 day, 1-2 days, 3-4 days, or 5-7 days). The total score is the sum of the 20 items. With cores ranging from 0 to 60; higher scores suggest greater levels of depression. Because Radloff (32) has suggested that the CES-D total score alone should usually be used as a general estimate of the degree of depressive symptoms, the CES-D total score was used as a psychological impairment predictor variable.

The Perceived Self-Efficacy (SE) Scale for People with Arthritis (20) consists of 3 subscales designed to ascertain a patient's perceived ability to deal with the consequences of arthritis symptoms. The SE pain subscale (PSE) consists of 5 items focused on patients' abilities to control arthritis pain. The SE function subscale (FSE) consists of 9 items that query patients about their degree of certainty that they can perform 9 daily living tasks without assistive devices or help from another person. The SE other symptoms subscale (OSE) consists of 6 items that examine the certainty with which patients believe they can control arthritis symptoms such as fatigue and "feeling blue." Subjects rate the degree to which they feel they can control the specific symptoms queried in each item on a corresponding visual analog scale. The scales range from 10, indicating "very uncertain," to 100, indicating "very certain." PSE, FSE, and OSE were all considered psychological impairment predictor variables.

Disability outcomes were measured using the HAQ (2), which is a self-report instrument designed to evaluate 8 categories of ADL: dressing and grooming, arising, eating, walking, hygiene, reach, grip, and outside activity. The HAQ has established validity and reliability (2, 35, 36) and has a demonstrated sensitivity to change (28, 29, 37). Each ADL category includes 2 or 3 items. Each item is rated as being completed without difficulty, with some difficulty, with much difficulty, or unable to do, and scored from 0 to 3, respectively. The score for each ADL category is determined by the highest score (i.e., most disability) for any item. The HAQ disability index, which ranged from 0 to 3, is calculated by adding the scores for each ADL category and dividing the number of ADL categories answered: the higher the disability index score, the greater the disability. The two disability outcome variables in this study were the HAQ time 1 disability index scores, which are reported as HAQ time 1 disability index for the time 1 acute status, and HAQ time 2 disability index for the followup future disability status.

Data analyses. Descriptive statistics were calculated for the total sample (n = 85) to ascertain the sample's characteristics and performance on the measures used in the study. Univariate comparisons consisted of Pearson product moment correlations to establish the strength and significance of the relationships among the predictor and outcome variables in the two models. A Bonferroni adjustment (38) was used because of the large number of correlations. Therefore, an unadjusted P value of 0.0005 was required for an alpha level of $P < 0.01$ (i.e., 0.01/19 comparisons = 0.0005). Variables were chosen for the model based on correlations >0.20 with one of the outcome variables. Because FSE, PSE, and OSE were highly correlated subscales of the same instrument, FSE was chosen for inclusion in the models, as it was the subscale that had the best conceptual fit with the HAQ.

Two models were then examined using the hierarchial regression. The more stable social and demographic variables (gender, age) were entered in block 1, the underlying disease variables (joint count, duration of RA) were entered in block 2, and the impairment variables of interest (KFT, pain perception, FSE, and CES-D) were entered in block 3. In model 2, the time 1 disability variable (HQ time 1) was also entered in block 3. Model 1 was designed to ascertain which variables at admission to the hospital (time 1, concurrent status) best accounted for concurrent functional disability, and model 2 was designed to ascertain which time 1 variables best predicted functional disability one year following discharge (time 2/future disability). Minimum tolerance of each variable entered into the model was then checked to detect multicollinearity. Scatterplots of the residuals for both models were then analyzed to determine if the distribution of the residuals was acceptable.

Results

Subject characteristics. Table 1 includes descriptive statistics of all variables considered for entry into the models for the original sample and study completers. Time 1 impairment measures indicated that the subjects exhibited moderate restrictions in joint mobility (KFT; mean 44.5); pain perception associated with the performance of functional takes listed on the HAQ was also moderate (mean 1.4); and the mean depression score on the CES-D was 18.1. Self-efficacy scores for pain (mean 53.7) function (mean 47.0), and other symptoms (mean 58.8) were in the middle range of the instrument, with self-efficacy for functional tasks being less than for control of pain symptoms or other symptoms. Based on the HAQ disability index, the RA subjects in this study exhibited moderate to severe disability during hospitalization (39) (HAQ time 1 disability index; mean 1.8) and the same level of disability at the 1-year followup (HAQ time 2 disability index; mean 1.5). The mean change score on the HAQ from time 1 to time 2 was 0.32 (SD 0.77), and the HAQ time 1 disability measure was significantly greater than that of the HAQ time 2 (t = 3.36, $P < 0.001$).

Relationships among variables. Zero-order correlations are presented in Table 2. After the Bonferroni adjustment 4 time 1 impairment variables (i.e., KFT, pain perception, FSE, and CES-D) significantly correlated with the HAQ time 1 disability measure. Two time 1 impairment measures (i.e., KFT and FSE) and the HAQ time 1 disability measure were significantly correlated with the HAQ time 2 disability measure.

Explained disability during time 1 (concurrent) status. Based on R values, on admission to the hospital for an acute episode the more stable social and demographic variables entering model 1 in block 1 (i.e., gender, age) accounted for approximately 20% of the variance in concurrent functional disability. In block 2, the addition of the disease variables helped explain another 11% of the variance. Block 3, which included two physical impairment variables (i.e., KFT, the amount of restricted joint mobility; and pain perception) and two psychological impairment variables

Continued

Box 6-7   PREDICTORS OF FUNCTIONAL DISABILITY IN PATIENTS WITH RHEUMATOID ARTHRITIS — CONT'D

(i.e., FSE, low self-efficacy for function, and CES-D, depression) explained the largest portion of the variance in concurrent functional disability at time 1 (Table 3). Based on the standardized regression coefficients (beta weights), in emerging order of appearance, only restricted joint mobility (KFT), followed by increased perception of pain and being female were independent variables that made statistically significant contributions in the total model.

Although subjects' low self-efficacy for function (FSE) and depression scores (CES-D) were significantly correlated with the HAQ time 1 disability measure, in the multivariate analysis they did not enter the model, which is consistent with the findings of others (16). Based on the beta

TABLE I   TIME 1 VARIABLE MEANS AND PERCENTAGES FOR THE ORIGINAL SAMPLE AND STUDY COMPLETERS*

	TIME 1 VALUES	
	ORIGINAL SAMPLE (N = 85)	STUDY COMPLETERS (N = 64)
Social and demographic variables		
Age, years[†]	61.5	61.3
Females, % [†]	82.0	81.0
Living alone, %	27.0	30.0
Married, %	58.0	56.0
Education Level		
<12 years	38.0	36.0
12 years, %	40.0	45.0
>12 years, %	22.0	19.0
Disease variables		
Duration of RA years[†]	16.4	16.1
1987 ACR criteria, mean	5.3	5.3
Joint count, mean[†‡]	23.0	22.3
RF late titer > 1:60, %	85.0	86.0
RF log latex[§]	2.7	2.6
Erosion-any site, %	46.0	50.0
Morning stiffness > 30 min., %	90.0	90.0
Impairment variables		
Keitel function test[†]	44.5	43.6
1Pain visual analog scale[†¶]	1.4	1.3
Self-efficacy pain#	53.7	53.1
Self-efficacy function[†]#	47.0	48.6
Self-efficacy other#	58.8	59.3
CES-D[†]	18.1	17.5
Disability outcome variables		
HAQ time 1 (concurrent)[†**]	1.8	1.8
HAQ time 2 (future)[†•]	—	1.5

*RA=rheumatoid arthritis; ACR=American College of Rheumatology (formerly the American Rheumatism Association); RF= rheumatoid factor; CES-D=Center for Epidemiologic Studies Depression Scale.
[†]Variables that met criteria for entry into the models.
[‡]Number of tender joints out of 30.
[§]Log base 10 of the RF latex titer.
[¶]Adapted Health Assessment Questionnaire (HAQ) pain visual analog scale.
#The Perceived Self-Efficacy Scale for People with Arthritis.
**HAQ disability index scores at time 1 and time 2.

BOX 6-7 PREDICTORS OF FUNCTIONAL DISABILITY IN PATIENTS WITH RHEUMATOID ARTHRITIS—CONT'D

TABLE 2 ZERO-ORDER CORRELATIONS OF STUDY VARIABLE (N = 85)*

	AGE	GENDER	LIVES ALONE	MARITAL STATUS	EDUCATION	OF RA	DURATION TOTAL	COUNT	ACR TITER	JOINT ACR7	RF ACR1	KFT	PAIN	PSE	FSE	OSE	CES-D	HAQ T1	HAQ T2
Age	1.00	—	—	—	—	—	—	—	—	—	—	—	—	—	—	—	—	—	—
Gender	0.16	1.00	—	—	—	—	—	—	—	—	—	—	—	—	—	—	—	—	—
Lives Alone	−0.37	−0.11	1.00	—	—	—	—	—	—	—	—	—	—	—	—	—	—	—	—
Marital Status	0.26	−0.15	0.20	1.00	—	—	—	—	—	—	—	—	—	—	—	—	—	—	—
Education	−0.45†	−0.20	0.08	−0.16	1.00	—	—	—	—	—	—	—	—	—	—	—	—	—	—
Duration of RA	0.27	−0.04	−0.17	0.17	−0.22	1.00	—	—	—	—	—	—	—	—	—	—	—	—	—
1987 ACR criteria	−0.10	−0.04	0.03	−0.06	0.01	−0.12	1.00	—	—	—	—	—	—	—	—	—	—	—	—
Joint Count	−0.88	−0.13	0.17	0.17	−0.20	0.06	0.02	1.00	—	—	—	—	—	—	—	—	—	—	—
RF latex titer	0.17	0.01	0.02	−0.19	0.11	0.12	−0.30	−0.15	1.00	—	—	—	—	—	—	—	—	—	—
Erosion (ACR7)	−0.23	0.02	0.11	−0.13	0.07	−0.08	−0.05	−0.12	0.23	1.00	—	—	—	—	—	—	—	—	—
Morning Stiffness (ACR1)	0.02	0.16	0.10	−0.08	0.05	−0.01	−0.05	−0.09	0.32	0.16	1.00	—	—	—	—	—	—	—	—
KFT	0.18	−0.15	−0.01	0.02	−0.16	0.27	0.18	0.23	−0.05	0.02	0.14	1.00	—	—	—	—	—	—	—
Pain Scale	−0.11	−0.31	0.20	0.01	−0.07	0.19	0.13	0.12	0.07	−0.02	−0.06	0.13	1.00	—	—	—	—	—	—
PSE	−0.21	−0.12	−0.05	0.11	0.16	−0.18	−0.10	−0.01	0.05	−0.19	−0.04	−0.35	−0.22	1.00	—	—	—	—	—
FSE	−0.21	0.19	0.15	−0.08	0.18	−0.28	−0.08	−0.12	0.08	−0.07	−0.01	−0.62†	−0.23	0.47†	1.00	—	—	—	—
OSE	−0.12	0.01	−0.03	0.12	0.19	−0.15	−0.07	−0.02	0.05	−0.12	−0.01	−0.21	−0.13	0.53†	0.46†	1.00	—	—	—
CES-D	−0.22	−0.22	0.01	−0.04	0.05	0.13	0.01	0.07	−0.02	0.01	−0.23	0.22	0.43†	−0.10	−0.17	−0.26	1.00	—	—
HAQ time 1‡	0.06	−0.39†	0.03	0.16	−0.14	0.35	0.02	0.23	−0.02	−0.02	−0.16	0.52†	0.55†	−0.26	−0.49†	−0.11	0.43†	1.00	—
HAQ time 2‡	0.26	−0.24	0.10	0.03	−0.15	0.31	0.04	0.22	0.06	0.06	−0.01	0.52	0.28	−0.38	−0.64†	−0.31	0.10	0.50†	1.00

*RA=rheumatoid arthritis; ACR=American College of Rheumatology (formerly the American Rheumatism Association); RF=rheumatoid factor; KFT= Keitel Function Test; Perceived Self-Efficacy Scales: PSE=Pain; FSE=Function; OSE=Other; CES-D=Center for epidemiologic Studies Depression Scale; HAQ= Health Assessment Questionnaire.

†P<0.01 with Bonferroni adjustment.

‡HAQ disability index scores at time 1 (concurrent) and time 2 (future).

Continued

BOX 6-7 PREDICTORS OF FUNCTIONAL DISABILITY IN PATIENTS WITH RHEUMATOID ARTHRITIS — CONT'D

coefficients, CES-D would have been the next variable to enter, but FSE would not have entered for another 4 steps, meaning that these two variables are still contributory factors for patients but not significant enough statistically to enter the model. Minimum tolerances of all variables in the model were within acceptable ranges, indicating that the contributions of the independent variables in the multivariate model were not unduly influenced by the other independent variables. The model 1 standardized residual was −0.002, and 99.9% of the residuals were within the 2 SD band, indicating an acceptable distribution of the residuals with no discernible pattern in the data.

Explained disability during time 2 (future disability) status. The R value was used to determine the collective contribution of time 1 social and demographic, disease, and impairment and disability variables for explaining future functional disability at time 2. The more stable time 1 social and demographic variables in block 1 (i.e., gender, age) accounted for approximately 16% of the variance in functional disability at time 2. In block 2, the addition of the time 1 disease variables helped explain another 8% of the variance. In block 3, four time 1 impairment variables (i.e., KFT, pain perception, FSE, and CES-D) and one disability variable (HAQ time 1) explained another 25% of the variance in future functional disability at time 2. The full model was significant ($P < 0.001$), meaning that data gathered at time 1 could explain 49% of the variance in functional disability at time 2 (future disability status). Based on the standardized regression coefficients (beta weights), however, in emerging order of importance, only low self-efficacy for function (FSE) and being older (age) made statistically significant contributions as independent variables in the total model (Table 4).

TABLE 3 REGRESSION ANALYSIS OF TIME 1 FACTORS CONTRIBUTING TO FUNCTIONAL DISABILITY AT TIME 1 (CONCURRENT) (N = 85)

	R2	CHANGE	BETA	t	F RATIO
Block 1: social and demographic variables					
Gender			−0.45	−4.31*	
Age			0.14	1.37	
Block 1 equation	0.20				9.47†
Block 2: social and demographic and disease variables					
Gender			−0.36	−3.5†	
Age			0.09	0.80	
Joint Count			0.26	2.65*	
Disease duration			0.18	1.66	
Block 2 equation	0.31	0.11			8.30†
Block 3: social and demographic, disease, impairment, and disability variables					
Gender			−0.18	−2.22‡	
Age			0.04	0.53	
Joint count			<0.01	0.08	
Disease duration			0.08	0.95	
CES-D§			0.11	1.38	
Self-efficacy scale-function			−0.02	−0.25	
Pain visual analog scale			0.36	4.26†	
Keitel function test			0.46	4.60†	
Model 1 equation	0.64	0.33			16.04†

*$P < 0.01$
†$P < 0.001$
‡$P < 0.05$
§ CES-D = Center for the Epidemiologic Studies Depression Scale.

Box 6-7 PREDICTORS OF FUNCTIONAL DISABILITY IN PATIENTS WITH RHEUMATOID ARTHRITIS—CONT'D

While the KFT and the HAQ time 1 disability measure significantly correlated with the HAQ time 2 disability measure, they were not significant variables in the multivariate model. Based on the beta coefficients, the KFT would have been the next item to enter the model, but HAQ time 1 would have been the last item to enter. Minimum tolerances of all variables in the model were within acceptable ranges, indicating that the contribution of the independent variables in the multivariate model were not unduly influenced by the other independent variables. The model 2 standardized residual was −0.007, and 100% of the residuals were within the 2 SD band, indicating an acceptable distribution of the residuals with no discernible pattern in the data.

DISCUSSION

After accounting for the effects of social, demographic, and disease variables, our findings suggest that it was restricted joint mobility, more than pain or being female, that contributed to concurrent functional disability of patients with RA in an acute episode severe enough to warrant hospitalization. Because the majority of the patients in the sample were admitted due to an exacerbation of their arthritis, and number of tender joints also entered the model, joint swelling and tenderness may have compounded joint mobility restrictions. In contrast to our findings, Ormel and colleagues (40) found that psychological factors such as motivation can be determinants of concurrent functional disability. Consistent with our findings, however, Hakala and colleagues (16) also found that the explanatory power of physical impairment measures for self-reported disability was significantly higher than for affective impairment measures.

For predicting future functional disability, a reversal occurred in the explanatory power of physical and psychological impairment variables in the sample. Our data indicate that two physical impairment variables (restricted joint mobility, increased perception of pain) and being female were the

TABLE 4	REGRESSION ANALYSIS OF TIME 1 FACTORS CONTRIBUTING TO FUNCTIONAL DISABILITY AT TIME 2 (FUTURE) (N = 64)				
	R2	R2 CHANGE	BETA	T	F RATIO
Block 1: social and demographic variables					
Gender			−0.30	−2.43*	
Age			0.32	2.56†	
Block 1 equation	0.16				5.30†
Block 2: social and demographic and disease variables					
Gender			−0.24	−1.98	
Age			0.29	2.23*	
Joint count			0.22	1.74	
Disease duration			0.15	1.15	
Block 2 equation	0.24	0.08			4.27†
Block 3: social and demographic, disease, impairment, and disability variables					
Gender			−0.08	−1.73	
Age			0.24	2.04*	
Joint count			0.11	0.98	
Disease duration			−0.03	−0.26	
CES-D			−0.05	−0.38	
Self-efficacy scale-function			−0.44	−3.34†	
Pain visual analog scale			0.09	.065	
Keitel function test			0.16	1.01	
HAQ time 1 disability indes			0.03	0.14	
Model 2 equation	0.59	0.25			5.35§

*P < .05.
†P < .01.
‡ CES-D=Center for the Epidemiologic Studies Depression Scale.
§ P < .001.

Continued

Box 6-7   PREDICTORS OF FUNCTIONAL DISABILITY IN PATIENTS WITH RHEUMATOID ARTHRITIS—CONT'D

most determining factors in predicting concurrent disability. However, no physical impairment variables and one psychological impairment variable (low-perceived self-efficacy for function), as well as being older, were the most significant factors in predicting future disability. It is likely that during an acute arthritis episode, the physical sequel of RA predominate in a disease process that occurs more frequently in women. Once health status becomes stabler or the chronic condition is reinstated, perceived self-efficacy to carry out daily activities, as well as the risks associated with aging with RA, emerge as more salient predictors of functional disability.

The perception of pain and its relation to disability may vary. Pain perception was associated with concurrent disability in our sample, but the experience of pain during the acute phase had little or no association with disability one year later. Similarly, while our sample as a whole had somewhat elevated depression scores at time 1 (concurrent status), depression had little association with disability during time 2 (future status). Our findings that time 1 elevated depression scores did not have an impact on future status are in agreement with those of Ahlmen et al (31), whose depression measure had little predictive power, and also with the findings of Serbo and Jajic (8), who ascertained that the influence of pain on task performance overshadowed that of depression. Further, our results are similar to other studies that reported the concurrent relationship of pain and disability (11,41) and only weak correlations between depression and disability (10,11,13). Our findings, however, are in contrast to those studies identifying pain as a predictor of disability at a later time (11,42).

Our sample differs from those in other studies because it includes data taken when the subjects were hospitalized during an acute phase of their disease process. The subjects in this study also reported more functional disability on admission to the hospital and at the 1-year followup than had been reported in other studies (2,6,10,11,13,16,28–30,36) as well as higher levels of depression (8,17). Time 1 data were collected within 3 days of admission to the hospital between 1989 and 1992. Because the HAQ asks patients about difficulty performing tasks during the previous week, an exacerbation of the disease process precipitating admission may account for the increased functional disability of the subjects at time 1. Although a lower level of disability was reported one year later at time 2, the improvement in this sample of adults whose disease process was so severe as to warrant hospitalization was minimal. Subjects' apprehension and discouragement with the disease process and their hospitalizations may also have accounted for the presence of elevated depression scores in the sample.

In summary, the time 1 model explained 64% of subjects' concurrent functional disability on admission to the hospital for an arthritis-related condition, and one demographic (gender), no disease, and two physical impairment variables (restricted joint mobility, increased perception of pain) made statistically significant contributions. The time 2 model, consisting of time 1 predictor variables, explained 49% of subjects' future functional disability at the 1-year followup. One demographic (age), no disease, and one psychological impairment (low self-efficacy for function) variable made statistically significant contributions. Although the subjects exhibited elevated depression scores, depression did not contribute to functional disability at the time of hospitalization or predict it at followup. Using the WHO model classification system, our results suggest that disability during hospitalization and at followup primarily reflects the combined influence of demographic characteristics and the consequences of the pathology of RA experienced as physical and psychological impairments.

References

1. World Health Organization. International classification of impairments, disabilities and handicaps. Geneva: World Health Organization; 1980.
2. Fries JF, Spitz P, Kraines RG, Holman HR. Measurement of patient outcomes in arthritis. *Arthritis Rheum* 1980;23:137-45.
3. Meenan RF, Gertman PM,, Mason JH. Measuring health status in arthritis: the Arthritis Impact Measurement Scales. *Arthritis Rheum* 1980;23:146-52.
4. Blalock SJ. Introduction. Special issue: health status assessment. *Arthritis Care Res* 1992;5:117-8.
5. Badley EM, Wagstaff S, Wood PHN. Measures of functional ability (disability) in arthritis in relation to impairment of range of joint movement. *Ann Rheum Sis* 1984;43:563-9.
6. Blalock SJ, Van H Sauter S, De Vollis RF. The Modified Health Assessment Questionnaire difficulty scale: a health status measure revisited. *Arthritis Care Res* 1990;3:182-8.
7. Eberhardt KB, Svensson B, Moritz U. Functional assessment of early rheumatoid arthritis. *Br J Rheumatol* 1988;27:364-71.
8. Serbo B, Jajic I. Relationship of the functional status, duration of the disease and pain intensity and some psychological variables in patients with rheumatoid arthritis. *Clin Rheumatol* 1991;10:419-22.
9. Kazis LE, Meenan RF, Anderson JJ. Pain in the rheumatic diseases: investigation of a key health status component. *Arthritis Rheum* 1983;26:1017-22.
10. Pock JR, Smith TW, Ward JR, Milano R. Disability and depression in rheumatoid arthritis: a multi-trait, multi-method investigation. *Arthritis Rheum* 1989;32:1100-6.
11. Wolfe, F, Cathey MA. The assessment and prediction of functional disability in rheumatoid arthritis. *J Rheumatol* 1991;18:1298-306.
12. Anderson KO, Keefe FJ, Bradley LA, McDaniel LK, Young LD, Turner RA, et al. Prediction of pain behavior and functional status of rheumatoid arthritis patients using medical status and psychological variables. *Pain* 1988;3:25-32.

Box 6-7 **PREDICTORS OF FUNCTIONAL DISABILITY IN PATIENTS WITH RHEUMATOID ARTHRITIS — CONT'D**

13. Hawley DJ, Wolfe F. Anxiety and depression in patients with rheumatoid arthritis: a prospective study of 400 patients. *J Rheumatol* 1988;15:932-41.

14. Katz PP, Yelin EH. Prevalence and correlates of depressive symptoms among persons with rheumatoid arthritis. *J Rheumatol* 1993;20:790-6.

15. Schiaffino KM, Revenson TA, Gibofsky A. Assessing the impact of self-efficacy beliefs on adaptation to rheumatoid arthritis. *Arthritis Care Res* 1991;4:150-7.

16. Hakala M, Niemenen P, Manelius J. Joint impairment is strongly correlated with disability measured by self-report questionnaires. Functional status assessment of individuals with rheumatoid arthritis in a population based series. *J Rheumatol* 1994;21:64-9.

17. Callahan LF, Kaplan MR, Pincus T. The Beck Depression Inventory, Center for Epidemiological Studies Depression Scale (CES-D), and General Well-Being Schedule Depression Subscale in rheumatoid arthritis: criterion contamination of responses. *Arthritis Care Res* 1991;4:3-11.

18. Blalock SJ, DeVellis RF, Grown GK, Wallston KA. Validity of the Center for Epidemiological Studies Depression Scale in arthritis populations. *Arthritis Rheum* 1989;32:991-7.

19. Foelker GA, Shewchuk RM. Somatic complaints and the CES-D. *J Am Geriatr Soc* 1992;40:259-62.

20. Lorig K, Chastain RL, Ung E, Shoor S, Holman HR. Development and evaluation of a scale to measure perceived self-efficacy in people with arthritis. *Arthritis Rheum* 1989;32:37-44.

21. Bandura A. Self-efficacy mechanism in human agency. *Am Psychol* 1982;37:122-47.

22. Pincus T, Callahan LF, Vaughn WK. Questionnaire, walking time and button test measures of functional capacity as predictive markers for mortality in rheumatoid arthritis. *J Rheumatol* 1987;14:240-51.

23. Rogers JC, Poole JL, Holm MB, Kwoh CK, Stofko LL. Assistive devices: prescriptions, patient education, patient perceptions [abstract]. *Arthritis Care Res* 1989;2:S11.

24. Holm MB, Rogers JC, Poole J, Kwoh CK, Stofko L. Relationship of pain, function, and self-efficacy [abstract]. *Arthritis Care Res* 1990;3:S20.

25. Rogers JC, Holm MB, Poole JL, Kwoh CK, Stofko L. Impairment and disability in arthritis patients [abstract]. *Arthritis Care Res* 1990;3:S20.

26. Arnett FC, Edworthy SM, Block DA, McShane DJ, Fries JF, Cooper NS, et al. The American Rheumatism Association 1987 revised criteria for the classification of rheumatoid arthritis. *Arthritis Rheum* 1988;31:315-24.

27. Eberl DR, Fasching V, Rahlfs V, Schleyer I, Wolf R. Repeatability and objectivity of various measurements in rheumatoid arthritis: a comparative study. *Arthritis Rheum* 1976;19:1278-86.

28. Bombardier C, Ware J, Russell IJ, larson M, Chalmers A, Read JL. Auranofin therapy and quality of life in patients with rheumatoid arthritis: results of a multicenter trial. *Am J Med* 1986;81:565-78.

29. Bombardier C, Raboud J. A comparison of health-related quality-of-life measures for rheumatoid arthritis research: the Auranofin Cooperating Group. *Control Clin Trials* 1991;12:243S-56S.

30. Kalla AA, Kotze TJ, Meyers OL, Parkyn ND. Clinical Assessment of disease activity in rheumatoid arthritis: evaluation of a functional test. *Ann Rheum Dis* 1988; 47:733-9.

31. Ahlmen M, Bjelle A, Sullivan M. Prediction of team care effects in outpatients with rheumatoid arthritis. *J Rheumatol* 1991;18:1655-61.

32. Radloff LS. The CES-D scale: a self-report depression scale for research in the general population. *Appl Psychol Meas* 1977;1:385-401.

33. Beck AT, Ward CH, Mendelson M, Mock J, Erbaugh J. An inventory for measuring depression. *Arch Gen Psychiatry* 1961;4:561-71.

34. Zung WWK. A self-rating depression scale. *Arch Gen Psychiatry* 1965;12:63-70.

35. Brown JH, Kazis LE, Spitz PW, Gertman P, Fries JF, Meenan RF. The dimensions of health outcomes: a cross-validated examination of health status measurement. *Am J Public Health* 1984;74:159-61.

36. Fries JF, Spitz PW, Young DY. The dimensions of health outcomes: the Health Assessment Questionnaire, disability and pain scales. *J Rheumatol* 1982;9:789-93.

37. Ward MM. Clinical Measures in rheumatoid arthritis: which are most useful in assessing patients? *J Rheumatol* 1993;21:17-27.

38. Shott S. Statistics for health professionals. Philadelphia: Saunders; 1990.

39. Wolfe F. 50 years of antirheumatic therapy: the prognosis of rheumatoid arthritis. *J Rheumatol* 1990;17 Suppl 22:24-32.

40. Ormel J, Von Korff M, Ustun B, Pini S, Korten A, Oldehinkel T. Common mental disorders and disability across cultures. *JAMA* 1994;272:1741-8.

41. Callahan LF, Brooks RH, Summey JA, Pincus T. Quantitative path assessment for routine care of rheumatoid arthritis patients, using a pain scale based on activities of daily living and a visual analog pain scale. *Arthritis Rheum* 1987;30:630-6.

42. Leigh JP, Fries JF. Predictors of disability in a longitudinal sample of patients with rheumatoid arthritis. *Ann Rheum Dis* 1992;51:581-7.

From Holm, M.B., Rogers, J.C., & Kwoh, C.K. (1998). Predictors of functional disability in patients with rheumatoid arthritis. *Arthritis Care and Research, 11* (5), 346-355.

By way of review, this study falls into the *quantitative research category* in that it involves an *association-oriented research strategy*. Within that strategy it represents the *predictive research method* and uses a *multiple-predictor design*. The defining *research procedures* include the following: the identification and measurement of three or more original dependent variables of interest, the calculation and display of a correlation matrix that shows the correlation coefficient for each pair of DVs, the subsequent specification of one of those original DVs as a CV, the further specification of two or more of the original DVs as PVs, the calculation of a beta weight for each of the two or more PVs, and the calculation of the multiple coefficient of determination (also known as the squared multiple correlation coefficient), or R^2. Through the use of its four tables, this article provides information on each of these research procedures.

This study focuses on a sample of 85 rheumatoid arthritis patients and tries to identify which of several factors or variables are most effective in predicting functional disability at two points in time: (a) concurrently while experiencing an acute episode–Time 1, and (b) in the future–Time 2. Functional disability, then, is the CV; however, it is considered as such in the context of each of the two points in time as just explained. For the purpose of this abbreviated critique, we will focus only on the Time 1 phase of the study.

The remaining variables are considered in the context of three clusters: (a) the social and demographic variables cluster that incorporates five variables, (b) the disease variables cluster that encompasses seven variables, and (c) the impairment–physical and psychological–variables cluster that spans six variables. A total of 18 original DVs, then, represent the collection of variables from which a subset of variables is named as PVs. (See Tables 1 and 2 in the article.)

From among the five social and demographic variables, two are investigated as PVs; among the seven disease variables, two are designated as PVs; and among the six impairment variables, four are explored as PVs. (See Table 3 in the article.)

Table 2 in the article displays the correlation matrix that allows us to examine the Pearson correlation coefficient for each possible pair of variables. For example, the correlation, r, between duration of rheumatoid arthritis and age is .27. The reference to these being *zero-order correlations* simply means that the correlation coefficient for a pair of variables has not been adjusted on a third variable as is the case

with a **partial correlation coefficient**. The $r = .27$ for duration of rheumatoid arthritis and age, then, does not reflect any type of adjustment in terms of the influence of some third variable being "partialed" out.

Table 3 displays the results of a multiple linear regression equation being "progressively built" in terms of the eight PVs previously cited and the one CV of functional disability at Time 1 (concurrent). The most relevant components of this table for our purposes are the columns designated beta, R^2, and R^2 change. To decipher what is going on here, let us focus initially on the first horizontal row designated as "Block 1: social and demographic variables."

First, this part of Table 3 shows that in the cluster of social and demographic variables, only two of the original five variables were investigated as PVs, namely, gender and age. The so-called beta weight, or regression coefficient, affiliated with the predictor variable of age, has a value of .14. This indicates that for each unit increase in age, the CV of functional disability increases by .14 of a unit, assuming that all other PVs are held constant. The $R^2 = .20$ for the so-called Block 1 equation simply means that at this stage of "progressively building" the regression equation, .20 proportion of the variance on the CV can be explained by the PVs of gender and age considered simultaneously. In other words, 20% of the variations in functional disability manifested in our sample of 85 patients can be explained, or accounted for, by the combined influence of gender and age.

Generalizing from what we have just said, then, you can consider the beta weight value for any given PV as representing the partial unit increase or decrease on the CV for each unit increase in the PV, assuming that the influence of all other PVs is held constant. The R^2 value for the regression equation at any given stage of development indicates the proportion of variability on the CV that can be explained by the combined influence of the several PVs in the equation at that stage.

Referring back to Table 3 in the article, the final horizontal row that refers to the "Model 1 equation" shows that .64 proportion of the variability on the CV of functional disability can be explained, or accounted for, by the combined influence of all eight PVs considered simultaneously. Based on what has just been said, as well as the earlier explanation of the meaning of each beta weight, it should be apparent that Table 3 allows us to examine the actual influence of each of the several PVs as they are "added" to the development of the multiple linear regression equation.

WHERE DO WE GO FROM HERE?

THE ASSOCIATION-ORIENTED RESEARCH STRATEGY: THE SECOND OF THREE VISITS IN OUR JOURNEY THROUGH THE "WONDERLAND" OF THE QUANTITATIVE RESEARCH CATEGORY

Assuming that you have persevered to this point, the marvels of the correlational and predictive research methods that constitute the association-oriented research strategy should be firmly implanted in your mind. The quantitative research category spans a total of three research strategies: difference-oriented, association-oriented, and descriptive-oriented. Having covered the first two of these in Chapters 5 and 6, the stage is now set for us to explore those research methods that define the descriptive-oriented research strategy.

NEXT STOP: THE DESCRIPTIVE-ORIENTED RESEARCH STRATEGY

Chapter 7 deals with the descriptive-oriented research strategy and the four research methods that define it: the single-case quantitative analysis method, the survey method, the naturalistic/structured observational method, and the case report method. Building on the details of what we have covered so far in the book, you will probably consider this next chapter to be comparatively easy. This is certainly not to short-change the potential value and sophistication of descriptive-oriented research, but simply to acknowledge that progress in our journey builds on what you have learned thus far. All learning to a large extent is cumulative and builds on prior knowledge obtained, particularly in areas that are as sequential and developmental as scientific research.

REFERENCES

Cozby, P. C. (2004). *Methods in behavioral research* (8th ed.). Boston: McGraw-Hill.

Goodwin, C. J. (2005). *Research in psychology: Methods and design* (4th ed.). Hoboken, NJ: John Wiley & Sons.

Gravetter, F. J., & Forzano, L. B. (2003). *Research methods for the behavioral sciences.* Belmont, CA: Thomson Wadsworth.

Harris, S. (1992). *Chalk up another one: The best of Sidney Harris.* New Brunswick, NJ: Rutgers University Press.

Healey, J. F. (2005). *Statistics: A tool for social research* (7th ed.). Belmont, CA: Thomson Wadsworth.

Holm, M. B., Rogers, J. C., & Kwoh, C. K. (1998). Predictors of functional disability in patients with rheumatoid arthritis. *Arthritis Care and Research, 11*(5), 346–355.

Jaccard, J., & Becker, M. A. (2002). *Statistics for the behavioral sciences* (4th ed.). Belmont, CA: Thomson Wadsworth.

Leise, C. M. (1993). The correlation between humor and the chronic pain of arthritis. *Journal of Holistic Nursing, 11*(1), 82–95.

Portney, L. G., & Watkins, M. P. (2000). *Foundations of clinical research: Applications to practice* (2nd ed.). Upper Saddle River, NJ: Prentice-Hall Health.

Rosnow, R. L., & Rosenthal, R. (2005). *Beginning behavioral research: A conceptual primer* (5th ed.). Upper Saddle River, NJ: Prentice-Hall.

ADDITIONAL RECOMMENDED RESOURCES

Burns, N., & Grove, S. K. (2003). *Understanding nursing research* (3rd ed.). Philadelphia: W. B. Saunders.

Domholdt, E. (2000). *Physical therapy research: Principles and applications* (2nd ed.). Philadelphia: W. B. Saunders.

Dryden, T., & Achilles, R. (2003). *Massage therapy research curriculum kit.* Evanston, IL: AMTA Foundation.

Hagino, C. (2003). *How to appraise research: A guide for chiropractic students and practitioners.* New York: Churchill Livingstone.

Shifren, K., Park, D. C., Bennett, J. M., & Morrell, R. W. (1999). Do cognitive processes predict mental health in individuals with rheumatoid arthritis? *Journal of Behavioral Medicine, 22*(6), 529–547.

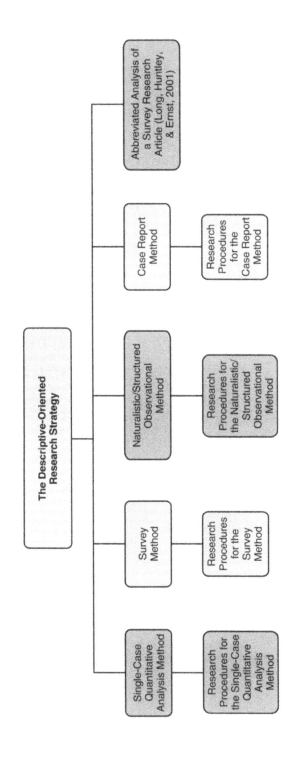

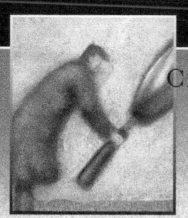

THE DESCRIPTIVE-ORIENTED RESEARCH STRATEGY

OUTLINE

OBJECTIVES

Upon completion of this chapter, the reader will have the information necessary to perform the following tasks:

1 List the four research methods that are included in the descriptive-oriented research strategy.

2 Identify and explain the five major research procedures that define the single-case quantitative analysis research method.

3 Recognize, or be able to provide, an example of a study illustrating the single-case quantitative analysis method.

4 Identify and explain the seven major research procedures that define the survey research method.

5 Recognize, or be able to provide, an example of a study illustrating the survey research method.

6 Identify and explain the eight major research procedures that define the naturalistic/structured observational research method.

7 Recognize, or be able to provide, an example of a study illustrating the naturalistic/structured observational research method.

8 Identify and explain the major characteristics of the case report research method and how it contrasts with the single-case quantitative analysis method.

9 Recognize, or be able to provide, an example of a study illustrating the case report research method.

10 Read and critique published research reports that exemplify the following research methods: the single-case quantitative analysis method, the survey method, the naturalistic/structured observational method, and the case report method.

KEY TERMS

Case report research method
Cluster sampling
Confirmatory single-case quantitative analysis
Descriptive-oriented research strategy
Exploratory single-case quantitative analysis
Naturalistic/structured observational
   research method

Observer bias
Passive observation/measurement
Probability sampling procedure
Quantitative research category
Simple random sampling
Single-case quantitative analysis
   research method

Stratified random sampling
Subject/participant reactivity
Survey research method

WHERE HAVE WE BEEN AND WHERE ARE WE NOW? THE CONNECTION

Our previous chapter provided an introduction to the second of three research strategies constituting the **quantitative research category**, namely, the association-oriented research strategy. We reviewed those research designs affiliated with the following two research methods: (a) the correlational method and (b) the predictive method.

Unlike the difference-oriented strategy (discussed in Chapter 5), the association-oriented research strategy does not involve any type of independent variable (IV) being manipulated as is typically the case in intervention studies. Instead, the focal point in Chapter 6 was on those research studies that examine two or more dependent variables (DVs) in an effort to unveil relationships that might exist. More to the point, the previous chapter investigated associations—typically in the form of co-relationships, or correlations—between or among two or more DVs.

This is the third of three chapters that constitute Part Three and that focus on the quantitative research category. In Chapter 7 we examine the **descriptive-oriented research strategy** and its *affiliated research methods* (Figure 7-1). This research strategy investigates one or more DVs with an eye toward characterizing, portraying, profiling, or describing the one or more DVs of interest. There is no attempt, however, to investigate relationships between or among the DVs when two or more are considered (as we did in the previous chapter). Furthermore, because no independent variables are involved, the issue of examining a relationship between an IV and a DV is nonexistent. Such an interest was the focal point in Chapter 5 when we considered the difference-oriented research strategy.

As we work our way through this chapter, it will be helpful to keep in mind the fact that research problem areas frequently have their origin in initial attempts to characterize, portray, profile, or simply describe one or more factors of interest. Once this is done, it is not uncommon for the research process

- **Quantitative Research Category**
  - • Difference-Oriented Research Strategy (Chapter 5)
    - • • True Experimental, or Randomized Controlled Trial, Method (treatment/intervention focused)
    - • • Quasi-Experimental Method (treatment/intervention focused)
    - • • Single-Case Experimental Method (treatment/intervention-focused)
    - • • Nonexperimental Comparative Groups Method (focus on previous/existing exposure and recent/present/future outcome)
  - • Association-Oriented Research Strategy (Chapter 6)
    - • • Correlational Method
    - • • Predictive Method
  - • **Descriptive-Oriented Research Strategy (Chapter 7)**
    - • • **Single-Case Quantitative Analysis Method**
    - • • **Survey Method**
    - • • **Naturalistic/Structured Observational Method**
    - • • **Case Report Method**

FIGURE 7-1 ■ The quantitative research category: Its affiliated research strategies and their variable control-driven methods (bold emphasis designates coverage in Chapter 7).

to then evolve to a consideration of associations that might exist between or among the DVs that earlier had only been described. This in turn will sometimes lead to difference-oriented studies that build on the earlier association-oriented and descriptive-oriented studies that started the process in the first place.

With this lead-in firmly in place, let us now review the following four research methods that define the association-oriented research strategy: (a) the *single-case quantitative analysis research method*, (b) the *survey method*, (c) the *naturalistic/structured observational method*, and (d) the *case report method*.

THE DESCRIPTIVE-ORIENTED RESEARCH STRATEGY: OVERVIEWING ITS AFFILIATED RESEARCH METHODS AND PROCEDURES

Four research methods define the descriptive-oriented research strategy addressed in this chapter. As mentioned earlier, the intent in this strategy is to characterize, portray, profile, or describe one or more DVs of interest without any particular view toward uncovering relationships when two or more variables are investigated.

Our discussion of these four research methods will *not* include, however, any identification of specific research designs under any given method. This is in keeping with the usual consideration of those methods falling under the descriptive-oriented research strategy. Individual research procedures, however, do define each of the four methods covered in this chapter and will be specified in each case.

The first of four methods we consider in this chapter is the **single-case quantitative analysis research method**. This method is similar to, yet distinct from, the single-case experimental method covered in Chapter 5. Likewise, this method is similar to, but somewhat different from, both (a) the *case report method*, which is the fourth of four covered in this chapter, and (b) the *case study method* addressed in the next chapter, which introduces the *qualitative research category*.

The second and third methods reviewed in this chapter are the *survey method* and the **naturalistic/ structured observational method**. Of particular interest regarding these two methods are recent efforts to document the extent to which complementary and alternative medicine (CAM) modalities– inclusive of therapeutic massage and bodywork–are

being appealed to in general (e.g., Eisenberg et al., 1998) and for what conditions (e.g., Long, Huntley, & Ernst, 2001).

Resources that may prove valuable in reinforcing the content of this chapter include the following: Ballinger, Yardley, and Payne (2004); Cozby (2004); Goodwin (2005); Polgar and Thomas (2000); Polit and Beck (2004); and Portney and Watkins (2000).

SINGLE-CASE QUANTITATIVE ANALYSIS METHOD

Figure 7-2 spotlights the *single-case quantitative analysis method* in the context of the descriptive-oriented research strategy.

An extremely valuable source for this method is an article by Hilliard (1993) in which single-case research methodology in general is discussed. In so doing, the article provides an overview of three specific research methods: the single-case experimental method (as covered in Chapter 5), the single-case quantitative analysis method (our present focus), and the case study method (to be covered in Chapter 8).

It will be easier to understand our present concern with the single-case quantitative analysis method if we reflect initially on our discussion in Chapter 5 of the single-case experimental method. You will recall that the single-case experimental method (a) focuses on one specific participant rather than a group of participants and (b) involves a manipulated IV in the form of a treatment or intervention. Differences on an outcome measure are examined across a baseline phase and at least one and perhaps more treatment phases, thereby qualifying it as a difference-oriented type of study. This single-case experimental method is typically used for hypothesis-testing purposes in the context of quantitative data having been collected.

In the instance of the single-case quantitative analysis method, the focus again is on a single participant rather than a group of participants. There is no direct manipulation of an IV; instead, the researcher engages in passive observation of

- Quantitative Research Category
  - • Descriptive-Oriented Research Strategy (Chapter 7)
    - • • **Single-Case Quantitative Analysis Method**
    - • • Survey Method
    - • • Naturalistic/Structured Observational Method
    - • • Case Report Method

FIGURE 7-2 ■ Spotlight on the single-case quantitative analysis research method in the context of the descriptive-oriented research strategy (bold emphasis designates coverage in this section).

what is occurring on one or more DVs as reflected in the quantitative data collected. Also, this method may be used for hypothesis-testing purposes, or it may generate hypotheses for future investigation. In the case of *hypothesis-testing purposes*, we might say that we are engaging in a **confirmatory single-case quantitative analysis**. In the case of *hypothesis generation*, we might view this type of study as an **exploratory single-case quantitative analysis**. Box 7-1 provides a bare bones summary of those research procedures essential to the single-case quantitative analysis method.

An illustration of the single-case quantitative analysis method could be a study of a single client's progress regarding levels of chronic fatigue and anxiety during semiweekly massage therapy treatments over a given period of several weeks. In this example, the interest is in documenting and describing the effect of the massage treatments on the two outcome measures mentioned for this particular client over a designated period of time (say, for example, 10 weeks). At the conclusion of the second semiweekly session each week, measures are taken on the two dependent variables, namely, the client's (a) level of chronic fatigue using a self-report 10-point scale and (b) level of anxiety using the Beck Anxiety Inventory. The weekly results are plotted for each outcome measure across the duration of the 10 weeks of treatment.

Notice in this illustration that baseline measures on chronic fatigue and anxiety are not recorded over a period of time prior to the massage intervention being introduced. The researcher is not interested in contrasting the measures of the two DVs before treatment and then again after treatment has started as would be the case in the simplest version of the single-case experimental method (i.e., the A-B design discussed in Chapter 5). Instead, what we have here is an effort to profile or characterize in quantitative terms the progress of the client on the two outcome measures over the duration of time that treatment is being received. Box 7-2 displays a hypothetical set of data that possibly could result if indeed the semiweekly massage treatments are generating the desired progressive results over the duration of 10 weeks.

SURVEY METHOD

The second of four research methods included in the descriptive-oriented strategy is the *survey method* as spotlighted in Figure 7-3.

This approach to quantitative research relies on a direct appeal to a population of people from whom the researcher wants input on one or more DVs. Goodwin (2005) characterizes survey research as entailing "a structured set of questions or statements given to a group of people to measure their attitudes, beliefs, values, or tendencies to act" (p. 402). Several CAM survey studies inclusive of manual therapy have been conducted on both the national and regional levels and synthesized in terms of their major findings (Wooton & Sparber, 2001). One study of particular note by Long, Huntley, and Ernst (2001) surveyed 223 professional organizations regarding which CAM therapies benefit which conditions.

The need, therefore, for massage therapists to be familiar with survey research procedures is indeed paramount. Included among these research procedures is a focus on a clearly defined population of individuals from whom information is needed regarding certain attitudes, beliefs, values, interests, behavioral tendencies, and demographic characteristics. This clearly defined population of potential research subjects must be appropriately sampled so that the data collected are generalizable back to the original accessible population. Decisions must also be made regarding the technique used for actually collecting the survey data. Possible options here include face-to-face interviews, phone surveys, electronic surveys via the Internet, and written surveys. In each case the value of the technique is largely dependent on the validity and reliability of the survey instrument used. Assuming that the data generated reflect an appropriately constructed instrument, attention must then be given to analyzing and presenting the data in a justifiable manner.

BARE BONES BOX 7-1

Essential Features of the Single-Case Quantitative Analysis Research Method

- Focus on a single participant rather than a group of participants
- No manipulation of an independent variable
- Instead, **passive observation/measurement** of one or more dependent variables as reflected in the quantitative data collected
- Considered a *confirmatory* single-case quantitative analysis if done for hypothesis-testing purposes
- Considered an *exploratory* single-case quantitative analysis if done for hypothesis-generating purposes

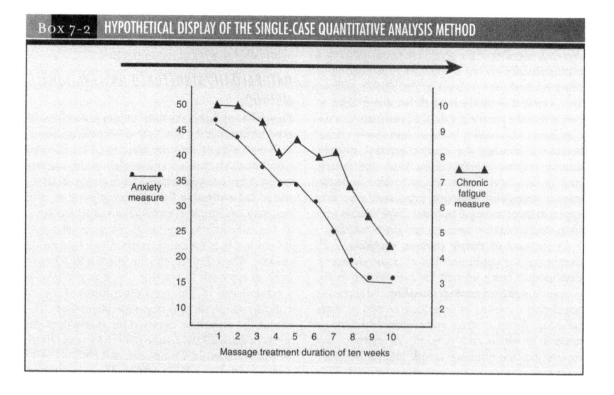

BOX 7-2 HYPOTHETICAL DISPLAY OF THE SINGLE-CASE QUANTITATIVE ANALYSIS METHOD

- Quantitative Research Category
  - Descriptive-Oriented Research Strategy (Chapter 7)
    - Single-Case Quantitative Analysis Method
    - **Survey Method**
    - Naturalistic/Structured Observational Method
    - Case Report Method

FIGURE 7-3 ■ Spotlight on the survey research method in the context of the descriptive-oriented research strategy (bold emphasis designates coverage in this section).

All of the preceding procedures must, of course, reflect the original research question that has prompted the survey study in the first place. The research question, in turn, gives rise to one of the study's two possible purposes: (a) an exploratory purpose with the intent of generating a database for decision making or hypotheses for future study and (b) a confirmatory function for hypothesis-testing purposes. Bare Bones Box 7-3 summarizes these several research procedures and their related issues essential to the survey research method.

Further clarifications regarding some of the above-mentioned essential features of the survey method are perhaps in order. For example, the derivation of a sample that is unbiased and representative of the

BARE BONES BOX 7-3

Essential Features of the Survey Research Method

- Investigator formulates a research question concerning one or more dependent variables that pertain to the attitudes, beliefs, values, interests, behavioral tendencies, and/or demographic characteristics of an identifiable population of interest.
- Method is typically used for *exploratory* purposes with the intent of generating (a) a database for decision making or (b) hypotheses for future study; however, it may be used in a confirmatory manner for hypothesis-testing purposes.
- Characteristics of the population of research subjects are clearly defined.
- A representative and unbiased sample of subjects is derived from the accessible population by one of several probability sampling procedures: simple random sampling, stratified random sampling, or cluster sampling.
- A survey technique for collecting the data is chosen from among several possibilities: face-to-face interviews, phone surveys, electronic surveys, and written surveys.
- Reflecting the survey technique chosen, an appropriate survey instrument is chosen or developed with a view toward acceptable validity and reliability.
- The survey data collected are analyzed and presented in a justifiable manner.

population of interest really calls for what is known as a **probability sampling procedure**. This means that each member of the accessible population has a mathematically known probability or likelihood of being selected for inclusion in the study's sample. This is critical in survey research because it helps to ensure that the sample is indeed representative of the population from which it came. And this is crucial because it elevates the study's external validity, thereby making generalizations from the sample back to the population more defensible. To implement a probability sampling procedure, one may appeal to three principal options: *simple random sampling*, *stratified random sampling*, and *cluster sampling*.

In the case of **simple random sampling**, each member of the population has an equal chance or likelihood of being selected for membership in the sample. In **stratified random sampling**, the accessible population is viewed as consisting of two or more subgroups, layers, or strata, and random selections are made from within each subgroup or stratum. This ensures that the resulting sample reflects the same subgroups or strata as exist in the population itself. In the case of a really huge population for which it might be impossible to obtain a complete listing of members, **cluster sampling** is typically used. In this approach, the population is viewed as being composed of clusters of subjects all having some characteristic in common, and the researcher randomly selects a given number of clusters from among the several possibilities. The members in the selected clusters then collectively constitute the study's sample.

Regarding the technique used for actually collecting the survey data, options available to the researcher include face-to-face interviews as well as surveying by phone, electronic means (e.g., the Internet), and written/printed forms. For each of these techniques, there is a reliance on an appropriate *survey instrument* on which the subjects' responses to the questions posed are recorded. Critical to this process is the establishment of the instrument's *validity* and *reliability*. The former attests to the fact that the instrument is indeed measuring what it claims to be measuring; the latter speaks to the issue of the instrument consistently measuring what it is measuring.

Assuming that the survey data are generated by an instrument that is both valid and reliable, it is then essential for the researcher to use appropriately chosen statistical techniques to analyze the data and present the results in a comprehensible manner.

As a final point to this section on the survey method, you may recall the study by Long et al. (2001) referenced earlier that surveyed 223 professional organizations on the issue of which CAM interventions

benefit which client conditions. This published study is used in the latter part of this chapter to illustrate an abbreviated analysis of survey research.

NATURALISTIC/STRUCTURED OBSERVATIONAL METHOD

Figure 7-4 spotlights the third of four research methods constituting the descriptive-oriented strategy.

Before delving into the features of the observational research method as intended in this chapter, we first need to make certain clarifications about the use of the expression "observational research" that one may encounter in various books and articles.

On occasion the expression *observational research* is used in a broad sense in contrast with *experimental research*. When this is done, the intent is to acknowledge an approach to research that does not involve a manipulated IV and many other forms of control typically affiliated with true experimentation. This use of the expression appears, for example, in the works of Katz (2001); Kazdin (2003); Menard (2003); Newman, Browner, Cummings, and Hulley (2001); and Stommel and Wills (2004). There is a certain amount of validity to this broad-based contrast in that studies that do not entail the manipulation of some type of treatment must rely in some way on observing what is happening in a research setting. To do so, however, paints with a rather broad brush the many types of research that are not experimental in nature. Consequently, this is not the way in which we are using the expression *observational research* in this chapter. Our use of the expression, as you will see shortly, is in a more specific sense than what has just been described.

Another clarification needed at the outset of this section pertains to a more limited use of the expression *observational research* that comes somewhat closer to our intended use. The more limited use referred to here involves the distinction between naturalistic observation and participant observation. *Naturalistic/structured* observational research is associated with the quantitative research category whereas *participant* observational research is more affiliated with

- • Quantitative Research Category
  - • • Descriptive-Oriented Research Strategy (Chapter 7)
    - • • • Single-Case Quantitative Analysis Method
    - • • • Survey Method
    - • • • **Naturalistic/Structured Observational Method**
    - • • • Case Report Method

FIGURE 7-4 ■ Spotlight on the naturalistic/structured observational research method in the context of the descriptive-oriented research strategy (bold emphasis designates coverage in this section).

the qualitative research category (see, for example, Ballinger, Yardley, & Payne, 2004; Brockopp & Hastings-Tolsma, 2003; Goodwin, 2005; Polgar & Thomas, 2000; Polit & Beck, 2004; Smith & Davis, 2003). Of the two, this section focuses on the naturalistic/structured type of observational research as belonging to the quantitative research category. Our treatment of participant observational research, however, is delayed until the next chapter where we address it under the qualitative research category.

The *observational research method*, understood for our purposes here as *naturalistic/structured observation*, tries to study the behavior of individuals (sometimes only one) as they act in their typical everyday environment or setting. The underlying purpose may be either exploratory or confirmatory regarding the study's hypothesis. The research procedures used here emphasize a highly objective description of what is observed by having the researcher function as a completely detached and neutral observer. This may be accomplished by ensuring that the study's subjects are not aware they are being observed or by the subjects being so accustomed (habituated) to the observer that they behave normally. Additional research procedures in this method include the investigator specifying in advance the one or more behaviors (DVs) to be observed, using predetermined forms/instruments for record keeping that yield numeric data, and sometimes employing more than one observer to ensure greater consistency of what is recorded.

Inherent in the naturalistic/structured observational method are potential difficulties relating to observer bias, subject/participant reactivity, and ethical concerns. As the expression denotes, **observer bias** involves the possibility that an observer's preconceived notions about the behavior being studied might influence the accuracy of what is observed and recorded. This bias can be minimized if the researcher provides precise operational definitions of the target behavior(s) and trains the observers beforehand to recognize the target behavior(s).

The potential problem of **subject/participant reactivity** involves the risk that those being observed might react atypically if they know they are being observed. To reduce this possibility, the researcher may use so-called unobtrusive measures of the target behavior (i.e., measures taken at a time and in such a way that the subject is unaware of being observed). Inconspicuous observers to whom the study's subjects are accustomed or habituated offer one possible route to unobtrusive measures. Hidden video or audio recorders as well as hidden observers are also typical means sometimes appealed to for

this purpose, although in these instances serious ethical issues must be considered. Though not always feasible or advisable, the use of these hidden means of observing subject behavior can at times be of potential benefit. At other times, variations in the use of these means can be appealed to such as circumstances wherein video or audio recorders are employed with the knowledge of the subjects, yet they are not openly visible to the subjects as a reminder of the recordings taking place.

Ethical concerns represent a third potential difficulty inherent in the observational method. For example, issues of privacy rights, informed consent on the part of the subjects, and the debriefing of subjects subsequent to the study naturally come to mind and must be accommodated. Appendix B addresses the ethical principles governing research in the behavioral and health sciences. The ethical principles relating to the concerns just acknowledged are discussed there.

Bare Bones Box 7-4 summarizes the several research procedures and issues just covered in

BARE BONES BOX 7-4

Essential Features of the Naturalistic/ Structured Observational Research Method

- Research question investigates one or more dependent variables in the form of the behavior of individuals as they act in their typical everyday environment or setting.
- Method is typically used for exploratory purposes with the intent of generating (a) a database for decision making or (b) hypotheses for future study; however, it may be used in a confirmatory manner for hypothesis-testing purposes.
- Focal point may be on an individual subject or on a group of subjects whose behavior in a typical setting or circumstance is of interest.
- Researcher ensures the detached and neutral observation of the subject(s) so as to safeguard a highly objective description of the target behavior.
- Researcher specifies in advance the one or more dependent variables to be observed in precise operational form.
- Predetermined forms/instruments are employed for record keeping that generates numeric data lending themselves to statistical analysis.
- One or more trained observers are used for the data recording of the target behavior so as to enhance the consistency of the measures taken.
- Potential difficulties regarding observer bias, subject reactivity, and ethical dilemmas are accommodated by way of established principles and procedures.

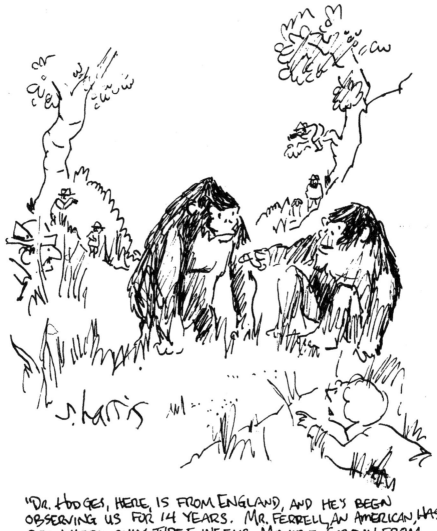

"DR. HODGES, HERE, IS FROM ENGLAND, AND HE'S BEEN OBSERVING US FOR 14 YEARS. MR. FERRELL, AN AMERICAN, HAS BEEN HERE ONLY THREE WEEKS. MONIQUE CORVEAU, FROM PARIS, HAS PRACTICALLY BEEN LIVING WITH US FOR ABOUT NINE YEARS..."

HUMOR BREAK ■ Precisely who is observing whom in this situation? (From Harris, S. [2004]. *Einstein simplified: Cartoons on science by Sidney Harris* [Rev. ed.]. New Brunswick, NJ: Rutgers University Press.)

conjunction with the naturalistic/structured observational research method.

CASE REPORT METHOD

The **case report research method** is closely related to both (a) the *single-case quantitative analysis method* discussed at the outset of this chapter and (b) the *case study method* covered in the next chapter under the qualitative research category. Let us first examine how the case report varies only slightly from the single-case quantitative analysis, and then we will project a more delayed discussion in the next chapter as to how the case report and case study methods are both similar and different.

We have already seen that in the instance of the single-case quantitative analysis method, certain features stand out among several. Specifically, the *focal point* is *not* on the manipulation of an IV in the form of a treatment to be contrasted with its earlier absence. The targeted treatment of interest is indeed acknowledged, but with more of an emphasis on the observation/measurement of one or more DVs as reflected in the quantitative data collected. Consequently, we have the expression single-case quantitative analysis method and the details of its essential features as displayed earlier in Bare Bones Box 7-1

In the instance of the case report method, however, the focal point instead is principally on a detailed description of the clinical practice itself that defines the treatment plan in the context of (a) the client's profile and (b) the supporting justification for the intervention selected. Against this backdrop, the report describes the sequence of clinical visits as well as the ongoing and final results of the treatment's effectiveness. The Massage Therapy Foundation (2004) provides a set of guidelines for structuring a case report that is accessible at http://massagetherapyfoundation.org/grants_education.html. Furthermore, resources by Domholdt (2000) and McEwen (2001) also provide valuable in-depth discussions of the case report method and its contrast with other single-case research methods.

In the context of this chapter, then, both the single-case quantitative analysis method and the case report method represent possibilities under the descriptive-oriented research strategy. Each is serving primarily a descriptive function, although with slightly different emphases. The case report can also be considered, however, in relation to the case study method covered in the next chapter under the qualitative research category. In Chapter 8, then, we will revisit the case report method for a further discussion regarding (a) the distinction between retrospective and prospective case reports and (b) the contrast between a case report and a case study.

The decision as to where to best position the discussion of the case report method is somewhat difficult. Differing views exist as to precisely where and how this method relates to other single-case research approaches. As already seen, it has certain characteristics and uses similar to the two other methods cited earlier and, hence, is appropriately positioned in this chapter as well as the next.

DETAILED SUMMARY

Figure 7-5 provides a detailed summary of the descriptive-oriented research strategy as well as its affiliated research methods that have been covered in this chapter.

- Quantitative Research Category
  - • Descriptive-Oriented Research Strategy (Chapter 7)
    - • • Single-Case Quantitative Analysis Method
    - • • Survey Method
    - • • Naturalistic/Structured Observational Method
    - • • Case Report Method

FIGURE 7-5 ■ Detailed summary of the descriptive-oriented research strategy and its affiliated research methods covered in Chapter 7.

ILLUSTRATION OF THE SURVEY RESEARCH METHOD: AN ABBREVIATED ("QUICKIE") ANALYSIS OF A COMPLETE RESEARCH ARTICLE

Box 7-5 contains the complete research article by Long, Huntley, and Ernst (2001) that illustrates the **survey research method**. These researchers investigated the issue of which CAM therapies benefit which conditions as reflected in the opinions of 223 professional organizations.

Based on your careful reading of the Long et al. (2001) study, we can now critique this research article in an abbreviated way. We will do so based on (a) our earlier discussions in this book of what constitutes the preliminary, introductory, method, results, discussion, and concluding sections of a research report and (b) the essential features of the survey research method as detailed in Bare Bones Box 7-3.

PRELIMINARY SECTION

The title of this article obviously shows that it is a report of a survey, thus indicating a descriptive-oriented study that falls within the quantitative research category. The major variables focus on CAM therapies and those client conditions that seem to benefit from the therapies. The study's participants are 223 professional organizations surveyed on the variables of interest.

The article's rather extensive abstract does a commendable job of synthesizing the major points of the study that cut across the main sections of the report, namely, the introduction, method, results, and discussion. Information appropriate to an abstract is provided in terms of the following: an implied research question, an implied exploratory interest in generating a database for decision-making purposes, number and types of participants, research method used, major variables, instrumentation in the form of a questionnaire, major findings in terms of broad descriptive analyses used, and conclusions.

Text continued on p. 139

BOX 7-5 WHICH COMPLEMENTARY AND ALTERNATIVE THERAPIES BENEFIT WHICH CONDITIONS? A SURVEY OF THE OPINIONS OF 223 PROFESSIONAL ORGANIZATIONS

L. Long, A. Huntley, E. Ernst
Department of Complementary Medicine, School of Postgraduate Medicine and Health Sciences, University of Exeter, UK

Summary.   With the increasing demand and usage of complementary/alternative medicine (CAM) by the general public, it is vital that healthcare professionals can make informed decisions when advising or referring their patients who wish to use CAM. Therefore they might benefit from advice by CAM-providers as to which treatment can be recommended for which condition. Aim: The primary aim of this survey was to determine which complementary therapies are believed by their respective representing professional organizations to be suited for which medical conditions. Method: 223 questionnaires were sent out to CAM organizations representing a single CAM therapy. The respondents were asked to list the 15 conditions they felt benefited most from their CAM therapy, the 15 most important contra-indications, the typical costs of initial and any subsequent treatments and the average length of training required to become a fully qualified practitioner. The conditions and contra-indications quoted by responding CAM organizations were recorded and the top five of each were determined. Treatment costs and hours of training were expressed as ranges. Results: Of the 223 questionnaires sent out, 66 were completed and returned. Taking undelivered questionnaires into account, the response rate was 34%. Two or more responses were received from CAM organizations representing twelve therapies: aromatherapy, Bach flower remedies, Bowen technique, chiropractic, homoeopathy, hypnotherapy, magnet therapy, massage, nutrition, reflexology, Reiki and yoga. The top seven common conditions deemed to benefit by all twelve therapies, in order of frequency, were: stress/anxiety, headaches/migraine, back pain, respiratory problems (including asthma), insomnia, cardiovascular problems and musculoskeletal problems. Aromatherapy, Bach flower remedies, hypnotherapy, massage, nutrition, reflexology, Reiki and yoga were all recommended as suitable treatments for stress/anxiety. Aromatherapy, Bowen technique, chiropractic, hypnotherapy, massage, nutrition, reflexology, Reiki and yoga were all recommended for headache/migraine. Bowen technique, chiropractic, magnet therapy, massage, reflexology and yoga were recommended for back pain. None of the therapies cost more than £60 for an initial consultation and treatment. No obvious correlation between length of training and treatment cost was apparent. Conclusion: The recommendations by CAM organizations responding to this survey may provide guidance to health care professionals wishing to advise or refer patients interested in using CAM. © 2001 Harcourt Publishers Ltd.

Introduction

Complementary/alternative medicine (CAM) is commonly used in many countries including the UK,[1] Germany,[2,3] USA[4,5] and Australia.[6] The incidence of CAM use by defined patient populations, e.g. those suffering from rheumatic diseases,[7] acquired immunodeficiency syndrome (AIDS)[8] dermatological conditions[9] or cancer,[10] has been relatively well established. Consumer's demand has led to considerable support for CAM to be provided by national healthcare systems (e.g.[11]). In the UK, 64% of people seeking CAM consult their general practitioner or hospital specialist first,[12] and 24% concurrently receive orthodox care.[13] It is vital that primary care physicians and other health care professionals can make informed choices when referring patients on to CAM providers. Yet they often feel uncertain as to which patients might benefit from which treatments. Various solutions have been sought for this problem. In an integrated healthcare practice in Glastonbury, UK, for instance, each CAM practitioner supplied a list of conditions for which they considered their therapy to be particularly appropriate.[14] This was deemed necessary, at least initially, as neither the CAM practitioners nor the doctors were familiar with one another's work.

There is a lack of reliable data for informing physicians on which CAM therapies are best suited for which conditions. This investigation is an attempt to start filling this gap. Its primary aim is to determine which forms of CAM are believed to be suited for which conditions by their respective professional organizations.

Methods

Five hundred and twenty six addresses of CAM organizations had been generated by the Department of Complementary Medicine at Exeter University. It included 364 addresses of all UK CAM organizations generated by a systematic survey sponsored by the UK Department of Health[15]. Furthermore it included 162 addresses from outside the UK which were compiled over 7 years at our Department. To the best of our knowledge it represents the most comprehensive address list of CAM organizations collected to date. There was no restriction regarding the professional status of practitioners represented by the CAM organizations. Of the 526 addresses, 303 were excluded because they did not correspond to organizations representing single therapies. Thus 223 questionnaires were sent out.

The confidential questionnaire was purpose-designed and asked what CAM therapy the organization represented. Our aim was to target organizations that represented a single CAM therapy but those that covered more than one therapy were asked to photocopy the form for each. The respondents were asked to list the top 15 conditions they felt benefited from their CAM therapy, the top 15 contra-indications, the typical costs of initial and any subsequent treatments and the average length of training (in hours) a fully qualified practitioner would require. Participants were asked to fill in as much of the form as they felt appropriate. A sample of the questionnaire is obtainable from the authors.

The questionnaires were sent out on 1st February 2000 and a reminder followed to nonrespondents 1 month later. Responses were collected until the closing date of 30 April 2000. All information was entered into Excel spread sheets and presented by descriptive statistics.

Only data from therapies for which we received two or more questionnaire responses were used in the present analysis. We determined those indications which CAM organizations thought benefited most from CAM therapies. Therapies were grouped into physical therapies, mind/body therapies or complementary medicines. By counting how frequently conditions of contra-indications were quoted, the top five of each were determined for each therapy. Treatment costs and hours of training were expressed as ranges.

Results

Of the 223 questionnaires sent out, 66 were received from separate addresses. Several organizations sent back more than one completed questionnaire (obviously completed by different individuals within that organization): this is not included in the response rate although all the data were pooled and used for analysis of conditions treated/contraindications etc. Twenty-six questionnaires were returned unopened, for responded by stating they did not wish to participate and four wrote to say that the questionnaire was not suitable/applicable for their organization. Thus the response rate was 34%. The range of CAM organizations contacted is listed in Table 1.

TABLE I LIST OF THERAPIES REPRESENTED BY COMPLEMENTARY AND ALTERNATIVE MEDICINE ORGANIZATIONS, RESPONDING TO SURVEY

THERAPY	QUESTIONNAIRES SENT OUT	RESPONSE
Acupuncture/TCM	20	1
Alexander technique	3	1
Aromatherapy	20	10
Art Therapy	2	1
Ayurvedic medicine	2	1
Bach flower remedies	5	2
Biodanza	1	1
Bowen technique	3	2
Chiropractic	10	2
Counselling & Psychotherapy	2	1
Herbal medicine	7	1
Homoeopathy	23	4
Hypnotherapy	11	5
Kinesiology	4	1
Magnet therapy	2	2
Massage	18	7
Music therapy	1	1
Neural therapy	4	1
Neuro-Linguistic Programming (NLP)	1	1
Nutrition	4	3
Osteopathy	3	1
Polarity	1	1
Radionics	2	1
Rebirthing	1	1
Reflexology	8	8
Reiki	3	2
Spiritual healing	1	1
Tai Chi	1	1
Yoga	5	2

Other therapies represented by professional organizations which were contacted but did not respond: Shamanic healing & counselling, Cranio sacral therapy, Ophthalmic Somatology, Dream analysis, Bioharmonics, Crystal therapy, Chelation therapy, Progressive relaxation, Colour therapy, Spa therapy, Temperature therapy, Oxygen therapy, Organ extract therapy.

Continued

Box 7-5 WHICH COMPLEMENTARY AND ALTERNATIVE THERAPIES BENEFIT WHICH CONDITIONS? A SURVEY OF THE OPINIONS OF 223 PROFESSIONAL ORGANIZATIONS—CONT'D

There were two or more responses from twelve therapies: aromatherapy ($n=11$), Bach flower ($n=2$), Bowen technique ($n=2$), chiropractic ($n=2$), homoeopathy ($n=4$), hypnotherapy ($n=5$), magnet therapy ($n=2$), massage ($n=8$), nutrition ($n=3$), reflexology ($n=11$), Reiki ($n=2$) and yoga ($n=2$).

When the answers from all the questionnaires were pooled, the most common conditions deemed to benefit from CAM, in descending order of frequency, were: anxiety/stress, headaches/migraine, back pain, respiratory problems including asthma, insomnia, cardiovascular problems and musculoskeletal problems. Table 2 lists the 25 most frequently cited conditions and the therapies advocated for treating them.

The answers to the questions of which individual therapies are deemed to benefit which condition are summarized in Tables 3, 4 & 5. Of the therapies with just two responses, no consensus was found in terms of the conditions treated and contra-indications and the limitations of these data must be noted. None of the therapies cost more than £60 for an initial consultation and treatment (Tables 3–5). There was no clear correlation between the length of training and cost of treatment.

Discussion

The rapid increase in public demand for CAM means that communication and co-operation with orthodox health services is increasingly desirable[16], especially considering that many patients use CAM concurrently with orthodox medicine[17]. Also, it is likely that the public will increasingly seek clarification on the limitations of the various CAM therapies. Indeed, a recent report to the UK Department of Health recommended that a clearer articulation of competence and limitations to treatment by CAM practitioners may be a basis for improved liaison with other health services and may lead to wider acceptance of their contribution.[18] Such an approach may also help to promote public confidence in CAM and provide information to doctors for assessing therapies or advising patients who wish to use CAM. To the best of our knowledge, this is the first survey of CAM organizations asking for their views on treatment benefit, safety and cost. Its results may provide a useful guide to healthcare professionals: they give some indication as to which conditions are most commonly being treated by CAM providers and which treatments might be best for which conditions.

The most obvious limitation of this survey is its low response rate. The explanation for this is probably complex and certainly speculative. Many forms of CAM (e.g. homeopathy, spiritual healing, Reiki) do not subscribe to the biomedical classification of diseases. Thus, these organizations would have had difficulties answering our questions, or felt they were not applicable. Similarly, some organizations representing the more established disciplines (e.g. chiropractic and osteopathy), may have considered their therapy to be mainstream rather than CAM. Other reasons may include a level of distrust and/or non co-operation with this type of survey which could be seen to define CAM usefulness solely in terms of conventional medical criteria. Furthermore, individualized approaches to treatment cannot be accurately reflected with this kind of survey, and CAM organizations may have felt that it could not fully represent what their therapy has to offer. Moreover the topic of our investigation may not have been thought of as important by some CAM organizations. Finally, writing to organizations is less likely to elicit a response than addressing individuals in person. Nevertheless, with 66 organizations replying, this is the largest survey of its kind and therefore a first step towards answering the questions we posed. Further surveys should perhaps not cover the entire scope of CAM, but focus on the most established complementary and alternative disciplines.[19]

It is widely accepted that CAM therapies can provide beneficial non-specific effects that are often associated with clinically relevant outcomes. But can they have specific effects beyond a placebo response? It is interesting to compare the results of our survey with the trial evidence regarding effectiveness for the three most frequently cited conditions found in this survey: stress/anxiety, headaches/migraine and back pain (Table 2). According to our results, aromatherapy, Bach flower remedies, hypnotherapy, massage, nutrition, reflexology, Reiki and yoga are all recommended for stress/anxiety (Table 2). There is supporting clinical evidence, of varying methodological quality, for all these therapies with the exception of Reiki (Table 6). The second most frequently cited condition emerging from our survey was headache/migrane, with aromatherapy, Bowen technique, chiropractic, hypnotherapy, massage, nutrition, reflexology, Reiki and yoga recommended as suitable treatments (Table 2). With the exception of Bowen technique and Reiki, all appear to be supported by clinical evidence (Table 7). Back pain is the condition that brings patients most frequently to try CAM (3) and, according to the present findings, the following treatments are recommended as promising: Bowen technique, chiropractic, magnet therapy, massage, reflexology and yoga (Table 2). Clinical trials have investigated the effectiveness of all these therapies for back pain, with the exception of Bowen technique (Table 8). Hence it appears that, in general, the recommendations by CAM organizations are supported by trial evidence.

In conclusion, this survey yields potentially useful data regarding the applicability of CAM in clinical settings. As a first step in bringing reliable information about CAM to the attention of health care professionals, this survey's findings may provide some guidance to those physicians wishing to advise or refer patients interested in using CAM.

Box 7-5 WHICH COMPLEMENTARY AND ALTERNATIVE THERAPIES BENEFIT WHICH CONDITIONS? A SURVEY OF THE OPINIONS OF 223 PROFESSIONAL ORGANIZATIONS—CONT'D

TABLE 2 TOP 25 MOST FREQUENTLY CITED CONDITIONS WITH THE THERAPIES ADVOCATED

COMMON CONDITIONS (IN ORDER OF MOST FREQUENTLY CITED)	AROMATHERAPY	BACH FLOWER	BOWEN	CHIROPRACTIC	HOMOEOPATHY	HYPNOTHERAPY	MAGNET THERAPY	MASSAGE	NUTRITION	REFLEXOLOGY	REIKI	YOGA
Anxiety/stress	×	×				×		×	×	×	×	×
Headaches/migraine	×			×		×	×	×	×	×	×	×
Back pain	×		×	×			×	×		×		×
Respiratory problems incl. asthma			×	×	×			×		×		
Insomnia										×	×	×
Cardiovascular problems incl. high blood pressure and circulatory problems				×			×	×	×	×	×	×
Musculoskeletal problems			×	×			×	×				
Menstrual/PMT	×									×		
Arthritis and Rheumatism	×		×		×	×	×	×	×	×		×
Depression	×	×	×		×	×	×	×	×	×	×	×
Skin problems incl. exzema	×				×	×		×				
Chronic fatigue/ME	×	×	×		×	×						
General mental stress			×			×	×					
Neck/shoulder pain				×				×			×	
Phobias/nervous habits			×			×		×				
IBS			×	×		×				×		
Sports injuries								×		×		
Sinus condition										×		
Hormonal problems						×				×	×	
Lack of confidence		×						×			×	
Constipation										×		
Trauma-emotional & physical		×				×				×		
Multiple sclerosis	×							×		×		×
Cancer	×	×						×		×	×	
HIV/AIDS	×	×						×		×		

Only therapies for which 2 or more responses were received were included in the table.

× = The therapy was recommended by at least one respondent.

Abbreviations: IBS = Irritable Bowel Syndrome. PMT = Premenstrual Tension. HIV = Human Immunodeficiency Virus. AIDS = Acquired Immunodeficiency Syndrome.

Continued

BOX 7-5   WHICH COMPLEMENTARY AND ALTERNATIVE THERAPIES BENEFIT WHICH CONDITIONS?
A SURVEY OF THE OPINIONS OF 223 PROFESSIONAL ORGANIZATIONS — CONT'D

TABLE 3   PHYSICAL THERAPIES

THERAPY [NO. OF QUESTIONNAIRES]	TOP 5 CONDITIONS TREATED	TOP 5 CONTRAINDICATIONS	TREATMENT COST FIRST* (£)	SUBSEQUENT (£)	RANGE OF HOURS OF TRAINING
Aromatherapy [11]	anxiety/stress musculoskeletal Insomia headaches/migraine hormonal problems	pregnancy recent surgery thrombosis fractures/wounds some medications	21–50	21–40	200–500
Reflexology [11]	headaches/migraine back pain musculoskeletal menstrual/PMT stress/mental	unstable pregnancy acute infections/fever deep vein thrombosis surgical/medical emergency veruccas/mycosis	11–30	11–30	100–500
Bowen technique [2]	no obvious trend, however, large number of musculoskeletal conditions quoted	no obvious trend, "no response to treatment" quoted twice	21–30	21–30	100–180
Massage [8]	stress & tension back pain headache & migraine neck/shoulder pain insomnia	contagious & infectious disease broken skin cancer exacerbation of chronic condition skin disease	11–50	11–50	100–1000
Chiropractic [2]	no obvious trend	no obvious trend	31–50	21–50	3000–5000

*Consultation and treatment.

TABLE 4   MIND/BODY THERAPIES

THERAPY [NO. OF QUESTIONNAIRES]	TOP 5 CONDITIONS TREATED	TOP 5 CONTRAINDICATIONS	TREATMENT COST FIRST* (£)	SUBSEQUENT (£)	RANGE OF HOURS OF TRAINING
Yoga [2]	no obvious trend	no obvious trend	5–40	5–20	500–5000
Hypnotherapy [5]	anxiety/stress phobias/nervous habits smoking lack of confidence depression	psychosis schizophrenia epilepsy some depressions influence of drugs/drink	31–50	31–50	300–1600
Reiki [2]	no obvious trend: pain, depression & stress quoted twice	no obvious trend, 1/2 respondees quoted "not applicable"	11–50	11–40	1000
Magnetic therapy [2]	no obvious trend: lower back pain cramps & aches quoted twice	no obvious trend, pace makers & pregnancy quoted twice	<10–40	<10–40	500

*Consultation and treatment.

BOX 7-5 WHICH COMPLEMENTARY AND ALTERNATIVE THERAPIES BENEFIT WHICH CONDITIONS? A SURVEY OF THE OPINIONS OF 223 PROFESSIONAL ORGANIZATIONS—CONT'D

TABLE 5 COMPLEMENTARY MEDICINES

THERAPY [NO. OF QUESTIONNAIRES]	TOP 5 CONDITIONS TREATED	TOP 5 CONTRAINDICATIONS	TREATMENT COST FIRST* (£)	SUBSEQUENT (£)	RANGE OF HOURS OF TRAINING
Bach flower [2]	no obvious trend	no obvious trend	<10–20	<10–20	12–100
Nutrition [3]	arthritis/rheumatism chronic fatigue/ME hypertension Candida ulcers	medical emergencies eating disorders chemotherapy antibiotic dependent steroid dependent	21–>60	11–40	100–3000
Homoeopathy [4]	conditions that can be regulated by the organism's life force/treated constitutionally presenting symptom, e.g. eczema, arthritis, menstrual symptoms, attention deficit disorder treated by treating the person and not the condition	medical emergencies indication for surgery no response oral medications contraindicated pregnancy if remedy is inappropriate for this condition	31–>60	10–50	500–3000

*Consultation and treatment.

TABLE 6 SUMMARY OF CLINICAL EVIDENCE FROM CONTROLLED CLINICAL TRIALS FOR THERAPIES RECOMMENDED FOR STRESS/ANXIETY

THERAPY	SUMMARY OF PUBLISHED CLINICAL EVIDENCE
Aromatherapy	A systematic review of aromatherapy[20] included six RCTs concerning the use of aromatherapy for anxiety and well-being. With one exception, they all suggest positive effects.
Bach flower remedies	Two controlled clinical trials exist testing the effectiveness of Bach flower remedies in the treatment of examination stress in university students.[21,22] Neither trial reported a significant specific effect of 'five flower remedies' on anxiety above placebo, although a non-specific beneficial effect for both treatment and placebo was observed.[22]
Hypnotherapy	Four controlled trials have found hypnotherapy to be beneficial for state anxiety,[23–26] although one crossover study produced a negative result.[27]
Massage	Six controlled trials[28–33] support beneficial effects of massage on anxiety.
Nutrition	A clinical trial showed that dietary supplements reduced anxiety, as measured in a quality of life scale, in dieting individuals when compared to placebo,[34] indicating possible benefits of nutrition for anxiety.
Reflexology	A single controlled trial showed that treatment with reflexology reduced anxiety in patients suffering from this condition.[35]
Yoga	Two clinical studies indicate a beneficial effect of yoga on stress management: a controlled trial showed beneficial effects of Sahaja yoga on stress management in patients with epilepsy,[36] while an uncontrolled study of one year's duration showed improvements in obsessive compulsive disorder in patients who practised yoga regularly.[37]

RCT= Randomized clinical trial

Continued

Box 7-5 WHICH COMPLEMENTARY AND ALTERNATIVE THERAPIES BENEFIT WHICH CONDITIONS?
A SURVEY OF THE OPINIONS OF 223 PROFESSIONAL ORGANIZATIONS—CONT'D

TABLE 7 SUMMARY OF CLINICAL EVIDENCE FROM CONTROLLED CLINICAL TRIALS FOR THERAPIES RECOMMENDED FOR HEADACHE/MIGRAINE

THERAPY	SUMMARY OF PUBLISHED CLINICAL EVIDENCE
Aromatherapy	One RCT on the effectiveness of topically applied peppermint oil for headaches reported significant analgesic effects compared to placebo.[38]
Chiropractic	A recent systematic review suggests that spinal manipulation has a useful effect on tension, cervicogenic and post-traumatic headaches, with five of the six studies reporting benefit.[39] Two studies showed positive effects of spinal manipulation on migraine,[40,41] although another study found no positive benefits above a control treatment.[42]
Hypnotherapy	Self-hypnosis appears to be more effective than waiting list control in the treatment of headache,[43] although it is unclear whether it is superior to other forms of relaxation. Different combinations of therapies including hypnotherapy have been compared to various control interventions in several trials[44,45] with favourable results.
Massage	One RCT showed beneficial effects of massage on migraine headaches,[46] while an uncontrolled study showed improvements in chronic tension headache in patients treated with massage.[47]
Nutrition	Nutrition has been shown to be important in the treatment of migraine, as the incidence of migraine is affected by food allergy in both children[48] and adults.[49]
Reflexology	Two trials support the use of reflexology for headache. A large observational study found that 81% of patients with headache were helped or cured at 3-months follow-up[50] while a single RCT showed a positive non-significant trend in the same condition.[51]
Yoga	Yoga, in addition to standard medication, produced significant reduction in headache activity when compared to standard medication alone in an RCT of subjects with mixed migraine and tension headache.[52]

RCT=Randomized clinical trial

TABLE 8 SUMMARY OF CLINICAL EVIDENCE FROM CONTROLLED CLINICAL TRIALS FOR THERAPIES RECOMMENDED FOR BACK PAIN

THERAPY	SUMMARY OF PUBLISHED CLINICAL EVIDENCE
Chiropractic	The evidence for chiropractic is generally positive although methodological flaws in most of the trials performed to date prevent definitive conclusions.[53]
Magnet therapy	A recent pilot study reported no benefits of the use of magnets in the treatment of chronic low back pain.[54]
Reflexology	There is no strong trial evidence in support of reflexology.[55]
Massage	While a review of clinical trials concluded that there is no strong trial evidence in support of massage therapy,[56] a recent positive RCT[57] supports the view that massage is beneficial for this condition.
Yoga	Data from clinical trials on yoga is promising,[58] but too scarce to allow any firm judgement.

RCT=Randomized clinical trial

Box 7-5   **WHICH COMPLEMENTARY AND ALTERNATIVE THERAPIES BENEFIT WHICH CONDITIONS? A SURVEY OF THE OPINIONS OF 223 PROFESSIONAL ORGANIZATIONS — CONT'D**

References

1. Ernst E, White A. The BBC survey of complementary medicine use in the UK. Complement Ther Med 2000; 8: 32–36.
2. Himmel W, Schulte M, Kochen MM. Complementary medicine: are patients' expectations being met by their general practitioners? *Br J Gen Pract* 1993; 43: 232–235.
3. Häusserman, D. Increased confidence in natural therapies. *Dtsch Arzt* 1997; 94: 1857–1858.
4. Astin JA. Why patients use alternative medicine. Results of a national study. *J Am Med Assoc* 1998; 279: 1548–1553.
5. Eisenberg E et al. Trends in alternative medicine use in the United States, 1990–1997. *J Am Med Assoc* 1998; 280: 1569–15751.
6. MacLennan AH, Wilson DH, Taylor AW. Prevalence and cost of alternative medicine in Australia. *Lancet* 1996; 347: 569–573.
7. Ernst E. Usage of complementary therapies in rheumatology: A systematic review. *Clin Rheumatol* 1998; 17: 301–305.
8. Ernst E. Complementary AIDS therapies: the good, the bad and the ugly. *Int J STD AIDS* 1997; 8: 281–285.
9. Ernst E. The usage of complementary therapies by dermatological patients: a systematic review. *Br J Dermatol* 2000; 142: 857–861.
10. Ernst E, Cassileth BR. The prevalence of complementary/alternative medicine in cancer. *Cancer* 1998; 83: 777–782.
11. Emslie M, Campbell M, Walker K. Complementary therapies in a local healthcare setting. Part I: Is there real public demand? *Complement Ther Med* 1996; 4: 39–42.
12. Thomas K, Fall M, Parry G, Nicholl J. National Survey of Access to Complementary Health Care via General Practice. SCHARR, University of Sheffield, 1995.
13. Moore J, Phipps K, Marcer D. Why do people seek treatment by alternative medicine? *Br Med J* 1985; 290: 28–29.
14. Welford R. Integrated healthcare in Glastonbury. *Holistic Health* 2000; 64: 6–9.
15. Mills S, Peacock W. Professional organization of complementary and alternative medicine in the United Kingdom 1997: a report to the Department of Health, Centre for Complementary Health Studies, University of Exeter.
16. Dickinson DPS. Complementary therapies in medicine: the patient's perspective. *Complement Ther Med* 1995; 3: 9–12.
17. Thomas K, Carr J, Westlake L, Williams BT. Use of non-orthodox and conventional health care in Great Britain. *Br Med J* 1991; 302: 207–210.
18. Mills S, Budd S. Professional organization of complementary and alternative medicine in the United Kingdom 2000. A second report to the Department of Health. The Centre for Complementary Health Studies, University of Exeter.
19. Zollman C, Vickers A. Users and practitioners of complementary medicine. *Br Med J* 1999; 319: 836–838.
20. Cooke B, Ernst E. Aromatherapy: a systematic review. Br J Gen Pract 2000; 50: 493–496.
21. Armstrong NC, Ernst E. A randomized, double-blind, placebo-controlled trial of Bach Flower Remedy. *Perfusion* 1999; 11: 440–446.
22. Walach H, Rilling C, Engelke U. Bach flower remedies are ineffective for test anxiety: results of a blinded, placebo-controlled, randomized trial. *Forsch Komplementärmed* 2000; 7: 55.
23. Moore R, Abrahamsen R, Brodsgaard I. Hypnosis compared with group therapy and individual desensitisation for dental anxiety. *Eur J Oral Sci* 1996; 104: 612–618.
24. Zeltzer L, LeBaron S. Hypnosis and nonhypnotic techniques for reduction of pain and anxiety during painful procedures in children and adolescents with cancer. *J Pediatr* 1982; 10: 1032–1035.
25. Boutin GE, Tosi DJ. Modification of irrational ideas and test anxiety through rational stage directed hypnotherapy. *J Clin Psychol* 1983; 39: 382–391.
26. Hurley JD. Differential effects of hypnosis. Biofeedback training, and trophotropic responses on anxiety, ego strength, and locus of control. *J Clin Psychol* 1980; 36: 503–507.
27. Van Dyck R, Spinhoven P. Does preference for type of treatment matter? A study of exposure in vivo with or without hypnosis is the treatment of panic disorder with agoraphobia. *Behav Modif* 1997; 21: 172–186.
28. Field T, Grizzle N, Scafidi F, Schanberg S. Massage and relaxation therapies' effects on depressed adolescent mothers. Adolescence 1996; 31: 903–911.
29. Field T, Ironson G, Scafidi F, Nawrocki T, Goncalves A, Burman I. Massage therapy reduces anxiety and enhances EEG pattern of alertness and math computations. *Int J Neurosci* 1996; 86: 197–205.
30. Field T, Morrow C, Valdeon C, Larson S, Kuhn C, Schanberg S. Massage reduces anxiety in child and adolescent psychiatric patients. *J Am Acad Child Adolesc Psychiatry* 1992; 31: 125–131.
31. Fraser J, Kerr JR. Psychophysiological effects of back massage on elderly institutionalised patients. *J Adv Nurs* 1993; 18: 238–245.
32. Hernandez-Reif M, Field T, Krasnegor J, Martinez E, Schwartzman M, Mavunda K. Children with cystic fibrosis benefit from massage therapy. *J Pediatr Psychol* 1999; 24: 175–181.

Continued

Box 7-5　WHICH COMPLEMENTARY AND ALTERNATIVE THERAPIES BENEFIT WHICH CONDITIONS? A SURVEY OF THE OPINIONS OF 223 PROFESSIONAL ORGANIZATIONS — CONT'D

33. Hernandez-Reif M, Field T, Krasnegor J, Theakston H, Hossain Z, Burman I. High blood pressure and associated symptoms were reduced by massage therapy. *Journal of Bodywork and Movement Therapies* 2000; 4:31–38.
34. Ussher JM, Swann C. A double blind placebo-controlled trial examining the relationship between Health-Related Quality of Life and dietary supplements. *Br J Health Psychol* 2000; 5: 173–187.
35. Thomas M. Fancy footwork. *Nursing Times* 1989; 85: 42–44.
36. Panjwani U, Gupta HL, Singh SH, Selvamurthy W, Rai UC. Effect of Sahaja yoga practice on stress management in patients of epilepsy. *Indian J Physiol Pharmacol* 1995; 39: 111–116.
37. Shannahoff-Khalsa DS, Beckett LR. Clinical case report efficacy of yogic techniques in the treatment of obsessive compulsive disorders. *Int J Neurosci* 1996; 85: 1–17.
38. Gobel H, Fresenius J, Heinze A, Dworschak M, Soyka D. Effectiveness of Oleum menthae piperitae and paracetamol in therapy of headache of the tension type. *Nervenarzt* 1996; 67: 672–681.
39. Vernon H, McDermaid CS, Hagino C. Systematic review of randomized clinical trials of complementary/alternative therapies in the treatment of tension-type and cervicogenic headache. *Complement Ther Med* 1999; 7: 142–155.
40. Nelson CF, Bronfort G, Evans R, Boline P, Goldsmith C, Anderson AV. The efficacy of spinal manipulation, amitriptyline and the combination of both therapies for the prophylaxis of migraine headache. *J Manipulative Physiol Ther* 1998; 21: 511–519.
41. Tuchin PJ, Pollard H, Bonllo R. A randomized controlled trial of chiropractic spinal manipulative therapy for migraine. *J Manipulative Physiol Ther* 2000, 23: 91–95.
42. Parker GB, Tupling H, Pryer DS. A controlled trial of cervical manipulation of migraine. *Aust NZ J Med* 1978; 8: 589–593.
43. Melis PM, Rooimans W, Spierings EL, Hoogduin CA. Treatment of chronic tension-type headache with hypnotherapy: a single-blind time controlled study. *Headache* 1991; 31: 686–689.
44. Ter Kuile MM, Spinhoven P, Linssen ACG, Zitman FG, Van Dyck R, Rooljmans HGM. Autogenic training and cognitive self-hypnosis for the treatment of recurrent headaches in three different subject groups. *Pain* 1994; 58: 331–340.
45. Reiche BA. Non-invasive treatment of vascular and muscle contraction headache: a comparative longitudinal clinical study. *Headache* 1989; 29: 34–41.
47. Puustjarvi K, Airaksinen O, Pontinen PJ. The effects of massage in patients with chronic tension headache. *Acupuncture and Electro-Therapeutics Research.* 1990; 15: 159–162.
48. Egger J, Carter CM, Wison J, Turner MW, Soothill JF. Is migraine food allergy? A double-blind controlled trial of oligoantigenic diet treatment. *Lancet* 1983; 2: 865–869.
49. Mansfield LE, Vanghan TR, Waller SF, Haverly RW, Ting S. Food allergy and adult migraine: double-blind and mediator confirmation of an allergic etiology. *Annals of Allergy* 1985; 55: 126–129.
50. Launso L, Brendstrup E, Arnberg S. An exploratory study of reflexological treatment for headache. *Altern Ther Health Med* 1999; 5: 57–65.
51. Lafuente A, Noguera M, Puy C, Molins A, Titus F, Sanz F. Effekt der Reflexzonenbehandlung and Fuß bezüglich der prophylaktischen Behandlung mit Flunarizin bei an Cephalgea-Kopfschmerzen leidenden Patienten. *Erfahrungsheilkunde* 1990; 2: 713–715.
52. Latha, Kaliappan KV. Efficacy of yoga therapy in the management of headaches. *J Indian Psychol* 1992; 10: 41–47.
53. Van Tulder MW, Koes BW, Bouter LM. Conservative treatment of acute and chronic nonspecific low back pain: a systematic review of the most common interventions. *Spine* 1997; 22: 2128–2156.
54. Callacott EA, Zimmerman JT, White DW, Rindone JP. Bipolar permanent magnets for the treatment of chronic low back pain: a pilot study. *JAMA* 2000; 283: 1322–1325.
55. Ernst E, Koder K. An overview of reflexology. *Eur J Gen Pract* 1997; 3: 52–57.
56. Ernst, E. Massage therapy for low pain: a systematic review. *J Pain Symptom Manage* 1999; 17: 65–69.
57. Preyde M. Effectiveness of massage therapy for subacute low-back pain: a randomized controlled trial. *Can Med Assoc J* 2000; 162: 1815–1820.
58. Nespor K. Psychosomatics of back pain and the use of yoga. *Int J Psychosomat* 1989; 36: 72–78.

From Long, L., Huntley, A., & Ernst, E. (2001). Which complementary and alternative therapies benefit which conditions? A survey of the opinions of 223 professional organizations. *Complementary Therapies in Medicine, 9,* 178-185.

INTRODUCTORY SECTION

The first paragraph of the introductory section cites 14 sources in a succinct effort to reference the relevant professional literature. This is accomplished quite well by an appeal to both a general overview as well as with citations that speak to specific features of the research problem investigated. Based on the aim statement, the research question can be inferred from this section's second paragraph as follows: Which CAM therapies are judged by their respective health care providers to be suited for which medical conditions?

The study's rationale likewise is given in the second paragraph by the acknowledgment of a paucity of reliable data for informed decision making regarding which CAM therapies are most appropriate for which health conditions. This rationale becomes a very good justification for the study's exploratory interest in generating a database that can be used for (a) encouraging more informed decision making by practitioners and (b) suggesting hypotheses for future study. The exploratory purpose of this study illustrates quite well the typical use of the survey research method, although the option always exists for a survey study to serve a confirmatory purpose in terms of hypothesis testing.

METHOD SECTION

The study's participants include 223 CAM organizations both in and outside the United Kingdom, each of which represents a single CAM therapy. An attempt was made to be as inclusive and exhaustive as possible where CAM professional organizations are concerned. The principal exclusion criterion was that of an organization not representing only a single therapy. The professional status of the practitioners represented by the CAM organizations was not used as an exclusion criterion. A power analysis was not used in view of the focus of including as many organizations as possible that met the study's criteria. Furthermore, the power analysis issue is somewhat moot given that the study's purpose did not include hypothesis testing.

The study's accessible population was a total of 526 CAM organizations both in and outside the UK. Once the inclusion and exclusion criteria were applied, 223 of the original 526 organizations remained and, thereby constituted the study's sample. The full contingent of the remaining 223 organizations was used as opposed to randomly selecting a subset of this group.

Because this study is descriptive oriented in nature and uses a survey method, no IV was investigated. Consequently, the issue of the assignment of subjects to two or more comparison groups is nonexistent here. This point is being made simply to contrast the nature of a descriptive-oriented research strategy with that of a difference-oriented one. In the latter case, of course, the assignment of subjects to levels of the IV is a major consideration.

The only explicit reference to an ethics-related issue is the characterization of the questionnaire used as being confidential and by implication the resulting data generated by the participants' responses. This appears sufficient for this type of study. No mention is made of the study's original proposal being critiqued by an institutional review board. We must hasten to acknowledge that the nature of the study obviously did not involve subjects who in any way could have been potentially at risk. Consequently, it is possible that the survey nature of the investigation was not viewed as necessitating a formal institutional review. That decision is usually a function of the rigor with which an institution chooses to exercise oversight regarding studies performed by its representatives.

The method section is appropriately explicit regarding the descriptive nature of the study. Furthermore, the survey method and its typical research procedures are detailed in such a way that either a full or partial replication could be performed by an interested researcher as a follow-up.

No IVs were present in this study to be manipulated. Only the two DVs of type of CAM therapy and condition benefited were identified and measured. Again, enough detail is provided on these issues to allow replication as a sequel.

The only instrument necessitated in this study was the questionnaire used by the participants to respond to the various categories cited by the researchers. It appears that the questionnaire was of the open-ended variety in that it required a response more involved than a simple yes or no answer. Specifically, the participants were asked to respond in terms of categories such as (a) the top 15 conditions presumably benefited from their CAM therapy, (b) the top 15 contraindications, (c) typical costs of initial and follow-up treatments, and (d) the mean length of training hours required of a fully qualified practitioner of a given CAM therapy. Readers of the article are invited to obtain a sample of this instrument from the authors. Beyond what has just been described, no further information was provided regarding the technical characteristics of the questionnaire. At the least, one might presume appropriate face validity of the instrument given its nature.

RESULTS SECTION

The data analysis techniques cited in the article appropriately involve descriptive statistics, inclusive of tabular presentations. Of particular value in this report are the several tables presented by means of Excel spreadsheets that summarize the results quite well. This appears consistent with the descriptive nature of the study and its affiliated research question. It is also consistent with the study's exploratory purpose for generating a database to enhance decision making and suggesting hypotheses for future study. Critical to a survey report is the presentation of data regarding the response rate; in this study, 34% of the 223 CAM organizations responded. Inferential statistics were not included due to the absence of any focus on hypothesis testing, confidence interval estimation, or effect size calculations.

DISCUSSION SECTION

The authors of this report acknowledge the low response rate of only 34% as being an obvious limitation of this survey. Furthermore, they speculate on at least six reasons why the response rate was only 34%. This is helpful in terms of (a) placing the current study in proper perspective and (b) rendering somewhat of an explanation of possible dynamics occurring between CAM and orthodox/conventional medicine. This part of the discussion is also helpful with respect to implications for future studies of a similar nature.

The authors also acknowledge that this study is the largest of its type and represents at least an initial step toward generating the type of database needed for enhanced decision making. They also discuss implications of the current study that might suggest to future researchers the need to focus on the most established CAM disciplines rather than try to cover the entire range.

Perhaps the most valuable and intriguing feature of the discussion section relates to the authors' consideration of whether CAM therapies can have specific effects—beyond a placebo response—that are consistent with clinical trial evidence. The researchers compare available clinical trial evidence for effectiveness with the survey's three most frequently cited conditions: stress/anxiety, headaches/migraines, and back pain. The authors conclude that in general it appears that the CAM organizations' recommendations are supported by clinical evidence.

The discussion section, then, succeeds in speaking to several important areas such as the following: limitations and delimitations of the study, interpretation of the findings in the context of the study's significance, and recommendations for the direction of future related research.

CONCLUDING SECTION

The article is extensively well referenced with a total of 58 bibliographic citations that provide the literature support for several themes addressed in the report's main body. Author affiliation and contact information are provided as is standard practice. Footnotes and appendixes do not appear, presumably because the various tables and accompanying labels are sufficiently embedded in the main body of the article.

WHERE DO WE GO FROM HERE?

This chapter concludes Part Three of the book wherein we addressed those three research strategies included in the quantitative research category: the difference-oriented, association-oriented, and descriptive-oriented research strategies. Major emphases throughout this introduction to quantitative research have spanned such themes as the objective nature of the research process, the varying degrees of control exercised in different types of quantitative studies, and the reliance on numeric or quantitative data.

Part Four of the book covers two additional research categories representing alternatives to the quantitative research category just concluded. In Chapter 8 we examine what is known as the *qualitative research category* and its affiliated *contextual/interpretive research strategy*. As the terms *qualitative, contextual,* and *interpretive* imply, the emphases in Chapter 8 will be on studies representing such themes as the subjective nature of the research process, interpretations of variables and their dynamics reflecting the context in which they occur, and the reliance on data that are verbal rather than numeric.

In Chapter 9 we consider what can be called the *integrative research category* and its affiliated *synthesis-oriented research strategy*. Here too the terms are suggestive of what this research category and its research strategy entail. The focal points in Chapter 9 will be on studies addressing the need to integrate or pull together already-established research findings from completed studies, synthesizing their methodologies and results into more understandable patterns, and completing these tasks with respect to both quantitative and qualitative studies already present in the professional literature.

REFERENCES

Ballinger, C., Yardley, L., & Payne, S. (2004). Observation and action research. In D. F. Marks & L. Yardley (Eds.), *Research methods for clinical and health psychology* (pp. 102–121). Thousand Oaks, CA: Sage.

Brockopp, D. Y., & Hastings-Tolsma, M. T. (2003). *Fundamentals of nursing research* (3rd ed.). Sudbury, MA: Jones and Bartlett.

Cozby, P. C. (2004). *Methods in behavioral research* (8th ed.). Boston: McGraw-Hill.

Domholdt, E. (2000). *Physical therapy research: Principles and applications* (2nd ed.). Philadelphia: W. B. Saunders.

Eisenberg, D. M., Davis, R. B., Ettner, S. L., Appel, S., Wilkey, S., Rompay, M. V., et al. (1998). Trends in alternative medicine use in the United States, 1990–1997 results of a follow-up national survey. *Journal of the American Medical Association, 280,* 1569–1575.

Goodwin, C. J. (2005). *Research in psychology: Methods and design* (4th ed.). Hoboken, NJ: John Wiley & Sons.

Harris, S. (2004). *Einstein simplified: Cartoons on science by Sidney Harris* (Rev. ed.). New Brunswick, NJ: Rutgers University Press.

Hilliard, R. B. (1993). Single-case methodology in psychotherapy process and outcome research. *Journal of Consulting and Clinical Psychology, 61*(3), 373–380.

Katz, D. L. (2001). *Clinical epidemiology & evidence-based medicine: Fundamental principles of clinical reasoning & research.* Thousand Oaks, CA: Sage.

Kazdin, A. E. (2003). *Research design in clinical psychology* (4th ed.). Boston: Allyn & Bacon.

Long, L., Huntley, A., & Ernst, E. (2001). Which complementary and alternative therapies benefit which conditions? A survey of the opinions of 223 professional organizations. *Complementary Therapies in Medicine, 9,* 178–185.

Massage Therapy Foundation. (2004). *Case report structure: Guidelines for educational institutions and students.* Evanston, IL: Massage Therapy Foundation. Retrieved August 17, 2004, from http://massagetherapyfoundation.org/grants_education.html.

McEwen, I. (Ed.). (2001). *Writing case reports: A how-to manual for clinicians* (2nd ed.). Alexandria, VA: American Physical Therapy Association.

Menard, M. B. (2003). *Making sense of research: A guide to research literacy for complementary practitioners.* Toronto: Curties-Overzet.

Newman, T. B., Browner, W. S., Cummings, S. R., & Hulley, S. B. (2001). Designing an observational study: Cross-sectional and case-control studies. In S. B. Hulley, S. R. Cummings, W. S. Browner, D. Grady, N. Hearst, & T. B. Newman, *Designing clinical research* (2nd ed.) (pp. 107–123). Philadelphia: Lippincott Williams & Wilkins.

Polgar, S., & Thomas, S. A. (2000). *Introduction to research in the health sciences* (4th ed.). Philadelphia: Churchill Livingstone.

Polit, D. F., & Beck, C. T. (2004). *Nursing research: Principles and methods* (7th ed.). Philadelphia: Lippincott Williams & Wilkins.

Portney, L. G., & Watkins, M. P. (2000). *Foundations of clinical research: Applications to practice* (2nd ed.). Upper Saddle River, NJ: Prentice Hall Health.

Smith, R. A., & Davis, S. F. (2003). *The psychologist as detective: An introduction to conducting research in psychology* (3rd ed.). Upper Saddle River, NJ: Pearson/Prentice Hall.

Stommel, M., & Wills, C. E. (2004). *Clinical research: Concepts and principles for advanced practice nurses.* Philadelphia: Lippincott Williams & Wilkins.

Wootton, J. C., & Sparber, A. (2001). Surveys of complementary and alternative medicine: Part I. General trends and demographic groups. *Journal of Alternative and Complementary Medicine, 7*(2), 195–208.

ADDITIONAL RECOMMENDED RESOURCES

Burns, N., & Grove, S. K. (2003). *Understanding nursing research* (3rd ed.). Philadelphia: W. B. Saunders.

Gillis, A., & Jackson, W. (2002). *Research for nurses: Methods and interpretation.* Philadelphia: F. A. Davis.

Hicks, C. M. (1999). *Research methods for clinical therapists: Applied project design and analysis* (3rd ed.). Philadelphia: Churchill Livingstone.

McBurney, D. H. (2001). *Research methods* (5th ed.). Belmont, CA: Wadsworth Thomson Learning.

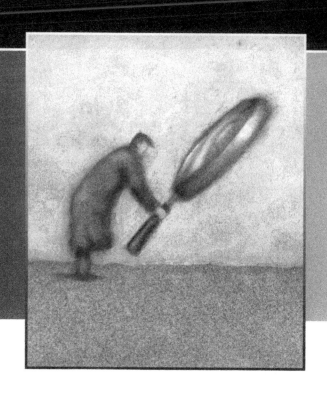

PART FOUR

QUALITATIVE AND INTEGRATIVE RESEARCH CATEGORIES: OPTIONS BEYOND THE QUANTITATIVE

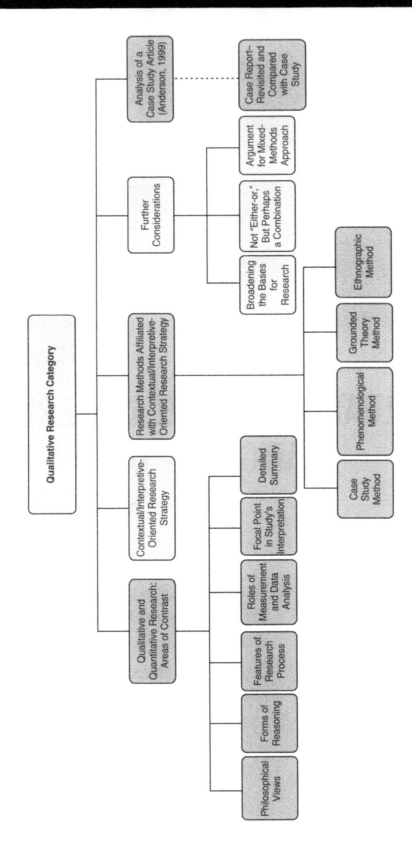

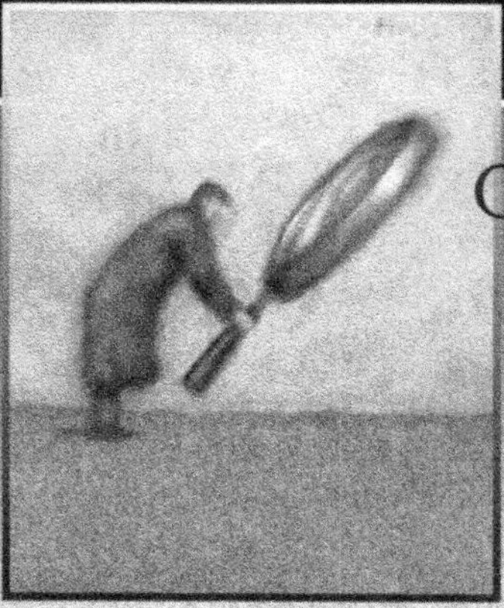

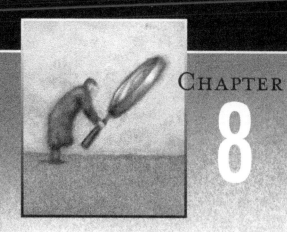

CHAPTER

8

THE QUALITATIVE RESEARCH CATEGORY AND ITS CONTEXTUAL/INTERPRETIVE-ORIENTED RESEARCH STRATEGY

OUTLINE

Where Have We Been and Where Are We Going? The Connection

The Qualitative Research Category: Areas of Contrast With Quantitative Research
- *Philosophical Views*
- *Forms of Reasoning*
- *Features of the Research Process*
- *Roles of Measurement and Data Analysis*
- *Focal Point in a Study's Interpretation*
- *Detailed Summary*

The Contextual/Interpretive-Oriented Research Strategy: Its Nature and Methods

Research Methods Affiliated With the Contextual/Interpretive-Oriented Research Strategy
- *Case Study Method*
- *Phenomenological Method*
- *Grounded Theory Method*
- *Ethnographic Method*

Further Considerations of the Contextual/Interpretive-Oriented Research Strategy
- *Broadening the Philosophical Perspectives and Methodological Options for Doing Research*
- *Not Simply an Either-Or, but Perhaps a Mixed/Blended/Combined Methods Approach*
- *The Argument for Blending or Combining the Quantitative and Qualitative Research Categories Into a Mixed-Methods Approach*

Illustration of the Case Study Method: An Analysis of a Complete Research Article
- *Focus of Critique Question 1: Clinical Problem via Research Question*
- *Focus of Critique Question 2: Rationale for Using a Qualitative Approach*
- *Focus of Critique Question 3: Context/Setting of the Case and Basis for Subject Selection*
- *Focus of Critique Question 4: Consideration Given to the Researcher's Perspective*
- *Focus of Critique Question 5: Detailed Description of Data Collection Methods*
- *Focus of Critique Question 6: Data Analysis Method and Quality Control*
- *Focus of Critique Question 7: Credibility and Clinical Importance of the Results*
- *Focus of Critique Question 8: Justification for the Conclusions Drawn*
- *Focus of Critique Question 9: Transferability of Study's Findings*

The Case Report: Revisited and Compared With the Case Study

Where Do We Go From Here?
- *Quantitative and Qualitative Categories Already in Place*
- *The Integrative Research Category (Chapter 9): Yet Another Option Beyond Quantitative and Qualitative Research*

KEY TERMS

Bounded system
Case entity
Case report research method
Case study research method
Collective case study
Constructivism
Contextual/interpretive-oriented
  research strategy
Emic
Ethnographic research method

Etic
Grounded theory research method
Inductive and deductive reasoning
Instrumental case study
Intrinsic case study
Methodological triangulation
Mixed/blended/combined methods
Numerical data
Participant observation
Participant-observer research

Phenomenological research method
Positivism
Postmodernism
Postpositivism
Prospective case report
Qualitative research category
Retrospective case report
Subjective and objective philosophical views
Symbolic interactionism
Verbal data

OBJECTIVES

Upon completion of this chapter, the reader will have the information necessary to perform the following tasks:

1 Characterize the qualitative research category.

2 Contrast the qualitative research category with the quantitative research category regarding the following areas: philosophical views, forms of reasoning, features of the research process, roles of measurement and data analysis, and focal point in a study's interpretation.

3 Identify and discuss the three major perspectives or contexts from which any qualitative study may be examined.

4 Identify and explain the name of the one research strategy orientation affiliated with qualitative research.

5 List the four research methods affiliated with the contextual/ interpretive-oriented research strategy.

6 Identify and explain the essential features that define the case study research method.

7 Recognize and apply the nine critical appraisal questions for critiquing qualitative research as suggested by Greenhalgh (2001).

8 Recognize, or be able to provide, an example of the case study method.

9 Identify and explain the essential features that define the phenomenological research method.

10 Recognize, or be able to provide, an example of the phenomenological method.

11 Identify and explain the essential features that define the grounded theory research method.

12 Recognize, or be able to provide, an example of the grounded theory method.

13 Identify and explain the essential features that define the ethnographic research method.

14 Recognize, or be able to provide, an example of the ethnographic method.

15 Discuss the distinctions between quantitative research and qualitative research with respect to the following:
   a. the philosophical perspectives of positivism, postmodernism, postpositivism, and constructivism;
   b. the methodological options that result from different philosophical perspectives.

16 Explain why the distinction between quantitative and qualitative research is not really an issue of "either-or."

17 Provide a sound argument in favor of a mixed-methods approach to doing research that blends or combines both quantitative and qualitative methodologies.

18 Read and critique published research reports that exemplify the following research methods: the case study method, the phenomenological method, the grounded theory method, and the ethnographic method.

19 Explain the similarities and differences between the case report method representing quantitative research and the case study method representing qualitative research.

20 Identify and characterize the third category of research that may be considered in addition to the quantitative and qualitative categories.

WHERE HAVE WE BEEN AND WHERE ARE WE GOING? THE CONNECTION

In Chapters 2 through 4 (Part Two) and Chapters 5 through 7 (Part Three), we examined the *quantitative research category* and its affiliated research strategies and methods. You may recall from our earlier discussions that quantitative research emphasizes such themes as the following: the objective nature of reality; a primarily deductive movement from theory to hypothesis to precise measurements; the control, manipulation, and measurement of appropriate variables in a study; investigator detachment so as to ensure an unbiased process; the measurement of clearly defined outcomes using valid and reliable instruments; the statistical analysis of the numeric data thus generated; and the interpretation of the study's results in the context of the existing literature in that research problem area.

In this chapter we consider an additional perspective on research known as the **qualitative research category**, its one affiliated *contextual/ interpretive-oriented research strategy*, and four related research methods: the *case study method*, the *phenomenological method*, the *grounded theory method*, and the *ethnographic method*. Once our coverage of the qualitative category is completed, we then consider the possibility of investigating any given research problem by making use of both quantitative and qualitative perspectives. Figure 8-1 displays the strategy and methods included in this chapter's coverage of the qualitative category.

This chapter details the areas of contrast between the quantitative and qualitative categories. As a general characterization, the qualitative research category emphasizes the following themes: the subjective and contextual nature of reality, a primarily inductive progression from observations to theory development, the absence of variables being controlled and manipulated in favor of processes being richly described, investigator immersion in the setting or

- Qualitative Research Category
  - Contextual/Interpretive-Oriented Research Strategy (Chapter 8)
    - Case Study Method
    - Phenomenological Method
    - Grounded Theory Method
    - Ethnographic Method

FIGURE 8-1 ■ The qualitative research category: Its affiliated research strategy and variable control-driven methods.

context of the study's participants, the recording of processes or phenomena using primarily verbal means, textual analyses of the verbal data thus generated, and the interpretation of the study's findings in the context of the participants' ascribed meanings and understandings.

THE QUALITATIVE RESEARCH CATEGORY: AREAS OF CONTRAST WITH QUANTITATIVE RESEARCH

The preceding paragraph captures several of the major features of the qualitative research category in that it speaks to many areas in which the qualitative approach represents an alternative to the quantitative perspective. These many areas, specifically, span such realms as *philosophical views, forms of reasoning, features of the research process itself*, the *roles of measurement and data analysis*, and the *focal point in a study's interpretation*. Let us examine each of these realms in greater detail.

PHILOSOPHICAL VIEWS

As elaborated on by Creswell (1998), in the *qualitative* research perspective, philosophical views on reality, truth, and values set the foundation for all that follows from a research methodology standpoint. Reality here is considered to be **subjective**, varied, based largely on how it is interpreted by a study's participants, and socially constructed. In the search for knowledge, researchers try to minimize as much as possible the gap or distance between themselves and the study's participants. This is done so as to increase the researchers' chances of accessing in a credible way the perceptions of the participants. In the realm of values, the qualitative research perspective hastens to acknowledge that biases are inevitably present, an important component of phenomena being studied, and reflective of the values operating in any given research context. They are not to be ignored, controlled, or denied; instead, they are to be embraced as part of the milieu or context that gives meaning to what is being studied.

The preceding is very much in contrast with what we have already seen in the *quantitative* tradition. For the quantitative researcher, reality is **objective**, essentially unchanging, not dependent on how it might be defined by one or more participants in a study, and "out there" in the physical universe to be discovered by empirical investigation. The researchers attempt to maintain a safe distance from the participants so as to minimize as much as possible any unintentional and unwanted influence between themselves and the participants, in either direction. Biases in a study, reflective of value orientations, are an ever-present concern and need to be controlled as much as possible so that the objectivity of the investigation is not compromised.

FORMS OF REASONING

Both Patten (2004) and Creswell (1998) discuss the reliance of qualitative researchers primarily on **inductive reasoning**. The qualitative category of research typically begins with an initial collection of verbal or image-based data by way of observation and other related means (such as interviews). Once these preliminary findings are in place, additional data are gathered that reflect and build on the initial data set. From there the researcher relies heavily on allowing a theory or explanation to emerge of the phenomena studied. In this sense, then, theory development occurs as a most desired focus as opposed to starting out beforehand with a theoretical formulation already in place and then proceeding to test it.

Here, too, is a contrast with the quantitative approach that starts with **deductive reasoning** and then eventually proceeds to induction. At the outset, quantitative researchers immerse themselves in the professional literature available in a given problem area. Included in this literature are already-proposed theories and the constructs on which they are built. The researcher relies on these theories and constructs as a basis for deducing a certain hypothesis or justified prediction of what should operationally follow from the theory. Numeric data are collected, statistically analyzed, and a decision made regarding the original hypothesis. To complete the circle, in a sense, the several measurements recorded in the study and the follow-up data analysis are then used inductively to inform the original theory or perhaps suggest the formulation of a new one.

FEATURES OF THE RESEARCH PROCESS

Lusardi (1999) provides one of the most extensive discussions available on the defining features of the qualitative research process. The focus here is on person-oriented processes and phenomena considered in a given social or cultural context.

The control and manipulation of variables are replaced in favor of processes and phenomena being observed and recorded by way of credible verbal or image-based descriptions. Inclusive understandings and explanations of whatever is being studied are encouraged from varied perspectives, without a predominant concern for generalizations. The researcher is an immersed participant-observer who tries to gain an insider's perspective. The research focus is holistic in nature and sensitive to unanticipated developments and interpretations. Research conclusions reflect to a large extent the authenticity and completeness of the data generated as well as the participants' confirmations of them.

Once again, the preceding paragraph is in contrast with the quantitative perspective that focuses on objectively measurable outcomes. The emphasis here is outcome or product oriented and usually avoids the context within which the study occurs. The control and manipulation of appropriate variables are critical, as is the measurement of outcomes in as valid, reliable, objective, and unbiased a manner as possible. The data thus generated are numeric in nature and analyzed statistically. Possible alternative explanations of study outcomes are controlled by way of the research design with a concern for protecting the study's internal validity. The generalizability, or the external validity, of the study is typically a concern and is addressed by way of appropriate sampling procedures. The researcher is objectively "detached" from the participants as well as the data generated and, consequently, is postured to provide an "outsider's" perspective that is unbiased. The research focus is, for the most part, considered "reductionistic" in that clearly defined components of the phenomenon being studied are usually segmented and controlled for investigative purposes. Research conclusions attempt to explain linkages and relationships among the variables studied.

ROLES OF MEASUREMENT AND DATA ANALYSIS

In yet another work by Creswell (2003), as well as the Lusardi (1999) contributions cited earlier, the measurement efforts in the qualitative realm are characterized as involving verbal and/or image-based data. The emphasis here is on both the researcher and the participant in a study providing credible descriptions and interpretations of phenomena that are rich in authenticity and personal meaning.

Textual, and at times image-based, analyses are conducted with a view toward interpreting with confidence the intent and underlying meaning of the process or phenomenon studied.

As seen before, in quantitative research a high premium is placed on the collection of **numerical data** by way of different measurement procedures that ensure validity and reliability. These two technical characteristics of the measuring instruments are typically demonstrated statistically. The data collection procedures are then followed by statistical analyses performed for the purpose of hypothesis testing, confidence internal estimation, and/or effect size calculations. This entire process of invoking both measurement and statistics as research tools reflects virtually everything said earlier about the nature of modern scientific methodology and the philosophical assumptions on which it is based.

FOCAL POINT IN A STUDY'S INTERPRETATION

The focal point in a qualitative study's interpretation has already been addressed somewhat by the resources cited and the ground covered thus far in this chapter. Perhaps the most pointed statement in this regard, though, is made by Creswell (2003), who states that "a qualitative approach is one in which the inquirer often makes knowledge claims based primarily on constructivist perspectives (i.e., the multiple meanings of individual experiences, meanings socially and historically constructed, with an intent of developing a theory or pattern)" (p. 18). The interpretation of a qualitative study, then, is in terms of understanding human behavior and interactions as reflections of both the participants' views and the sociocultural context within which they occur.

In the quantitative realm, though, the "approach is one in which the investigator primarily uses postpositivist claims for developing knowledge (i.e., cause and effect thinking, reduction to specific variables and hypotheses and questions, use of measurement and observation, and the test of theories)" (Creswell, 2003, p. 18). This leads to interpretations in quantitative studies that involve descriptions, explanations, and predictions of clearly defined variables rooted in objective facts. In so doing, sociocultural contexts and the subjective perceptions of both the researcher and the participant are intentionally minimized (if indeed factored in at all).

DETAILED SUMMARY

Having just highlighted the major contrasts between the quantitative and qualitative research categories, let us now examine a more detailed summary of the various points on which each category represents an alternative to the other. Several resources, beyond the ones we have already seen, are available for doing this (e.g., Burns & Grove, 2003; Christensen, 2004; and Flick, 2002); however, the source most highly recommended here for this purpose is Gillis and Jackson's (2002) effort as shown in Table 8-1.

TABLE 8-1	DETAILED SUMMARY OF THE CONTRASTS BETWEEN QUANTITATIVE AND QUALITATIVE RESEARCH
Quantitative	*Qualitative*
Single reality	Multiple realities
Reality is objective	Reality is socially constructed
Reality is context free	Reality is context interrelated
Reductionistic	Holistic
Strong theoretical base	Strong philosophical perspective
Reasoning is deductive and inductive	Reasoning is inductive
Cause-and-effect relationships are the bases of knowledge	Discovery of meaning is the basis of knowledge
Tests theory	Develops theory
Theory developed *a priori*	Theory development during study
Measurement of variables	Meaning of concepts
Outcome oriented	Process oriented
Control important	Control unimportant
Precise measurement of variables	Rich descriptions
Basic element of analysis is numbers	Basic element of analysis is words
Generalization	Uniqueness
Control of error	Trustworthiness of findings
Concepts of Rigor in Quantitative and Qualitative Research	
Validity	Credibility (authenticity)
Generalizability (external validity)	Transferability (fittingness)
Reliability	Dependability (auditability)
Objectivity	Confirmability

From Gillis, A., & Jackson, W. (2002). *Research for nurses: Methods and interpretation*. Philadelphia: F. A. Davis. pp. 182, 215.

THE CONTEXTUAL/INTERPRETIVE-ORIENTED RESEARCH STRATEGY: ITS NATURE AND METHODS

Our coverage of the qualitative research category so far has focused on many specific aspects of this particular view of the research process. Included under this research category is the generic **contextual/interpretive-oriented research strategy**. Soon we will be examining the four research methods that fall under this research strategy. Before examining them, however, it will be helpful for us to consider a diagram developed by Flick (2002) that does an excellent job of portraying the three major perspectives or contexts from which any qualitative study may be viewed (Box 8-1).

As illustrated, the three major perspectives or contexts from which any qualitative study may be examined include (a) the *subjects or participants* actually involved in the study, (b) the nature of the *interaction and discourses* that occur between or among the participants, and (c) the *sociocultural context* in which the phenomena under investigation occur. Superimposed on these three realms are all of the features of the qualitative research category that we discussed earlier and contrasted with the quantitative approach. Foremost in this array of features, though, are the subjective nature of reality as constructed by the individual, the immersion of the researcher in the process and setting, and the eventual discovery of meaning as it unfolds.

Each of the four research methods that we are to cover in the qualitative research category addresses in some manner the perspectives or context just summarized. Those methods include the case study

method, the phenomenological method, the grounded theory method, and the ethnographic method.

RESEARCH METHODS AFFILIATED WITH THE CONTEXTUAL/INTERPRETIVE-ORIENTED RESEARCH STRATEGY

CASE STUDY METHOD

By way of an introductory overview, Figure 8-2 spotlights the **case study research method,** which is the first of four methods affiliated with the contextual/interpretive-oriented research strategy.

Recall the distinction we made earlier among the three types of single-case research methodology: the (a) single-case experimental method, (b) the single-case quantitative analysis method, and (c) the case study method (Hilliard, 1993). Chapter 5 addressed the *single-case experimental method* as one option for implementing a difference-oriented research strategy. Chapter 7 covered the *single-case quantitative analysis method* as one alternative for

- Qualitative Research Category
  - • Contextual/Interpretive-Oriented Research Strategy (Chapter 8)
    - • • **Case Study Method**
    - • • Phenomenological Method
    - • • Grounded Theory Method
    - • • Ethnographic Method

FIGURE 8-2 ■ Spotlight on the case study research method in affiliation with the contextual/interpretive-oriented research strategy (bold emphasis designates coverage in this section).

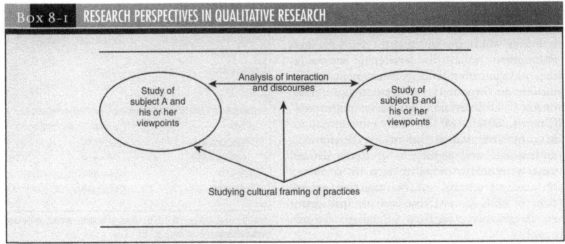

BOX 8-1   RESEARCH PERSPECTIVES IN QUALITATIVE RESEARCH

From Flick, U. (2002). *An introduction to qualitative research.* Thousand Oaks, Ca.: Sage. p. 25.

implementing a descriptive-oriented research strategy. This chapter, therefore, completes the needed coverage of single-case research methodology suggested by Hilliard by addressing the third of these three options, the case study method.

Another clarification in terminology is critical here before we delve into the specifics of the case study method. As Domholdt (2000) pointed out:

> Sometimes the terms "case report" and "case study" are used interchangeably as labels for systematic descriptions of practice. However, the term "case study" is also used, particularly by qualitative researchers, to describe a more complex analysis of . . . a single case within its organizational, social, or environmental context. For [our purposes], the term case report will refer to descriptions of clinical practice . . . and case study will refer to the more complete descriptions typical of research in the qualitative tradition. (p. 148)

With this reminder of the important distinction between a case report and a case study in place, we now move on to the initial focus of this chapter, the case study research method. Please note, however, that in the latter part of this chapter we will analyze a research article illustrating the case study method. Upon completing that analysis, we will return to the case report method briefly to elaborate more extensively on how these two approaches to a case compare.

The starting point in the case study research method is a research question of the following general form: What does an intensive description and analysis reveal about a **case entity** of interest, considered in its context and reflected by way of multiple sources of data? As implied by this generic research question, several considerations come into play when using the case study method. One such consideration at the outset is the characterization of precisely what a case study represents.

As indicated by Christensen (2004) and Creswell (1998), a *case study* is a comprehensive description and analysis of a single individual, organization, issue, activity, event, or program that reflects context-rich information gleaned from multiple sources such as observations, interviews, reports, documents, test results, multimedia materials, and archival records. The focus of the study (i.e., the *case*) is considered to be "bounded" by certain time and place "boundaries" or delimitations. An example here might be a study bounded by either a single program in a given location (i.e., a within-site study) or several programs positioned in diverse locations (i.e., a multisite study).

Robert Stake (as cited in Christensen, 2004; and Creswell, 1998) has proposed three types of case studies: intrinsic, instrumental, and collective case studies. An **intrinsic case study** provides an in-depth description of a specific entity–be that entity an individual, organization, issue, activity, event, or program of interest–so as to acquire a more insightful understanding of the uniqueness of that particular case. An **instrumental case study** is an intensive analysis of a specific entity–typically an issue or event–so as to refine or alter a theoretical explanation of the issue or event. This is done not so much for the insight gained about the specific case at hand, but rather to better understand the larger issue or event of which the case studied is only one manifestation. The specific case studied, then, literally becomes an instrument for illustrating and elaborating on the issue or event. The **collective case study** examines intensively not one but several entities, for example, several individuals, with a view toward gaining insight into the phenomenon represented across the several cases. This is the primary objective in the collective case study, and not simply a better understanding of only one individual.

Regardless of which of the three types of case studies one implements, the context of the case is critical. We are referring here to the actual setting or milieu of the case, be it a physical, social, cultural, historical, or economic setting. It is in this context that the dynamics of the entity being studied must be characterized and interpreted.

Our earlier characterization of the case study method acknowledged multiple sources of data collection options. These included observations, interviews, reports, documents, test results, multimedia materials, and archival records. The analysis performed on the data collected can be either a *holistic analysis,* in that it reflects the entire case, or an *embedded analysis* of only a particular aspect of the case (cf. Creswell, 1998). Bare Bones Box 8-2 displays the several features of the case study method as one way of implementing a contextual/interpretive-oriented research strategy.

Hypothetical illustrations of various therapeutic massage and related health science research areas to which the case study method might be applicable include the following: a massage therapist who has recently entered private practice after 12 years as head of a hospital-based massage program that has downsized, a pain management clinic with five massage therapists on staff who are trying to coordinate their diverse modality specialties with the varied

BARE BONES BOX 8-2

Essential Features of the Case Study Research Method

- Formulation of a research question of the following basic form: What does an intensive description and analysis reveal about a case entity of interest, considered in its context and reflected by way of multiple sources of data?
- Identification of a case entity as a single individual, organization, issue, activity, event, or program of interest
- Identification of a case entity as being bounded by certain time and place boundaries or delimitations
- Illustration of a case as a **bounded** system: within-site study as bounded by a single program in a given location or multisite study as bounded by several programs positioned in diverse locations
- Existence of three types of case studies: intrinsic case study so as to acquire more insight regarding the uniqueness of a particular case, instrumental case study so as to refine or alter a theoretical explanation of an issue or event, and collective case study of several case entities so as to gain insight regarding the phenomenon represented across the several cases
- Importance of the context of the case — that is, the actual setting or milieu of the case, be it a physical, social, cultural, historical, or economic setting
- Reliance on multiple sources of data collection options, including observations, interviews, reports, documents, test results, multimedia materials, and archival records

BARE BONES BOX 8-3

Critical Appraisal Checklist for Critiquing Qualitative Research (Greenhalgh, 2001, pp. 170–178)

Question 1. Did the paper describe an important clinical problem addressed via a clearly formulated question?

Question 2. Was a qualitative approach appropriate?

Question 3. How were (a) the setting and (b) the subjects selected?

Question 4. What was the researcher's perspective and has this been taken into account?

Question 5. What methods did the researcher use for collecting data and are these described in enough detail?

Question 6. What methods did the researcher use to analyze the data and what quality control measures were implemented?

Question 7. Are the results credible and, if so, are they clinically important?

Question 8. What conclusions were drawn and are they justified by the results?

Question 9. Are the findings of the study transferable to other clinical settings?

From Greenhalgh, T. (2001). *How to read a paper: The basics of evidence based medicine* (2nd ed.). London: BMJ Books.

client conditions treated, and the contributions of the massage therapist component of a sports medicine team at a intercollegiate track and field championship meet. Two other relevant examples are the progress of a client with fibromyalgia who is approaching the end of a two-month massage intervention program and the impact of massage therapists working with burn victims in three hospitals located in a large metropolitan area.

In addition to the sources already cited in this section, other important references that may expand our treatment of the case study research method include the following: Ballinger, Yardley, and Payne (2004); Cozby (2001); Goodwin (2005); Kazdin (2003a, 2003b, 2003c); Lukoff, Edwards, and Miller (1998); Smith (1988); Stake (1995); and Yin (1989).

Before leaving this section, please note that later in this chapter we provide an illustration of a case study by way of a complete research article authored by Anderson (1999). The full text of this case study

is accompanied by an analysis or critique consistent with the evaluative guidelines proposed by Greenhalgh (2001) and discussed next.

In an invaluable resource by Trisha Greenhalgh, the aforementioned author discusses the advisability of, and the history surrounding, the development of an all-encompassing critical appraisal checklist appropriate to critiquing qualitative research. The resulting checklist represents her efforts in tandem with those of several of her colleagues (as cited by Greenhalgh, 2001, pp. 170–178) and is synthesized in Bare Bones Box 8-3.

PHENOMENOLOGICAL METHOD

Figure 8-3 spotlights the **phenomenological research method**, which represents the second of four methods included within the contextual/interpretive-oriented research strategy.

In phenomenological research, the basic research question asked is the following: What is the meaning of the lived experience of each participant in the study? Several important considerations drive any investigation of this type of question. One of these considerations is an ongoing interdependency

- Qualitative Research Category
  - • Contextual/Interpretive-Oriented Research Strategy (Chapter 8)
    - • • Case Study Method
    - • • **Phenomenological Method**
    - • • Grounded Theory Method
    - • • Ethnographic Method

FIGURE 8-3 ■ Spotlight on the phenomenological research method in affiliation with the contextual/interpretive-oriented research strategy (bold emphasis designates coverage in this section).

or interaction between the person and the environment. The world and the individual mutually shape each other in a unique fashion. As expressed by Burns and Grove (2003):

> *The person is situated as a consequence of being shaped by his or her world and thus is constrained in the ability to establish meanings by language, culture, history, purposes, and values. . . . Situated means that the place of a person in the world shapes them in ways that limit their thinking and behavior. Each person has only situated freedom, not total freedom. . . . Not only is the world of each person different, but each person's concerns are qualitatively different. The body, world, and concerns, which are unique to each person, are the context within which that person can be understood. (p. 360)*

Another consideration central to phenomenological research is the concept that a study's participant is the only reliable source of insight regarding the meaning of that person's lived experience—no one else. The participant interprets his or her behavior or experience for the researcher, and the researcher in turn must interpret the explanation provided by the participant. A dynamism or interplay occurs between the two, thereby necessitating trust, authenticity, and dependability among all concerned.

Yet another important feature of phenomenological research is the typical reliance on in-depth interviews. This method of collecting **verbal data** is the means for moving from simply a participant's initial description of an experience to some sense of the meaning or interpretation of what has been described. The in-depth interview allows for the type of two-way exchange between participant and researcher that makes possible the exploration of underlying interpretations. This provides both parties with the chance for elaboration and correction as needed, thereby helping to ensure the credibility of what is eventually reported.

Data collection methods other than the in-depth interview used in phenomenological research include audiotaped conversations as well as written anecdotes of personal experiences. Regardless of the means used to collect the verbal data, the essential criterion for determining its appropriateness is the richness of the personal account of the experience being studied. This is a prerequisite for being able to bridge the gap between a mere description of an experience and an authentic interpretation of the experience's meaning.

All of the above-cited features of the phenomenological method suggest a strategic role for the researcher in terms of transforming information. This transformation is of the participant's personal description of a particular phenomenon as a lived experience into a form that is publicly understandable and helpful. In this regard, Streubert and Carpenter (1995) proposed five steps that the researcher must take in completing this transformational task: (a) converting the experiences of the participant into language; (b) translating the specifics of what is seen and heard into a viable portrayal of the original experience; (c) relating what is understood about the phenomenon being studied to those essential features constituting the original experience; (d) documenting the phenomenon's essential features as a reflection of not only the participant's descriptions/actions, but also the researcher's understanding of the experience; and (e) finalizing the written document into an exhaustive description that clarifies the preceding steps and ensures accuracy and richness. Bare Bones Box 8-4 summarizes the several features of the phenomenological research method as an approach to doing qualitative research.

BARE BONES BOX 8-4

Essential Features of the Phenomenological Research Method

- Formulation of a research question of the following basic form: What is the meaning of the lived experience of each participant in the study?
- Recognition of an ongoing interdependency or interaction between the person and the environment
- Identification of the participant as the only reliable source of insight regarding the meaning of that person's lived experience—no one else's
- Reliance on in-depth interviews as the typical method for collecting the study's verbal data
- Possible use of other data collection methods such as audiotaped conversations and written anecdotes of personal experiences
- Identification of the researcher's strategic role as that of transforming information.

Hypothetical illustrations of various therapeutic massage research problems to which the phenomenological method might be applied include the lived experiences of individuals in the following situations: massage therapy students in the clinical phase of their Swedish massage course who are working on clients for the first time; adults with hyperactivity and attention deficit disorders who are completing their first month of semiweekly massage treatments; paralegals in a corporate law setting who are just starting a workplace stress reduction program inclusive of chair massage; and lifelong, incessant smokers who are in a smoking cessation program using therapeutic massage. Other examples are as follows: fibromyalgia patients in the latter phase of a massage intervention program with a particular focus on sleep disorder and chronic fatigue experiences; law school aspirants practicing self-massage as a test anxiety intervention while preparing for the Law School Admissions Test; and traffic accident victims of whiplash as they conclude the final week of a month-long massage treatment regimen.

Beyond the Burns and Grove (2003) and Streubert and Carpenter (1995) sources cited earlier in this section, other valuable references that may elaborate on our treatment of phenomenological research include the following: Christensen (2004); Domholdt (2000); Giorgi and Giorgi (2003); Morse and Field (1995); and Polit, Beck, and Hungler (2001).

GROUNDED THEORY METHOD

Figure 8-4 spotlights the **grounded theory research method**, which is the third of four methods covered in our treatment of the contextual/interpretive-oriented research strategy.

The starting point in the grounded theory research method is a research question of the following general or basic form: What is the theory or abstract framework (schema) that explains an experience or phenomenon in a particular setting?

Whereas the phenomenological method emphasizes the meaning of an experience or phenomenon

- Qualitative Research Category
  - • Contextual/Interpretive-Oriented Research Strategy (Chapter 8)
    - • • Case Study Method
    - • • Phenomenological Method
    - • • **Grounded Theory Method**
    - • • Ethnographic Method

FIGURE 8-4 ■ Spotlight on the grounded theory research method in affiliation with the contextual/interpretive-oriented research strategy (bold emphasis designates coverage in this section).

for one or more individuals, the focal point of the grounded theory method is on rendering a conceptual or theoretical model that *explains* a phenomenon (Creswell, 1998). Typically, the phenomenon under study is both relevant to and problematic for the participants in a study. Once this problem is defined, the researcher employing this method tries to uncover the process used by the participants either to cope with or resolve the difficulty (Polit et al., 2001).

As noted by Burns and Grove (2003), "grounded theory has been used most frequently to study areas in which little previous research has been conducted and to gain a new viewpoint in familiar areas of research" (p. 363). Furthermore, in elaborating on why the term *grounded* is used in the expression *grounded theory,* these authors explain that a theory developed from using this method is rooted (or *grounded*) most directly in the data and insights from which it (the theory) is derived.

One of the key features of grounded theory research is **symbolic interactionism**, a notion identified by Morse and Field (1995) as the foundational base for grounded theory. This construct of symbolic interactionism has its origins in the work of Mead (1934), has been related to health science research (Chenitz & Swanson, 1986), and is succinctly explained by Burns and Grove (2003) as follows:

Symbolic interaction theory explores how people define reality and how their beliefs are related to their actions. Reality is created by attaching meanings to situations. Meaning is expressed in such symbols as words, religious objects, and clothing. These symbolic meanings are the basis for actions and interactions. However, symbolic meanings are different for each individual, and we cannot completely know the symbolic meanings of another individual. In social life, meanings are shared by groups and are communicated to new members through socialization processes. Group life is based on consensus and shared meanings. Interaction may lead to redefinition and new meanings and can result in the redefinition of self. Because of its theoretical importance, the interaction is the focus of observation in grounded theory research. (p. 363)

Beyond the features of grounded theory research already cited, several other considerations or procedures are critical to this methodology. Streubert and Carpenter (1995) have noted that researchers in this tradition do not begin with a theory. Rather, they proceed from the generation of data to the identification of essential constructs reflecting the collected data. From these data and constructs, the theoretical explanation of the phenomenon under study emerges. This process is carried out by an appeal to the following five procedures: (a) *Data* relevant to the phenomenon being studied are *generated* by such means as interviews, field notes, documents, journals, participant observation, and professional literature. These data are then *analyzed*. (b) Responding to the data generation and analysis, the researcher identifies recurring processes, themes, and concepts that emerge from the data. This *concept formation* effort suggests patterns that are operative in helping participants cope with the problem at hand. (c) The emerging processes, themes, concepts, and patterns identified in the concept formation stage are then elaborated on by way of *concept development*. This occurs in a threefold way by reducing the explanatory constructs to the most prevalent, selectively reviewing the literature relating to these most prevalent explanatory constructs, and selectively examining the existing data as well as possibly new data to confirm the earlier explanatory constructs that were identified. (d) The concept development effort provides the context for the emergence of the *core variable* or construct. This is the factor that seems to account most extensively for the pattern(s) of behavior most defining in the phenomenon being studied. (e) The core variable identification effort thus sets the stage for refinements that eventually move the process from a descriptive to a *theoretical level of explanation grounded in the original data*.

Beginning with the type of research question most compatible with the grounded theory method and proceeding through the five procedures just cited, Bare Bones Box 8-5 summarizes the essential features of this method.

Examples of hypothetical research problems to which the grounded theory method might be applied include attempts to provide data-based explanations of the following: an inconsistent compliance rate among clients at a pain management clinic regarding prescribed self-care hydrotherapy and stretching regimens, decisions by former massage therapy clients to discontinue their reliance on therapeutic massage as a preferred complementary and alternative medicine (CAM) intervention of choice, decisions by journal editors that contribute to the paucity of qualitative research articles in prominent journals for the manual therapy sciences, pain management efforts among carpal tunnel syndrome sufferers immediately prior to starting massage treatments, and the dynamics among family members of a patient recovering from bilateral hip replacement surgeries.

In addition to the sources already referenced in this section, other valuable materials that may add

---

BARE BONES BOX 8-5

Essential Features of the Grounded Theory Research Method

- Formulation of a research question of the following basic form: What theory or abstract framework (schema) explains an experience or phenomenon in a particular setting?
- Focus is on a conceptual or theoretical model that explains a phenomenon both relevant to, and typically problematic for, the participants in the study.
- Researcher attempts to uncover the process useful to participants in coping with or resolving the difficulty.
- Most applicable to areas characterized by a paucity of previous research or to established research areas necessitating new viewpoints.
- Foundational construct is that of social interactionism, which explores how people define reality and how their beliefs relate to their behavior.
- Research activities progress interactively from data generation/analysis to construct identification to theoretical formulation via five steps.
- Five aforementioned steps include data generation and analysis, concept formation, concept development, emergence of core variable, and formulation of theoretical explanation of the targeted phenomenon.
- Resulting emergent theory is rooted or grounded in the original data.

---

to this chapter's coverage of the grounded theory method are as follows: Chamberlain, Camic, and Yardley (2004); Domholdt (2000); Gillis and Jackson (2002); and Henwood and Pidgeon (2003).

ETHNOGRAPHIC METHOD

The fourth of four research methods included under the contextual/interpretive-oriented research strategy is the ethnographic method spotlighted in Figure 8-5.

- Qualitative Research Category
  - • Contextual/Interpretive-Oriented Research Strategy (Chapter 8)
    - • • Case Study Method
    - • • Phenomenological Method
    - • • Grounded Theory Method
    - • • **Ethnographic Method**

FIGURE 8-5 ■ Spotlight on the ethnographic research method in affiliation with the contextual/interpretive-oriented research strategy (bold emphasis designates coverage in this section).

In the **ethnographic research method**, the generic research question investigated is of the following type: How is human behavior to be understood and interpreted given the cultural context in which it is embedded?

Christensen (2004) noted that a basic theme in ethnographic research is that a culture (i.e., ways of life of a group of people reflecting patterns of behavior and customs) inevitably evolves if the group of individuals remains together long enough. Accordingly, ethnographic research seeks to understand and interpret these patterns of behavior and customs that define the way of life of a people. In doing so, a so-called *emic* approach might be taken that studies behavior from within the culture as opposed to an *etic* strategy of studying behaviors from outside and investigating cross-cultural similarities and differences (Burns & Grove, 2003).

Regardless of the approach taken, be it *emic* or *etic*, two additional features of ethnographic research include participant observation of long duration and in-depth interviewing. Christensen (2004) observes that although in-depth interviews are indeed used in these types of studies, participant observation has become the more extensively employed means of investigating the group of interest.

The expression *participant observation* implies the role of researcher as instrument (Streubert & Carpenter, 1995). This suggests quite directly the principal role assumed by an investigator in identifying, interpreting, and analyzing a given culture. The researcher is an *instrument* in the sense of observing and collecting cultural data. More specifically, the researcher *observes* in the context of actually becoming a participant in the cultural setting under study; hence, the expression **participant observation** or **participant-observer research**.

With somewhat more detail, R. Gold in the late 1950s (as cited in Ballinger, Yardley, & Payne, 2004, p. 107) "described four levels of interaction between the researcher/observer and the observed: 'complete participant,' 'participant-as-observer,' 'observer-as-participant,' and 'complete observer.'" These distinctions are pointed out here simply to acknowledge the possible range of involvement that a researcher functioning in a given culture may have on the participant-to-observer continuum.

Along with the features of ethnographic research already cited, other characteristics of this research method are the fieldwork and cyclic nature of data collection/analysis aspects (Streubert & Carpenter, 1995). Quite obviously, the fieldwork aspect indicates that the researcher operates in the place

where the culture of interest is (i.e., in the "field"). The cyclic nature of data collection/analysis suggests that due to the seemingly boundless similarities and differences in human experience, the ethnographic researcher must continually revisit these variances with a recognition that one really never exhaustively describes behavior embedded in any culture. Bare Bones Box 8-6 displays in summary form the several essential features of the ethnographic method for doing qualitative research.

Possible examples of research problems in the massage therapy profession to which the ethnographic method might be applied are as follows: the reluctance to touch—even appropriately—in American society; cross-cultural differences in receptivity to massage; reservations about massage in nonregulated regions, states, or provinces; cross-cultural differences in pain perception; cross-cultural differences in CAM usage; and interpretations of therapeutic massage in the allopathic professional culture.

Additional resources on the ethnographic research method beyond those already cited include the following: Brockopp and Hastings-Tolsma (2003); Burns and Grove (2003); Creswell (1998); Domholdt (2000); Gillis and Jackson (2002); McBurney (2001);

BARE BONES BOX 8-6

Essential Features of the Ethnographic Research Method

- Formulation of a research question of the following basic form: How is human behavior to be understood and interpreted given the cultural context in which it is embedded?
- Culture is a basic theme — that is, ways of life of a group of people reflecting patterns of behavior and customs.
- Behavior is studied from within the culture (i.e., *emic* approach) or from outside the culture with cross-cultural interests (i.e., *etic* approach).
- Reliance is primarily on participant observation and in-depth interviews for data collection purposes
- Participant observation implies the role of researcher as instrument — that is, researcher observes in the context of becoming a participant in the culture; hence, the expression participant-observer research.
- Four levels of interaction exist between the researcher/observer and the observed: complete participant, participant-as-observer, observer-as-participant, and complete observer.
- Researcher operates in the field (i.e., the place where the culture of interest exists).
- Data collection/analysis is cyclic and continual in nature due to boundless similarities and differences in human experience.

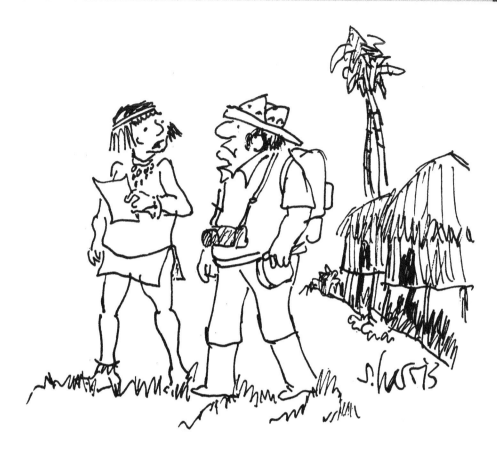

"You can't build a hut, you don't know how to find edible roots and you know nothing about predicting the weather. In other words, you do *terribly* on our IQ test."

HUMOR BREAK ■ Just as the ethnographic researchers have been saying all along! (From Harris, S. [1991]. *"You want proof? I'll give you proof!"*: More cartoons from Sidney Harris. New York: W. H. Freeman.)

Polgar and Thomas (2000); Roper and Shapira (2000); and Smith and Davis (2003).

FURTHER CONSIDERATIONS OF THE CONTEXTUAL/ INTERPRETIVE-ORIENTED RESEARCH STRATEGY

BROADENING THE PHILOSOPHICAL PERSPECTIVES AND METHODOLOGICAL OPTIONS FOR DOING RESEARCH

Parts Two and Three of this book (Chapters 2 through 7) covered the quantitative research category and its three affiliated research strategies: difference-oriented, association-oriented, and descriptive-oriented. The philosophical basis or perspective underlying quantitative research is known as **postpositivism**, a less extreme view of reality, truth, and values than its historical predecessor, **positivism**.

This chapter spans the qualitative research category, its one affiliated strategy designated as the contextual/interpretive-oriented research strategy, and the four corresponding research methods: case study, phenomenological, grounded theory, and ethnographic. The philosophical view underlying qualitative research is known as **constructivism**, a less extreme view of reality, truth, and values than its own historical successor, **postmodernism**.

This tedious distinction between the two philosophical worldviews underlying quantitative research and qualitative research is being made simply because they drive the methodologies that define quantitative research and qualitative research. These distinctions in philosophical perspectives and research methodologies are developed by Denzin (1996) and Denzin and Lincoln (1994), and they are discussed at length by Miller, Hengst, and Wang (2003) in very succinct ways.

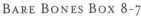

BARE BONES BOX 8-7

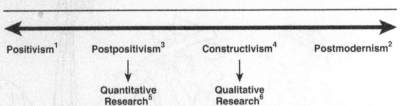

Philosophical Perspectives and Their Corresponding Implications for the Research Process and Categories

Positivism[1] Postpositivism[3] Constructivism[4] Postmodernism[2]

Quantitative Research[5]   Qualitative Research[6]

[1] Naive realist position holds that there is a reality out there that can be studied objectively and understood (Denzin & Lincoln, as cited by Miller et al., 2003).

[2] Radical doubt position counters the naive realist view in that "there can never be a final, accurate representation of what is meant or said, only different textual representations of different experiences" (Denzin, 1996, p. 132, as quoted by Miller et al., 2003).

[3] "Postpositivism rests on the assumption that reality can never be fully apprehended, only approximated. Postpositivists use multiple methods to capture as much of reality as possible; emphasize the discovery and verification of theories; and apply traditional evaluative criteria, such as validity" (Miller et al., 2003, p. 220, citing Denzin & Lincoln).

[4] Constructivism is defined as involving "a relativist ontology (there are multiple realities), a subjective epistemology (knower and subject create understandings), and a naturalistic (in the natural world) set of methodological procedures" (Denzin & Lincoln, 1994, p. 13, as quoted by Miller et al., 2003).

[5] Quantitative research category is rooted philosophically in postpositivism.

[6] Qualitative research category is rooted philosophically in constructivism.

With these resources in mind, Bare Bones Box 8-7 provides a summary of the philosophical continuum that has positivism and postmodernism at the two extreme poles, and postpositivism and constructivism at the more middle-ground positions. This summary also attempts to characterize the implications that exist for the range of research methodologies surveyed in Chapters 2 through 8.

There is no justifiable reason why a researcher should have to be restricted to either of these two philosophical perspectives and their corresponding research categories. Why not allow both to be in consideration as one tries to decide which research approach is better suited to the research problem and question at hand?

NOT SIMPLY AN EITHER-OR, BUT PERHAPS A MIXED/BLENDED/COMBINED METHODS APPROACH

Accordingly, the issue for the researcher is not an either-or deliberation, but rather the possibility of using two or more research methods from the quantitative *and* qualitative categories. This is commonly referred to as taking a **mixed/blended/combined methods** approach to addressing the research question. It is also variously known in the professional literature as a blended-methods or combined-methods approach. Excellent resources for the

mixed-methods approach include the works of Creswell (2003), Flick (2002), Johnstone (2004), Morse (1991), and Thomas (2003).

Morse (1991) elaborates on a mixed-method, combined quantitative-qualitative methodology, using the expression **methodological triangulation** to designate "the use of at least two methods, usually qualitative and quantitative, to address the same research problem" (p. 120). Flick (2002), likewise, discusses *triangulation* as different research perspectives being combined and supplemented, thereby expanding the focus on the research problem.

THE ARGUMENT FOR BLENDING OR COMBINING THE QUANTITATIVE AND QUALITATIVE RESEARCH CATEGORIES INTO A MIXED-METHODS APPROACH

The rationale or justification for using a blended/combined/mixed/triangulated research approach was touched on in the preceding section. To elaborate somewhat, though, the insights offered by both the postpositivist and constructivist philosophical perspectives potentially can enrich the investigation of a given problem area by allowing the researcher to be more inclusive rather than exclusive where worldviews are concerned. Also, this increased inclusiveness plays out well in terms of more methodological options available to the investigator so that the research problem may be approached from complementary—rather than competing—strategies.

Our earlier display of the research universe in Chapter 1 (see Figure 1-1) can now be reconfigured to reflect the notion of quantitative and qualitative research being combined. Figure 8-6 displays not only the quantitative, qualitative, and integrative research categories as existing separately, but also the quantitative and qualitative realms overlap to constitute a blended- or mixed-research possibility.

ILLUSTRATION OF THE CASE STUDY METHOD: AN ANALYSIS OF A COMPLETE RESEARCH ARTICLE

Box 8-8 contains the complete research article by Anderson (1999) that illustrates the case study research method. This researcher investigated the dynamics present when a team of six practitioners representing different mainstream or alternative medicine healing traditions convened to examine, diagnose, and prescribe for a patient suffering from chronic, severe, treatment-resistant back pain. Of concern was the extent to which members of an

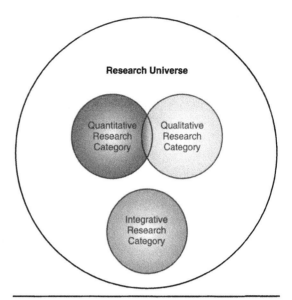

FIGURE 8-6 ■ The research universe: quantitative, qualitative, and integrative research categories as well as the mixing or blending of the quantitative and qualitative (overlapping or intersection of quantitative and qualitative). *Note:* The small section showing the overlapping, or intersection, of the quantitative and qualitative categories represents the mixing or blending of the two categories.

BOX 8-8   A CASE STUDY IN INTEGRATIVE MEDICINE: ALTERNATIVE THEORIES AND THE LANGUAGE OF BIOMEDICINE

Robert Anderson, M.D., Ph.D., D.C.

Abstract

In this case study, a diverse panel of 6 practitioners of mainstream and/or alternative medicine plus a moderator convened as an experiment in practicing integrative medicine to examine, diagnose, and prescribe for a patient suffering from chronic, severe, treatment-resistant back pain. Although panel members represented a wide range of theories of health and healing, they were able to communicate easily with one another by limiting themselves to the scientific language of biomedicine. From the perspective of medical anthropology, this can be interpreted as an unplanned and unconscious process of cultural imitation in a medical marketplace in which cultural differentiation formerly prevailed. Although the shift from differentiation to imitation was limited in this experiment to the sharing of a single language of discourse and to recommendations of mutually compatible treatment options, it raises an important question. With the institutionalization of integrated medical practice, will alternative medical systems survive only if they are stripped down to being no more than alternative therapeutic modalities?

Working Together

In less than decade, an unprecedented openness to radical change has witnessed the establishment of many new programs designed to encourage and institutionalize the sharing of patients across the historically unbridgeable medico-political chasm that used to, and often still does, rigidly separate physicians and surgeons from practitioners of alternative medicine (Angell and Kassirer, 1998). This new way of practicing is often referred to as integrative medicine.

The integrated medicine centers one reads about are usually associated with medical schools and well-known medical centers such as the Cedars-Sinai Medical Center in Los Angeles, the Stanford University Medical Center, and the UCLA Center for East-West Medicine. Little attention has been given to grass-roots efforts, locally driven without the benefits of special funding and well-paid staff. I report here on one such bootstrap operation. Known as the Health Medicine Forum (HMF), it has been meeting since 1996 at John Muir Medical Center in Walnut Creek, California. The HMF is directed by a specialist in internal medicine who himself shifted to an alternative way of practicing medicine by emphasizing nutritional

Text continued on p. 166

BOX 8-8   A CASE STUDY IN INTEGRATIVE MEDICINE: ALTERNATIVE THEORIES AND THE LANGUAGE OF BIOMEDICINE—CONT'D

and lifestyle counseling. From 3 to 6 medical doctors and about 50 to 75 unorthodox practitioners now meet monthly and in an annual summer convention to investigate how they might create new options for healing by learning to work together on a basis of mutual understanding and respect. Although the eventual goal is to share patients, the major effort to date has been to demonstrate what each kind of practitioner might contribute if they were to share responsibility for care of the sick.

As a way to demonstrate how motivated practitioners reliant on local, private initiative are beginning to work toward integrating their practices, I report on one of these meetings in which a 35-year-old white female supermarket clerk suffering from chronic, severe, treatment-resistant low back pain was examined and evaluated by each of 6 different practitioners who then formed a panel, moderated by the director, to discuss her health problems before an audience of 40 other practitioners and the patient herself. Because this was exploratory, all were providing volunteer expertise. On the panel (in addition to the moderator) were an orthopedic surgeon; a physician boarded in family medicine who specializes in a form of alternative, nonsurgical practice known as orthopedic medicine, which includes the practice of spinal manipulation and prolotherapy (the administration of sclerosant injections to create an inflammatory response); a psychologist specializing in biofeedback; a chiropractor; a practitioner of traditional Chinese medicine (TCM) who emigrated from China less than 2 years earlier; and a body worker. The purpose was to allow each of the 6 to explain what he or she might offer this patient if they were to collaborate.

As a medical anthropologist, I have been a member of the HMF since shortly after it was founded. I believe that an anthropologist has a contribution to make when practitioners who specialize in different healing traditions meet together to explore how they can coexist to the benefit of themselves and of people in need of healthcare. I offer this case study in order to raise one main question that must be answered if integrative medicine is to become a reality. How can practitioners share a patient if they evaluate and diagnose in terms of explanatory models (EMs) that constitute radically different alternatives to one another?

Discourse in the Shared Idiom of Biomedicine

The potential for ideological confrontation over differing medical theories was inherent in this meeting. Yet, dialogue among practitioners proceeded smoothly. Alternative theories were not contested. In fact, they were not even discussed as part of what panel members shared or disputed with one another. In a couple of instances when elements of non-main-stream or non-Western theory did surface, they were allowed to stand without comment, unchallenged and ignored.

Rather than confrontation, every one of the panel members discussed diagnosis in terms of a biomedical conceptualization of the anatomy, physiology, and tissue pathology involved in this case of spine-related pain and disability.

Orthopedic medicine, orthopedic surgery, and psychology

The orthopedic physician, who presented the patient as one he had been treating with only limited success, and the orthopedic surgeon who spoke after him, set the stage for this acceptance of the medical EM when they each stated that, as medical doctors, they were in agreement on a diagnosis of ligamental instability in the right sacroiliac joint compounded by secondary effects including trochanteric bursitis and emotional instability. The psychologist, whose EM resonates comfortably with that of mainstream medical practice, also accepted that diagnosis.

Chiropractic

Just over a century ago, chiropractic was founded on the basis of a competing EM, which doctors and chiropractors disputed fiercely for most of the twentieth century (Keating, 1990; Anderson, 1997). Chiropractors taught that back pain and other diseases result from misalignments (subluxations) of the spine, and therefore, that the only treatment needed for many diseases was to skillfully and precisely determine the direction and force needed for a hands-on thrust to re-position a subluxated vertebra and relieve nerve pressure. Most chiropractors have moved away from the limitations of this overly simplistic explanation, having adapted and modified the original paradigm so that it is consistent with current explanations based on medical anatomy and physiology (Haldeman, 1992).

The chiropractor on the panel, as part of his training, completed courses in both medical and chiropractic subjects. It is not surprising then, that he demonstrated an easy familiarity with medical thinking and obviously experienced no difficulty in agreeing that the basic pathology was a strain of the sacroiliac ligaments. He did offer a further chiropractic point of view, but it was justified by biomechanical reasoning consistent with the findings of scientific anatomy.

Chinese medicine

In discussing this patient, the doctor from the Peoples' Republic of China did not say anything at all about meridians, Qi, the law of five elements, yin and yang, or any of the other defining concepts of Chinese medicine that he would undoubtedly have invoked were he discussing the case with other practitioners of Chinese medicine. Nor did any member of the panel or audience ask him to do so. Contemporary practitioners of TCM, like chiropractors, complete courses in medical subjects as part of their training, whether in China, North America, or elsewhere. This practitioner was obviously accustomed to providing a biomedical rationale for how he practices, and did so with ease.

The TCM practitioner did deviate markedly from the medical paradigm, and from orthodox theory in TCM as well, when he explained that the patient was a scorpion/ox and therefore was romantic, with an emotional need to allow herself to sing, as he put it. He also located the pain between the kidneys, which, he said, are like 2 generators, left and right, male and female, their interaction producing bioelectricity. He clearly considered the astrological concept and the concept of gendered kidneys as an energy generator significant, but made no attempt to explain why, and no one queried him on either issue. The TCM practitioner also accepted the challenge to be one of healing painful ligaments in the sacroiliac spine, conceptualized in Western rather than traditional Chinese anatomic terms.

Body Work

The next practitioner spoke without direct reference to any alternative system of thought. She stated that she had a background in body work of all kinds, including Eastern and Western, and that she currently does "Berry Work," (a version of body work taught by Lauren Berry, now deceased). I learned later as part of my one-on-one follow-up with panel members that she was also trained in Chinese medicine and practiced as a licensed acupuncturist. In her presentation on the panel, she explained her thinking almost solely in terms of basic anatomy and physiology. The one exception was a passing reference to energy that implied a nonbiomedical concept of vital energy or a system of thought alternative practitioners, including those in Chinese medicine, often refer to as energetics. This practitioner agreed completely that the culprit was sacroiliac strain.

In summary, the biomedical paradigm, drawing on basic clinical sciences, was used by every panel member as a minimal shared language of discourse they all easily accessed for characterizing this patient's health problems. Specific explanatory concepts from alternative medical systems were not articulated. Nor, it would appear, were they felt to be required in order to confer as colleagues. By this acquiescence, however, they inadvertently colluded, apparently without awareness, in a remarkable shift from an approach in which each might offer an alternative medical paradigm of diagnosis and treatment to proposals of isolated therapy modalities wrenched free of theoretical justifications other than those of biomedicine.

Providing Care is What Counts

Without being instructed in advance on how they were to proceed, the attention of the panel members spontaneously oriented to treatment options rather than explanatory models, beginning with the orthopedic physician who spoke of the multiple treatments he had already provided for this patient, including analgesic medications and an injection of the sacroiliac joint with an anesthetic-cortico-steroid medication: both standard medical procedures. The injection resulted in complete but temporary relief of all pain symptoms, which confirmed the diagnosis but did not provide a cure. Although the patient's pain appeared to be about 30% less than it was at the start 6 months earlier, she was not progressing and was therefore invited by her doctor to participate in this experimental program as a free service so that the two of them could learn what other practitioners might have to offer.

As will become clear in what follows, successful communication among practitioners stood in contrast to a communication breakdown between each of the practitioners and the patient. This breakdown was not distinctive for involving alternative healthcare providers. On the contrary, it instantiated an all too familiar inability of patients to know what doctors are talking about when medical terminology is used and the pace of explanation is rapid. Probably all of the members of the panel are experienced in avoiding this kind of failure in daily practice, but under the circumstances of that evening, they tended to address each other and the audience rather than the patient who, in a sense, was merely one among many in attendance.

The HMF now convenes two integrated panels a week, but communication with patients appears to be less of a problem than it was in this case, in part because outside observers are no longer admitted, and in part because panel members, based on this case study, have been alerted to the importance of making themselves intelligible to each patient.

As concerns the participation of panel members, while it is true that discussions of theory did not occupy them, it is equally true that each one evaluated treatment options on the basis of divergent theories and training. As the orthopedic physician put it in his opening remarks, neurologists tend to treat nerves, chiropractors tend to treat spinal joints, and prolotherapists tend to inject ligaments.

Orthopedics

That comment was prescient, starting with the orthopedic surgeon, whose first thought was whether surgery might produce a definitive curve. He determined, however, that it was not appropriate in this case, so that option was immediately disregarded.

In its place he recommended an assortment of conservative treatment options widely applied in his profession. Interestingly, although he characterized the bursitis as probably a reaction to the primary lesion at the SI joint, his first thought was that he would aggressively treat it with corticosteroid injections, backed up with manual stretching of the overlying iliotibial band. For the sacroiliac joint as such he recommended a vigorous physical therapy program, including coaching in posture and movement (stabilization of the lower back). He also thought she should be enrolled in a weight reduction program, because she had become somewhat obese.

Among other things, he said he would prescribe an "antipsychotic." (That choice of words was unfortunate. His reference was to a class of drugs known as tricylic antidepressants, which are widely prescribed by psychiatrists for nonpsychotic as well as psychotic patients suffering from depression.

Continued

They are often prescribed for back pain patients in small amounts because they have the paradoxical effect of reducing pain. In addition, that class of drugs may improve sleep, which is often disturbed and nonrestorative in back pain patients. They may also diminish depression, which is a common comorbidity of long-lasting back pain, even though the standard dosage for back pain is much less than that normally prescribed by psychiatrists for the treatment of depression as such.)

The Patient's Response
A year and a half after she had been interrogated, examined, diagnosed, and advised by the panelists, I met with the patient in her home to talk with her about how she had responded that evening and what she had experienced in the months that followed. Our conversation was recorded on audiotape. In this open-ended questioning I particularly wanted to know whom if anyone, she had turned to for further care.

In discussing the recommendations of the surgeon, she remembered being distracted by the mention of surgery and horrified that he seemed to consider her psychotic. No doubt for those reasons, she was quite unable to recall any of his recommendations relating to injections, physical therapy, and weight reduction. "What he said didn't really make a lot of sense," she confided. "He didn't really get to know me, I didn't value his opinion much."

Part of the social dynamics of the evening for all participants was that they oscillated between speaking to the patient and addressing their remarks to fellow practitioners on the panel and in the audience (between speaking plain English and speaking in medical terms). The surgeon was well understood by all of the practitioners, several of whom particularly acknowledged that his brief history and rapid physical examination demonstrated enormous diagnostic skill that they admired and respected. Evidently, his success in dialoguing with practitioners was achieved at the cost of a failure to communicate effectively with the patient in that particular encounter.

Chiropractic
As he picked up the microphone, the chiropractor began by acknowledging that the surgeon's recommendations were worth considering, but then contributed recommendations of his own that he preferred. The patient should be enrolled in a low-stress, gentle breathing exercise program, he suggested. As another possibility, he might refer her for Alexander training (in posture and movement) so that she could learn to reduce strain when walking, getting up from chairs, and so on. In particular, he recommended a method of pressuring and stretching of muscles to free them from possible adhesions, a practice known as myofascial release.

In addition, he explained that from "a chiropractic perspective" one does not adjust a hypermobile joint such as the patient's right sacroiliac. Adjusting allows a joint to move more freely, so it only makes a lax joint worse to manipulate it. However, the body seems to compensate for hypermobility in one of the joints of the spine or pelvis by developing compensatory hypomobility (tightness or bracing) elsewhere. To restore normal dynamics to the spine as a unified entity, the hypomobile joints alone should be adjusted.

Finally, drawing on chiropractic teachings on the importance of proper nutrition, including trace elements, for musculoskeletal and whole body health he would evaluate her need for nutritional supplements, including vitamins.

The patient's response
From prior experience with chiropractors, the patient was well disposed to these recommendations, although she understood very little about them. As with the surgeon, they were addressed to the audience, and not meaningfully to her. What she came away with was limited to the feeling that this chiropractor might help her with spinal adjustments.

In the months that followed, the chiropractor was the only practitioner she went to for treatment additional to that of the orthopedic physician, who was her primary provided for this work-related injury. As we shall see, she was very interested in seeking treatment from some of the others, but to do so was never a realistic possibility. Her medical bills were paid by workman's compensation insurance, and the only practitioners who could be reimbursed under that scheme were medical and chiropractic doctors. Her limited personal finances allowed for none of the other possibilities that were of interest to her.

Chinese medicine
The practitioner of TCM offered no criticism of the preceding medical and chiropractic recommendations, but clearly had priorities of his own. He recommended acupuncture, adding that in his view the patient would not respond well to that treatment until she was prepared for it by achieving emotional release.

In addition, this practitioner said that the patient needed to change her diet completely. In Chinese medical thought, an emphasis on diet is not exceptional. Two medical anthropologists concluded from their research in Hong Kong that, "If there is one thing universal in Chinese medicine, classical or folk, professional or self-managed, that one thing is diet therapy. Modification of food patterns is part of medication, not to be separated from the use of drugs" (Anderson and Anderson, 1975; p 143). It is unusual in Chinese medical practice, however, that the recommendation be in favor of a strictly vegetarian diet, which this doctor advocated with passion for ethical as well as dietary reasons.

The patient's response

The recommendation for acupuncture went unnoticed, no doubt because it was offered only as a passing comment and without explanation of how it might impact on chronic pain. What impressed the patient was what she interpreted as the recommendation that she might be cured by shifting to a vegetarian diet. She was skeptical of that implied claim and was, in any case, totally unwilling to remove meat from her diet. She did acknowledge, though, that she needed to give attention to her diet.

The body worker

Until this moment, all of the panelists spoke from a sitting position at the speaker's table, but that staging suddenly changed as the body worker, microphone in hand, suddenly rose to her feet to say, "I agree with everything you said about her, *and I would teach her how to breathe* (speaker's emphasis). She does not know how to breathe, and until she learns how, she can't manage her own pain." "That's true," the Chinese doctor interjected, while the chiropractor nodded in agreement.

"The pain in the sacroiliac joint," she continued, "is an excess pain. That means I would not directly massage it, which would only make it worse. Massaging it made it worse when I examined her (and administered a trial of massage). And the reason it made it worse is, it's like pouring oil on fire. When you have a lot of energy in something and you massage it, then what happens is that instead of making it better it makes it worse."

Although theorized in energetic terms, her recommendation was consistent with that of the chiropractor, who for biomechanical reasons would not adjust the joint. However, where he would adjust related hypomobility in other joints, she took the position that for the pain to abate, new breathing techniques would be required. "I teach a class on pain management at a private hospital, and one of the main things I teach is how to breathe, and how to count while they are breathing so that they can get their pain under control. I would teach her how to work on herself so she could help me to heal her. Then after we got the pain a little better, then I would start rearranging her muscle structure so that the 'chief pathway' [not explained] could open. The work I do is Berry Work, which actually repositions and realigns the muscles. (Note the similarity to myofascial release recommended by the chiropractor.) It doesn't break them down like Rolfing does, though, but is a similar thing. It repositions the muscles through occasional movement."

In addition, she would refer the patient to someone else for a vigorous stretching and strengthening program known as Pilates work, or alternatively she would refer for training in a Chinese form of movement and meditation known as Qigong.

Finally, the body worker introduced a theme that all of the others eventually were to come together on. What she should do would depend on the patient's interests and motivation. "I would communicate with her to find out who she can work with, including for the emotional stuff — find that person — she needs to be able to express herself — to have fun. There's a kid inside there who wants to get out."

The patient's response

In talking with her months later, I found that the patient consistently remembered one main recommendation from each practitioner and tended to ignore or forget all the others. What she remembered from the body worker was that she needed to learn how to breathe. She wished she could have been taught that, but assumed that the cost would not be reimbursed and therefore gave it no further thought. As a compromise, she attempted on her own initiative to change her breathing habits, but without notable success.

Psychology

Finally, the biofeedback specialist offered his suggestions. "Using a bunch of equipment I don't carry in my back pocket," he said, "I would look at muscle fatigue, especially on the right side, and some compensating muscle action on the left side. Secondly, I would look at what happens cortically. Many with fibromyalgia have problems not supposed to be neurologically centered — a lot of high amplitude, low frequency activity that's monitorable in the cortex — and that can be inhibited with biofeedback training."

He then added, "I know it's not popular, but I would suggest real aggressive passivity: about 6 weeks in bed." (This recommendation appealed to no one, and was challenged by the surgeon). After extended immobilization, he would want her to get into a strengthening program and to be coached in ways to pace herself at work so that she wouldn't further injure herself.

The patient's response

What she recalled from the psychologist's recommendations was not biofeedback, about which she understood nothing, but that he would order bedrest for a month or two. That is exactly what she would have liked, but workman's compensation would not authorize it and her employer insisted that she return to work, so it was never an option.

Continued

BOX 8-8   A CASE STUDY IN INTEGRATIVE MEDICINE: ALTERNATIVE THEORIES AND THE LANGUAGE OF BIOMEDICINE—CONT'D

In sum, the treatment suggestions for this patient were quite numerous. They included steroid injections, stretching of tendons, posture and movement training, antidepressive medication, a weight reduction program, prolonged bed rest, an exercise program (including Pilotes or Qigong), Alexander training, myofascial release, Berry work, spinal adjustment, nutritional supplements, a vegetarian diet, acupuncture, psychological counseling, coaching in how to breathe, biofeedback, and learning to pace herself in order to move within the constraints of a disability.

Uniting Behind a Plan

At this point, as participants confirmed when I spoke with them afterwards, we were all quite overwhelmed by the many different possibilities proposed as treatment options. "How," the moderator asked, "are we going to work together as a team?"

The consensus was that the patient herself, in consultation with her attending physician, would have to decide which recommendations she should follow. A week or two later, she and her doctor agreed that she might profit from additional chiropractic care, which she subsequently received for several weeks. With her spine thus 'tuned up', as one observer put it, her doctor then administered a series of sacroiliac injections of a caustic (sclerosant) agent that appears to strengthen and toughen ligaments (see Klein and Eek, 1997). When I interviewed her I found that she had responded well to the prolotherapy, although she still experienced moderate intermittent pain after clerking for several hours at the checkout counter to the supermarket where she was employed. Her family life had returned to normal and her job responsibilities on the whole were easier because her employer had replaced some of her clerking duties with office work. She is very pleased with her experience in integrated medicine.

Sometimes all Medicine is Alternative

In the management of chronic low back pain, mainstream medical approaches, surgical and nonsurgical alike, often fail or are of uncertain value (Deyo, 1991; Tollison et al., 1989, p 63; Postacchini et al., 1988). The scientific literature on treatment efficacy is suggestive rather than definitive, because back pain is a category of diseases rather than a firm diagnosis (van Tulder et al., 1997). As concerns treatments recommended by this panel, spinal manipulative therapy performed by chiropractors or orthopedic physicians has been shown to result in quicker recoveries for patients with acute or chronic nonspecific low back pain involving dysfunctional vertebral joints, but no trial has targeted sacroiliac dysfunction as such (Anderson et al., 1992; Mead et al., 1995). Some empirical studies suggest that acupuncture may be beneficial for musculoskeletal pain but again, sacroiliac problems are not specifically identified (National Institutes of Health, 1997). Although many other recommendations made by the panel for the management of generic back pain sound reasonable on logical grounds, no solid evidence supports any of them unequivocally.

However, it should also be noted that research has not demonstrated that the recommended treatments are useless or harmful. The one exception is prolonged bed rest, which would only be suitable for someone in extreme pain, which was not true of this patient (Bigos et al., 1994).

Because the voiced recommendations of the panel were couched in general terms, some would need to be evaluated in greater detail if they were to be implemented. One must be alert to the possibility that, just as with prescribed drugs, certain herbs, vitamins, and dietary regimes can be harmful. For example, comfrey is an herb that can be taken internally for back pain, but it is dangerous because it can harm the liver (Anderson, 1992). Similarly, when recommending vitamins, overdosing with oil-soluble vitamins such as vitamin E can cause sickness and death. Again, in working out dietary regimes, extreme vegetarian diets can lead to pernicious anemia.

More precisely, as concerns this case study, no medical, surgical, or alternative research provides scientific guidelines for the treatment of chronic or recurrent sacroiliac instability, although a single case study of treatment with sclerosant injections does provide one example prior to this one of achieving a good outcome for a patient (Frost, 1994). Where efficacy cannot be demonstrated for any one form of treatment, every form of treatment that clearly does no harm becomes an alternative one may want to consider.

Alternative Theories: Do They Matter?

Ideally, all members of the HMF are expected to make themselves knowledgeable about the diverse theories and methods that inform each of the alternative approaches represented in their association. However, as this case study demonstrates, it is quite possible to collaborate in the absence of such understandings because, under the impact of globalization, the biological sciences widely if not universally provide a shared basis for discourse that is adequate, if not perfect, for integrated practice. Moreover, I would postulate that for mutuality to work, differing explanatory models must not be allowed to become symbols of confrontation and differentiation, as predictably happens when interaction is based on competition rather than collaboration.

The example of the HMF panel described here can be taken as indicative of what may be occurring on a widespread basis. It seems to document a shift from alternative medical systems as we have known them in the past toward a future in which highly divergent underlying theoretical bases may become increasingly subsumed as variations or versions of basic biomedicine with its foundations in scientific anatomy, physiology, and pathology. Alternative systems may well survive in integrated settings, in other words, as treatment modalities, as alternative therapies, but not as highly

Box 8-8	A CASE STUDY IN INTEGRATIVE MEDICINE: ALTERNATIVE THEORIES AND THE LANGUAGE OF BIOMEDICINE — CONT'D

differentiated ways of conceptualizing ill health and healing. If they are to survive as unique medical systems, as truly different paradigms, perhaps they must be practiced in a competitive environment rather than one of integrated medicine.

Whether it is better to work toward integration and imitation or toward competition and differentiation is an issue that would take us beyond what can be attempted in this article.

Acknowledgments

I am grateful to the following for helpful contributions, comments, criticism, corrections, and suggestions relating to an earlier draft of this paper: Richard Gracer, MD, Colette De-Vore, Lac, Len Ochs, PhD, Len Saputo, MD, Craig Weinston, DC, three anonymous reviewers, and the patient, who shall also remain anonymous. Responsibility for any remaining errors or problems, of course, rests with me alone.

References

Anderson, EN, Anderson ML. 1975. Folk dietetics in two Chinese communities, and its implications for the study of Chinese medicine. In: Kleinman A, Kunstadter P, Alexander ER, Gale JL (eds). Medicine in Chinese Cultures: Comparative Studies of Health Care in Chinese and Other Societies. DHEW Publication No. (NIH) 75–6531, Washington, DC: U.S. Government Printing Office, 1974:143–175.

Anderson R. Comfrey in the Chinese Materia Medica. Asian Medicine Newsletter 1992;(2):7–11.

Anderson R. Is chiropractic mainstream or alternative? A view from medical anthropology. In: Advances in Chiropractic. Vol 4. (An Official Publication of the American Chiropractic Association) St. Louis: Mosby, 1997:555–578.

Anderson R, Meeker WC, Wirick BE, Mootz RD, Kirk DH, and Adams A. A meta-analysis of clinical trials of spinal manipulation. J Manipulative Physiol Ther 1992;15:181–194.

Angell M, Kassirer JP. Alternative medicine — The risks of untested and unregulated remedies. N Engl J Med 1998;339:839–841.

Bigos S, Bowyer O, Braen G. Low pack problems in adults, clinical practice guideline No. 14. AHCPR Publication No. 95-0642. Rockville, MD: Agency for Health Care Policy and Research, Public Health Service, U.S. Department of Health and Human Services, December, 1994.

Deyo RA. Fads in the treatment of low pack pain. N Engl J Med 1991;324:1039–1040.

Frost WW. Case study: Sacro-iliac problems and the benefit of prolotherapy over time. J Orthop Med 1994;16.

Haldeman S. Principles and Practice of Chiropractic. 2nd ed. Norwalk, CT: Appleton & Lange, 1992.

Keating JC Jr. Rationalism, empiricism and the philosophy of science in chiropractic. Chiropractic History 1990;10:23–30.

Klein RG, Eek BCJ. Prolotherapy: An alternative approach to managing low back pain. J Musculoskeletal Med 1997;14:45–59.

Mead TW, Dyer S, Browne W, Frank AO. Randomised comparison of chiropractic and hospital outpatient management for low back pain: Results from extended follow up. Br Med J 1995;311:349–351.

National Institutes of Health. Consensus Development Conference Statement: Acupuncture. November 3–5. Revised Draft, 11/5/97. 1997:1–17.

Postacchini F, Facchini M, Palieri P. Efficacy of various forms of conservative treatment in low back pain: A comparative study. Neuro-Orthopedics 1988;6:28–35.

Tollison CD, Kriegel ML, Satterthwaite JR. Comprehensive treatment of acute and chronic low back pain: A clinical outcome comparison. Orthop Rev 1989;18:59–64.

van Tulder MW, Koes BW, Bouter LM. Conservative treatment of acute and chronic nonspecific low back pain: A systematic review of randomized controlled trials of the most common interventions. Spine 1977;22:2128–2156.

Address reprint requests to:
Robert Anderson, M.D., Ph.D., D.C.
Professor of Anthropology
Mills College
5000 MacArthur Boulevard
Oakland, CA 94613

From Anderson, R. (1999). A case study in integrative medicine: Alternative theories and the language of biomedicine. *The Journal of Alternative and Complementary Medicine, 5*(2), 165-173.

integrative medicine team can coexist to the benefit of themselves and of people in need of health care.

Based on your careful reading of the Anderson (1999) article, let us now critique this research study. In so doing, we will rely on our previous discussions in this chapter of the case study method, with particular attention to the essential features of a case study as summarized in Box 8-2. Also, we will rely on Greenhalgh's (2001) critical appraisal checklist for critiquing qualitative research as shown in Box 8-3 and repeated in this section.

FOCUS OF CRITIQUE QUESTION 1: CLINICAL PROBLEM VIA RESEARCH QUESTION
Did the paper describe an important clinical problem addressed with a clearly formulated question?

The abstract and the "Working Together" section of the article address a generic clinical problem as well as related issues. The generic problem seems to deal with the extent to which members of a multidisciplinary integrative medicine team can coexist to the benefit of not only themselves, but, more important, the people needing their health care services.

One related issue appears to focus on the advisability of moving from professional cultural differentiation to cultural imitation favoring both the language of biomedicine and only mutually compatible treatment options. Another related issue seems to be a potential scaling down of alternative medical systems in the face of integrated medicine becoming institutionalized.

The clinical problem and related issues just mentioned could possibly generate two or more research questions. In fact, the abstract ends with a question regarding the impact of institutionalized integrative medicine on alternative systems. The concluding sentence of the "Working Together" section, however, offers a research question more in keeping with the clinical problem when it asks, "How can practitioners share a patient if they evaluate and diagnose in terms of explanatory models (EMs) that constitute radically different alternatives to one another?" Based on this research question, a reader should indeed have a sense of what themes to anticipate in the remainder of this case study.

FOCUS OF CRITIQUE QUESTION 2: RATIONALE FOR USING A QUALITATIVE APPROACH
Was a qualitative approach appropriate?

This study ventures into a comprehensive description and analysis of (a) the dynamics of a small professional organization (in the form of six members

from the Health Medicine Forum–HMF) and (b) the professional activity of collaborating in an integrative way to examine, diagnose, and prescribe for a patient with severe chronic back pain. The research objective is obviously to explore, interpret, and better understand the clinical issue at hand. This is all done in the context of a medical setting involving health care professionals representing diverse specialties in both allopathic and alternative traditions. Accordingly, for these as well as several other reasons still to be cited, the choice of a qualitative study in this instance is indeed justified.

FOCUS OF CRITIQUE QUESTION 3: CONTEXT/SETTING OF THE CASE AND BASIS FOR SUBJECT SELECTION
How were (a) the setting and (b) the subjects selected?

The setting represents a grassroots effort and organization (the HMF) aimed at implementing a local bootstrap attempt to provide integrative medical services. The HMF is characterized as encompassing three to six medical doctors as well as 50 to 75 alternative medicine practitioners who meet on a regular basis. Their overall objective is to explore possible innovative options for healing by learning to collaborate on a basis of reciprocal understanding and respect.

The panel of six health care professionals–moderated by the HMF's director– were volunteers from the larger organization who examined and evaluated one 35-year-old female patient suffering from chronic back pain. The panel discussed the patient's case before 40 other practitioners and the patient herself. A principal objective here was to provide each panelist with the opportunity to explain what he or she might be positioned to offer this patient if indeed they were to collaborate.

The subject/patient was invited to participate as a free service due to her lack of progress over the preceding six months. The attending orthopedic physician (and member of the panel) indicated to the patient that this program could allow both of them to learn what other practitioners might have to offer in the way of treatment.

FOCUS OF CRITIQUE QUESTION 4: CONSIDERATION GIVEN TO THE RESEARCHER'S PERSPECTIVE
What was the researcher's perspective and has this been taken into account?

The researcher–as a medical anthropologist–actually asserts his belief that his area of expertise has the potential to contribute substantially to the professional setting and task described in this case. Specifically, he maintains that an integrative medical setting in which professionals with diverse specialties are trying to collaborate on a medical case can indeed benefit by (a) posing certain relevant questions and issues and (b) exploring them in an interactive and open manner.

Part of the researcher's perspective that comes through in the form of the research question concerns the potential difficulty of diverse EMs when integrative practitioners try to collaborate on a case. One can almost detect the researcher's reservation regarding just how well this type of collaboration can succeed for all concerned. This, of course, becomes a catalyst for precisely the type of open investigation undertaken here.

Perhaps the most revealing display of the researcher's perspective appears in the final summarizing paragraph of the "Discourse in the Shared Idiom of Biomedicine" section. It seems that the author's choice of words here suggests a passion and preconceived perspective that anticipated, and indeed would have welcomed, more explanations from the alternative therapists in keeping with their alternative medical orientations. Instead, as the author notes, "they inadvertently colluded, apparently without awareness, in a remarkable shift from an approach in which each might offer an alternative medical paradigm of diagnosis and treatment to proposals of isolated therapy modalities *wrenched* [emphasis added] free of theoretical justifications other than those of biomedicine" (p. 167).

FOCUS OF CRITIQUE QUESTION 5: DETAILED DESCRIPTION OF DATA COLLECTION METHODS
What methods did the researcher use for collecting data and are these described in enough detail?

The author specifies several methods used to collect the verbal data in this case study. Those methods included the following: panel members' individual presentations directed to other members, the patient, and an audience of 40 other practitioners; discussion among members; the researcher's observations of the presentations and discussions; the researcher's one-on-one interview with each panel member as a follow-up to the discussions; and the researcher's open-ended and audiotaped interview with the patient a year and a half after the panel discussion and deliberation occurred. As evidenced by the author's characterization of the

discussions and interviews, perhaps the most pervasive method used was that of the researcher documenting the verbal exchanges along with a critique of (a) his own reactions as an observer and (b) the patient's reactions to what each of the six panel members contributed. Each of these data collection methods was described in sufficient detail.

FOCUS OF CRITIQUE QUESTION 6: DATA ANALYSIS METHOD AND QUALITY CONTROL
What methods did the researcher use to analyze the data, and what quality control measures were implemented?

The researcher apparently relied largely on his observations as described earlier, but he made an important decision to corroborate them by way of subsequent interviews with each of the six panel members as well as the patient. The data collected were verbal in nature and, accordingly, subject to idiosyncratic interpretations on the part of the researcher. The corroboration via interviews, then, was critical to ensure as much as possible the accuracy of what the researcher had observed and interpreted. These procedures appear to have been followed systematically across all six panel members. The researcher, therefore, seems to have engaged not only in a detailed content analysis of the various verbal exchanges, but also in an attempt to ensure a valid interpretation.

Although these approaches protect somewhat the quality of the data collected and analyzed, there is no mention in the report of another researcher being involved in the verbal content analysis of the exchanges among the six panel members and patient. Even with the researcher's attempt at corroboration via interviews, quality control would have been further enhanced if a second observer had been used. This would have allowed for an analysis across the two observers of the verbal data generated in the study, thereby elevating the accuracy of what was observed and its interpretation. We must quickly note, however, that in qualitative research one has to be cautious about *not* assuming that there is only one right or correct way to interpret what has been observed.

A final consideration regarding the data analysis and quality control issues is the account given by the author in the "Uniting Behind a Plan" section. There the author discusses (a) the consensus reached by the panel members regarding a treatment plan and (b) the subsequent improvement in the patient's condition. With both of those factors considered, it appears that the process of integrative medical collaboration was informative and successful as evidenced primarily by the benefit that accrued to the patient.

FOCUS OF CRITIQUE QUESTION 7: CREDIBILITY AND CLINICAL IMPORTANCE OF THE RESULTS

Are the results credible and, if so, are they clinically important?

The credibility of the results rests to a large extent on two major procedures: the researcher's systematic approach to analyzing the content of the verbal exchanges and the actual citing of actual quotes from the panel members and the patient. This allows the reader to consider not only the researcher's interpretation of matters, but also the actual verbal statements made and upon which the interpretation is based.

The clinical importance of the results can hardly be disputed given the professional consensus reached by the panel of diverse members and, more important, the subsequent improvement in the patient's condition. Also, as concluded by the author in the "Sometimes All Medicine Is Alternative" section, "when efficacy cannot be demonstrated for any one form of treatment, every form of treatment that clearly does no harm becomes an alternative one may want to consider" (p. 172). On more than one point, then, the results of this case study do indeed suggest a level of clinical importance potentially helpful to practitioners.

FOCUS OF CRITIQUE QUESTION 8: JUSTIFICATION FOR THE CONCLUSIONS DRAWN

What conclusions were drawn, and are they justified by the results?

The author implies that the conclusions of this case study extend far beyond the specifics of the case per se. Referring back to a theme developed in an earlier section of this chapter, we might consider the case reported on here to be an example of an instrumental case study. This is so because the emphasis in the report is not restricted to the specific case at hand, but rather is geared to understanding at a higher level the larger issue or event of

which the case studied is only one manifestation. Accordingly, the author makes the following observations in the final section of the report:

I would postulate that for mutuality to work, differing explanatory models must not be allowed to become symbols of confrontation and differentiation, as predictably happens when interaction is based on competition rather than collaboration.

The example of the HMF panel described here can be taken as indicative of what may be occurring on a widespread basis. It seems to document a shift from alternative medical systems as we have known them in the past toward a future in which highly divergent underlying theoretical bases may become increasingly subsumed as variations or versions of basic biomedicine with its foundations in scientific anatomy, physiology, and pathology.

Whether it is better to work toward integration and imitation or toward competition and differentiation [emphasis added] is an issue . . . beyond what can be attempted in this article. (p. 172)

The results conveyed in this case study seem to justify the conclusions reached by the author. This is said not only regarding the eventual improvement in the patient's presenting signs and symptoms of chronic back pain, but also at a more global level regarding the process of integrative medical collaboration and its implications for CAM practitioners.

FOCUS OF CRITIQUE QUESTION 9: TRANSFERABILITY OF STUDY'S FINDINGS

Are the findings of the study transferable to other clinical settings?

The author seems to suggest the transferability of this study's findings to a certain degree by virtue of his observation that the example of the HMF presented here may indicate developments in integrative medicine on a widespread basis. Presumably, the intent of this study as an instrumental case study would encourage its transferability. A more strategic factor, though, in this regard really has to do with the sampling issue in the study. The author did not really address this issue extensively. What we do know, however, is that the panel of six members and the patient in this case represent a voluntary subset of the HMF's ongoing integrative medical collaboration. More information, therefore, would really be needed to assert with confidence the true extent of the study's transferability.

THE CASE REPORT: REVISITED AND COMPARED WITH THE CASE STUDY

Having just completed an analysis of the Anderson (1999) case study, let us now revisit the comparison that can be made between a *case study* and a *case report*.

At the outset of this chapter, we briefly pointed out that single-case research methodology can be viewed as spanning three different types: (a) the single-case experimental method, (b) the single-case quantitative analysis method, and (c) the case study method (Hilliard, 1993). The single-case experimental method was discussed earlier (Chapter 5) as one way of implementing a difference-oriented research strategy; the single-case quantitative analysis method was presented as one option for descriptive-oriented studies (Chapter 7); and in this chapter the case study method was explored as one possibility for doing qualitative research.

As we also saw earlier in Chapter 7, the case report relates to the organizational scheme we are using in that it is actually a method affiliated with the *descriptive-oriented research strategy*. We could easily allow our Chapter 7 coverage of case reports to suffice. Instead, by revisiting the **case report research method** now, it enables us to perhaps better understand the similarities and differences between it and the case study method.

With all of those reasons in place, let us now return to one of our sources cited earlier in characterizing the case report method (Dumholdt, 2000). Whereas the case study is a more complete coverage typical of the qualitative research category as we have seen in this chapter, the case report provides a focused description of clinical practice, which can be developed from either a retrospective perspective or a prospective view. As distinguished by Dumholdt (2000):

> **Retrospective case reports** *are developed when a practitioner realizes that there are valuable lessons to be shared from a case in which the . . . therapy episode has been completed.* **Prospective case reports** *are developed when a practitioner, on initial contact with a patient or sometime early in the course of treatment, recognizes that the case is likely to produce interesting findings that should be shared. When a case report is developed prospectively, there is the potential for excellent control of measurement techniques and complete description of the treatments and responses as they unfold. Unfortunately, the prospective case report suffers from the possibility that the case was managed*

> *differently from usual because of the desire to publish the results in the future* (emphasis added). *(p. 148)*

It is important to note, too, that a case report may be used, retrospectively or prospectively, not only regarding clinical practice, but also with respect to educational or administrative practices.

Regarding the format of a case report, the generic coverage found in more standard research articles is appropriate here in that introductory, method, results, and discussion sections typically allow for the practice features to be adequately reported. McEwen's (2001) "Writing Case Reports" manual is a helpful resource that includes, among many valuable features, a detailed checklist organized around those components essential to a comprehensive case report. The essential components identified by McEwen include the following: an *introductory section*; a *case description section* spanning subject description/history, systems review, examination, evaluation, diagnosis, prognosis, and intervention; an *outcomes section*; and a *discussion section*.

WHERE DO WE GO FROM HERE?

QUANTITATIVE AND QUALITATIVE CATEGORIES ALREADY IN PLACE

Chapter 8 has provided information on the qualitative research category, which represents an alternative—and potentially a complement—to the quantitative research emphasis of Chapters 2 through 7. Each of these two research categories is affiliated with a certain philosophical perspective and corresponding research methodologies. These two research categories represent the preponderance of published studies available in the professional literature spanning the health and behavioral sciences, although admittedly the quantitative category has been more prevalent and extensive. There is evidence, however, that qualitative research is becoming more recognized for its own unique contributions as well as for its potential to expand our repertoire of research options (cf. Creswell, 1998, 2003; Flick, 2002).

THE INTEGRATIVE RESEARCH CATEGORY (CHAPTER 9): YET ANOTHER OPTION BEYOND QUANTITATIVE AND QUALITATIVE RESEARCH

The second of two chapters constituting Part Four of the book, Chapter 9 presents yet another research category in addition to the quantitative and qualitative ones described thus far. Chapter 9 focuses on what may be labeled the *integrative research category* in that it covers a research strategy oriented toward synthesizing previously completed studies whether they occurred in the quantitative or qualitative tradition. The six research methods that will be discussed provide the means for integrating or synthesizing the efforts of earlier researchers.

REFERENCES

Anderson, R. (1999). A case study in integrative medicine: Alternative theories and the language of biomedicine. *Journal of Alternative and Complementary Medicine, 5*(2), 165–173.

Ballinger, C., Yardley, L., & Payne, S. (2004). Observation and action research. In D. F. Marks & L. Yardley (Eds.), *Research methods for clinical and health psychology* (pp. 102–121). Thousand Oaks, CA: Sage.

Brockopp, D. Y., & Hastings-Tolsma, M. T. (2003). *Fundamentals of nursing research* (3rd ed.). Toronto: Jones & Bartlett.

Burns, N., & Grove, S. K. (2003). *Understanding nursing research* (3rd ed.). Philadelphia: W. B. Saunders.

Chamberlain, K., Camic, P., & Yardley, L. (2004). Qualitative analysis of experience: Grounded theory and case studies. In D. F. Marks & L. Yardley (Eds.), *Research methods for clinical and health psychology* (pp. 69–89). Thousand Oaks, CA: Sage.

Chenitz, W. C., & Swanson, J. M. (1986). Qualitative research using grounded theory. In W. C. Chenitz & J. M. Swanson (Eds.), *From practice to grounded theory: Qualitative research in nursing* (pp. 3–15). Menlo Park, CA: Addison-Wesley.

Christensen, L. B. (2004). *Experimental methodology* (9th ed.). Boston: Pearson/Allyn & Bacon.

Cozby, P. C. (2001). *Methods in behavioral research* (8th ed.). Boston: McGraw-Hill.

Creswell, J. W. (1998). *Qualitative inquiry and research design: Choosing among five traditions.* Thousand Oaks, CA: Sage.

Creswell, J. W. (2003). *Research design: Qualitative, quantitative, and mixed methods approaches* (2nd ed.). Thousand Oaks, CA: Sage.

Denzin, N. K. (1996). The epistemological crisis in the human disciplines: Letting the old do the work of the new. In R. Jessor, A. Colby, & R. A. Shweder (Eds.), *Ethnography and human development: Context and meaning in social inquiry* (pp. 127–151). Chicago: University of Chicago Press.

Denzin, N. K., & Lincoln, Y. S. (Eds.). (1994). *Handbook of qualitative research.* Thousand Oaks, CA: Sage.

Domholdt, E. (2000). *Physical therapy research: Principles and applications* (2nd ed.). Philadelphia: W. B. Saunders.

Flick, U. (2002). *An introduction to qualitative research* (2nd ed.). Thousand Oaks, CA: Sage.

Gillis, A., & Jackson, W. (2002). *Research for nurses: Methods and interpretation.* Philadelphia: F. A. Davis.

Giorgi, A. P., & Giorgi, B. M. (2003). The descriptive phenomenological psychological method. In P. M. Camic, J. E. Rhodes, & L. Yardley (Eds.), *Qualitative research in psychology: Expanding perspectives in methodology and design* (pp. 243–273). Washington, DC: American Psychological Association.

Goodwin, C. J. (2005). *Research in psychology: Methods and design* (4th ed.). Hoboken, NJ: John Wiley & Sons.

Greenhalgh, T. (2001). *How to read a paper: The basics of evidence based medicine* (2nd ed.). London: BMJ Books.

Harris, S. (1991). *"You want proof? I'll give you proof!": More cartoons from Sidney Harris.* New York: W. H. Freeman and Company.

Henwood, K., & Pidgeon, N. (2003). Grounded theory in psychological research. In P. M. Camic, J. E. Rhodes, & L. Yardley (Eds.), *Qualitative research in psychology: Expanding perspectives in methodology and design* (pp. 131–155). Washington, DC: American Psychological Association.

Hilliard, R. B. (1993). Single-case methodology in psychotherapy process and outcome research. *Journal of Consulting and Clinical Psychology, 61*(3), 373–380.

Johnstone, P. L. (2004). Mixed methods, mixed methodology health services research in practice. *Qualitative Health Research, 14*(2), 259–271.

Kazdin, A. E. (2003a). Drawing valid inferences from case studies. In A. E. Kazdin (Ed.), *Methodological issues & strategies in clinical research* (3rd ed.), (pp. 655–669). Washington, DC: American Psychological Association.

Kazdin, A. E. (Ed.). (2003b). *Methodological issues & strategies in clinical research* (3rd ed.). Washington, DC: American Psychological Association.

Kazdin, A. E. (2003c). *Research design in clinical psychology* (4th ed.). Boston: Allyn & Bacon.

Lukoff, D., Edwards, D., & Miller, M. (1998). The case study as a scientific method for researching alternative therapies. *Alternative Therapies in Health and Medicine, 4*(2), 44–52.

Lusardi, P. T. (1999). Selecting a research design: Quantitative versus qualitative. In J. A. Fain (Ed.), *Reading, understanding, and applying nursing research: A text and workbook* (2nd ed.) (pp. 191–218). Philadelphia, PA: F. A. Davis.

McBurney, D. H. (2001). *Research methods* (5th ed.). Belmont, CA: Wadsworth/Thomson Learning.

McEwen, I. (Ed.). (2001). *Writing case reports: A how-to manual for clinicians* (2nd ed.). Alexandria, VA: American Physical Therapy Association.

Mead, G. H. (1934). *Mind, self and society.* Chicago: University of Chicago Press.

Miller, P. J., Hengst, J. A., & Wang, S-H. (2003). Ethnographic methods: Applications from developmental cultural psychology. In P. M. Camic, J. E. Rhodes, & L. Yardley (Eds.), *Qualitative research in psychology: Expanding perspectives in methodology and design* (pp. 219–242). Washington, DC: American Psychological Association.

Morse, J. M. (1991). Approaches to qualitative-quantitative methodological triangulation. *Nursing Research, 40*(1), 120–123.

Morse, J. M., & Field, P. A. (1995). *Qualitative research methods for health professionals* (2nd ed.). Thousand Oaks, CA: Sage.

Patten, M. L. (2004). *Understanding research methods: An overview of the essentials* (4th ed.). Glendale, CA: Pyrczak.

Polgar, S., & Thomas, S. A. (2000). *Introduction to research in the health sciences* (4th ed.). St. Louis: Churchill Livingstone.

Polit, D. F., Beck, C. T., & Hungler, B. P. (2001). *Essentials of nursing research: Methods, appraisal, and utilization* (5th ed.). Philadelphia: Lippincott Williams & Wilkins.

Roper, J. M., & Shapira, J. (2000). *Ethnography in nursing research*. Thousand Oaks, CA: Sage.

Smith, R. E. (1988). The logic and design of case study research. *The Sport Psychologist, (2)*, 1–12.

Smith, R. A., & Davis, S. F. (2003). *The psychologist as detective: An introduction to conducting research in psychology* (3rd ed.). Upper Saddle River, NJ: Pearson/Prentice-Hall.

Stake, R. E. (1995). *The art of case study research*. Thousand Oaks, CA: Sage.

Streubert, H. J., & Carpenter, D. R. (1995). *Qualitative research in nursing: Advancing the humanistic perspective*. Philadelphia: J. B. Lippincott.

Thomas, R. M. (2003). *Blending qualitative & quantitative research methods in theses and dissertations*. Thousand Oaks, CA: Corwin Press, A Sage Publications Company.

Yin, R. K. (1989). *Case study research: Design and method*. Newbury Park, CA: Sage.

ADDITIONAL RECOMMENDED RESOURCES

Bailey, D. M. (1997). *Research for the health professional: A practical guide* (2nd ed.). Philadelphia: F. A. Davis.

Camic, P. M., Rhodes, J. E., & Yardley, L. (Eds.). (2003). *Qualitative research in psychology: Expanding perspectives in methodology and design*. Washington, DC: American Psychological Association.

Denzin, N. K., & Lincoln, Y. S. (Eds.). (2000). *Handbook of qualitative research* (2nd ed.). Thousand Oaks, CA: Sage.

Fain, J. A. (1999). *Reading, understanding and applying nursing research: A text and workbook* (2nd ed.). Philadelphia: F. A. Davis.

Grbich, C. (1999). *Qualitative research in health*. Thousand Oaks, CA: Sage.

Greenhalgh, T., & Taylor, R. (1997). How to read a paper: Papers that go beyond numbers (qualitative research). *BMJ, 3,* 743.

Huberman, A. M., & Miles, M. B. (2002). *The qualitative researcher's companion*. Thousand Oaks, CA: Sage.

Kopala, M., & Suzuki, L. A. (Eds.). (1999). *Using qualitative methods in psychology*. Thousand Oaks, CA: Sage.

Morse, J. M. (2003a). A review committee's guide for evaluating qualitative proposals. *Qualitative Health Research, 13*(6), 833–851.

Morse, J. M. (2003b). The adjudication of qualitative proposals. *Qualitative Health Research, 13*(6), 739–742.

Morse, J. M. (2004). Qualitative significance. *Qualitative Health Research, 14*(2), 151–152.

Penrod, J. (2003). Getting funded: Writing a successful qualitative small-project proposal. *Qualitative Health Research, 13*(6), 821–832.

Peters, J., Charles-Edwards, I., & Franck, L. S. (2004). Exploring issues of parental consent to research: A case-study approach. *British Journal of Nursing, 13*(12), 740–743.

Polit, D. F., & Beck, C. T. (2004). *Nursing research: Principles and methods* (7th ed.). Philadelphia: Lippincott Williams & Wilkins.

Schwandt, T. A. (2001). *Dictionary of qualitative inquiry* (2nd ed.). Thousand Oaks, CA: Sage.

Young, B., Dixon-Woods, M., & Heney, D. (2003). Managing communication with young people who have a potentially life threatening chronic illness: Qualitative study of patients and parents. *BMJ, 326,* 305–308.

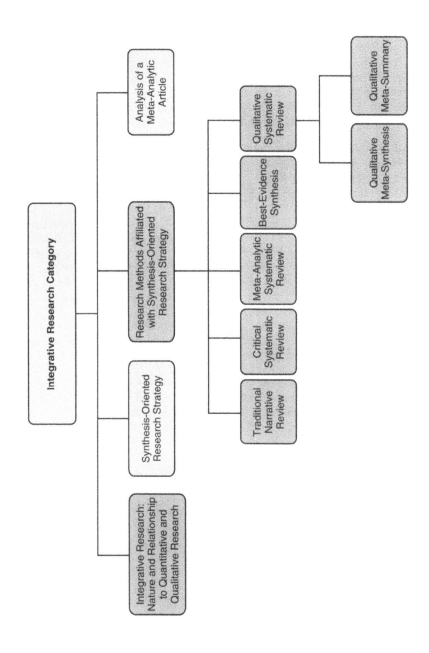

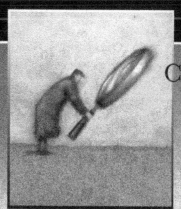

9

THE INTEGRATIVE RESEARCH CATEGORY AND ITS SYNTHESIS-ORIENTED RESEARCH STRATEGY

OUTLINE

OBJECTIVES

Upon completion of this chapter, the reader will have the information necessary to perform the following tasks:

1 Characterize the integrative research category.

2 Explain the nature of the integrative research category as well as its relationship to both the quantitative and qualitative research categories.

3 Identify and explain the name of the one research strategy orientation affiliated with integrative research.

4 List the six research methods affiliated with the synthesis-oriented research strategy.

5 Identify and explain the essential features that define the traditional narrative review method.

6 Recognize, or be able to provide, an example of the traditional narrative review method.

7 Identify and explain the essential features that define the critical systematic review method.

8 Recognize, or be able to provide, an example of the critical systematic review method.

9 Identify and explain the six sequential steps essential to performing a meta-analysis.

10 Identify and explain the essential features that define the meta-analytic systematic review method.

11 Recognize, or be able to provide, an example of the meta-analytic systematic review method.

12 Recognize and apply the 10 critical appraisal questions for critiquing a meta-analytic systematic review study.

KEY TERMS

A priori criteria
Best-evidence principle
Best-evidence synthesis research method
Classification and coding
Common scale or metric
Critical systematic review research method
Effect size

Integrative research category
Interpretive syntheses of data
Meta (as a prefix)
Meta-analysis
Meta-analytic systematic review research method
Primary analysis

Qualitative meta-summary research method
Qualitative meta-synthesis research method
Qualitative systematic review research methods
Secondary analysis
Synthesis-oriented research strategy
Topical or thematic summaries or surveys of data
Traditional narrative review research method

13 Identify and explain the essential features that define the best-evidence synthesis method.

14 Recognize, or be able to provide, an example of the best-evidence synthesis method.

15 Discuss the relatively recent need for qualitative researchers to address the integrative research category.

16 Characterize the nature of qualitative systematic review methods, and identify the various names or terms used to designate these methods.

17 Identify and explain the essential features that define
(a) the qualitative systematic review methods in general,
(b) the qualitative meta-synthesis method, and (c) the qualitative meta-summary method.

18 Recognize, or be able to provide, examples of the qualitative meta-synthesis method and the qualitative meta-summary method.

19 Read and critique a published research report that exemplifies the meta-analytic systematic review method.

WHERE HAVE WE BEEN AND WHERE ARE WE NOW? THE CONNECTION

Chapters 2 through 8 covered two of the three categories of research, the quantitative and qualitative research categories. We have seen that different philosophical perspectives come into play where these two research categories are concerned. Also, as a consequence of different philosophical perspectives, different research methodologies result and find their place within either the quantitative or qualitative realm. Taken together, the quantitative and qualitative approaches to doing research constitute the bulk of the research literature currently available to professionals. And as the information technology revolution has demonstrated, the sheer number and volume of research documents available even in highly specialized areas can be quite intimidating and an understandable cause for concern.

The third category of research, however, is intended to render the ever-increasing number of research documents appearing in the professional literature more manageable. This is accomplished by way of the **integrative research category**. This research category's principal function is quite literally to integrate or compile in various ways the accumulation of studies in a given area. Chapter 9, therefore, focuses on this research category and its one affiliated research strategy: the synthesis-oriented research strategy and those several research methods that it encompasses.

THE INTEGRATIVE RESEARCH CATEGORY: ITS NATURE AND RELATIONSHIP TO QUANTITATIVE AND QUALITATIVE RESEARCH

This third possible research category considered in this chapter provides massage therapists and related

- Integrative Research Category
  - • Synthesis-Oriented Research Strategy
    - • • Traditional Narrative Review Method
    - • • Critical Systematic Review Method
    - • • Meta-Analytic Systematic Review Method
    - • • Best-Evidence Synthesis Method
    - • • Qualitative Systematic Review Methods
      - • • • Qualitative Meta-Synthesis Method
      - • • • Qualitative Meta-Summary Method

FIGURE 9-1 ■ The integrative research category: Its affiliated research strategy and variable control-driven methods.

health science professionals with an approach to integrating the vast accumulation of research studies available. Presumably, this will allow the efforts of earlier researchers to have more of a collective impact than would be the case if only individual studies were considered.

Regardless of the health or behavioral science arena in which one works, keeping abreast of the numerous studies has become a daunting task. This research category, though, brings into play a strategy oriented toward synthesizing previously completed studies whether they occurred in the quantitative or qualitative tradition. And as we will see shortly, the research methods involved represent a broad range of options that examine the earlier studies with varying degrees of detail and precision.

Figure 9-1 provides a display of our planned coverage for this chapter, inclusive of the synthesis-oriented research strategy as well as the six research methods that fall under it.

THE SYNTHESIS-ORIENTED RESEARCH STRATEGY: ITS NATURE AND METHODS

The actual integration of previous research into a more manageable and meaningful form in a given area of interest is actually brought about by the act of synthesizing. The research strategy used here is oriented toward synthesizing the accumulation of earlier studies on several varied features. These include such areas as the research problems investigated, populations studied, size of samples derived, methodologies used, degrees of control exerted, data collection instruments employed, data analyses

completed, interpretations rendered, conclusions drawn, and needed areas of research recommended.

To accomplish these tasks, the **synthesis-oriented research strategy** provides investigators with the option of six research methods. These include the following: the traditional narrative review, the critical systematic review, the meta-analytic systematic review, the best-evidence synthesis, the qualitative meta-synthesis, and the qualitative meta-summary. Admittedly, the terminology here may seem somewhat alien and intimidating. Many themes from our earlier coverage of quantitative and qualitative research will serve you well as we work our way through these methodological options.

Let us now move on to the first of six research methods that gives life to the synthesis-oriented research strategy: the traditional narrative review method.

RESEARCH METHODS AFFILIATED WITH THE SYNTHESIS-ORIENTED RESEARCH STRATEGY

TRADITIONAL NARRATIVE REVIEW METHOD

Figure 9-2 spotlights the **traditional narrative review research method** in the context of those six methodological approaches to synthesizing already-completed research.

Different terminology has been used to designate this particular research method. Integrated literature review, conceptual review, theoretical review, and selective narrative review are among the possibilities. Perhaps the most prevalent expression consistent with current usage, though, is that of traditional narrative review method. This has certainly been the case in those efforts by authors who contrast the several varieties of systematic reviews with the presumed *nonsystematic* narrative reviews (cf. Cook, Mulrow, & Haynes, 1998; Onyskiw, 1996; and Slavin, 1986, 1995).

The traditional narrative review is conducted with a view toward identifying, categorizing, analyzing, and synthesizing the efforts of earlier investigators who completed independent studies. The interest here is in characterizing the current state of knowledge in a given research area. This is accomplished to a certain extent by this method providing a selective—though not necessarily exhaustive—coverage of previous independent studies germane to a given research problem. As indicated by Cook et al. (1998) and Bangert-Downs (1995), those research topics or needs most amenable

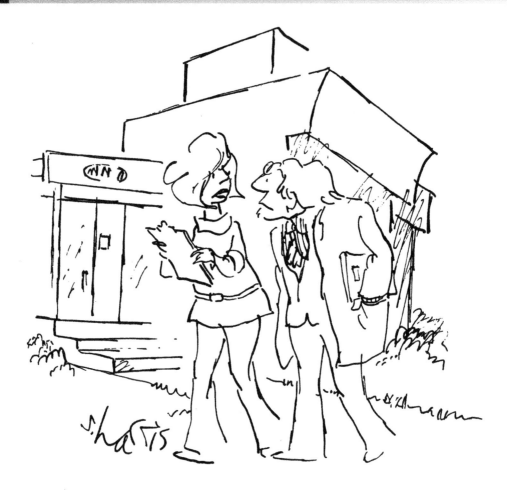

"GRANTED, WE HAVE TO DO THE RESEARCH. AND WE CAN DO SOME RESEARCH ON THE RESEARCH. BUT I DON'T THINK WE SHOULD GET INVOLVED IN RESEARCH ON RESEARCH ON RESEARCH."

HUMOR BREAK ■ Doing some "Research on the Research" may be one way to think about the methods presented in this chapter. (From Harris, S. [2004]. *Einstein simplified: Cartoons on science by Sidney Harris* [Rev. ed.]. New Brunswick, NJ: Rutgers University Press.)

- Integrative Research Category
  - • Synthesis-Oriented Research Strategy
    - • • **Traditional Narrative Review Method**
    - • • Critical Systematic Review Method
    - • • Meta-Analytic Systematic Review Method
    - • • Best-Evidence Synthesis Method
    - • • Qualitative Systematic Review Methods
      - • • • Qualitative Meta-Synthesis Method
      - • • • Qualitative Meta-Summary Method

FIGURE 9-2 ■ Spotlight on the traditional narrative review method in affiliation with the synthesis-oriented research strategy (bold emphasis designates coverage in this section).

to narrative reviews include portrayals of the history or development of a problem area, descriptions of encouraging developments if the available research is sparse or limited by faulty methodologies, and efforts to conceptually integrate two or more previously unrelated fields of inquiry.

This type of review may focus largely on original data-based studies wherein numerical and/or verbal data were collected and analyzed. One illustration of this type of traditional narrative review is a report by Callaghan (1993), in which studies pertaining to the role of massage in the management of the athlete are synthesized. The synthesis provided by Field (1998) is another example, in which the effects of massage therapy were reviewed across various populations and client conditions.

The traditional narrative review, however, is not limited to synthesizing only past data-based studies. It can include studies primarily conceptual or theoretical in nature that inform a chosen research problem area. An example of this possibility is a report by Schaefer (2003), in which sleep disturbances and fibromyalgia (FM) are linked. Selective literature pertinent to this research area is reviewed from a conceptual/theoretical view with a chosen emphasis on such themes as the epidemiology of FM, circadian cycles, the bases for the FM and sleep disturbance linkage, recommendations for nursing research, and implications for practice. Similar illustrations of this approach to doing a traditional narrative review are presented in a report by Davis (2003), in which improved sleep is postulated to reduce arthritis pain, as well as in a review by Tiidus (1997), which explores manual massage and muscle function recovery following exercise.

In addition to the research mentioned, Slavin (1995) cited other essential features of the traditional narrative review method as including a reliance—as the name implies—on a narrative summary of the procedures and results of various studies that address a focused problem area. This is done to formulate conclusions across the various studies and, thereby, perhaps inform the theory surrounding the problem area. Slavin also pointed out that narrative reviews optimally have the potential to provide insight regarding those mechanisms underlying the results of individual studies. Furthermore, " the intelligent narrative reviewer . . . might form theory-based categories of studies and compare their findings, and might thereby come up with conclusions that no individual study could have supported, suggesting new avenues for research as well as summarizing the current state of the art" (p. 9).

Potential drawbacks to the traditional narrative review include the fact that they are seldom exhaustive in their coverage of studies that exist in a given research problem area, a limitation already cited in this section. Also, the possibility always exists for bias on the part of the researcher regarding decisions as to which studies to include in the review. This difficulty is frequently driven by the absence of definite inclusion and exclusion criteria that would otherwise ensure a more unbiased selection of studies for examination. A further limitation that usually surrounds the traditional narrative review is the lack

of a standard and systematic way of ascribing weights to different study features, thereby making it difficult and potentially inconsistent in deciding on which studies the bulk of the research evidence rests. Finally, although narrative reviews may have value in giving a broad-based perspective on a topic, they are considerably less useful in providing detailed quantitative insight on specific clinical issues. These and other related imitations of the traditional narrative review are discussed further by Cook et al. (1998) and Slavin (1986, 1995).

The traditional narrative review, then, has an array of potential benefits to the research community as well as recognized limitations that need to be considered. Box 9-1 summarizes the essential features of this methodological approach to synthesizing previously completed studies available in the professional literature.

CRITICAL SYSTEMATIC REVIEW METHOD

The **critical systematic review research method** is the second of six research methods under the synthesis-oriented research strategy as spotlighted in Figure 9-3.

The expression "systematic review" in the context of research syntheses is defined by Cook et al. (1998) as entailing "the application of scientific strategies, in ways that limit bias, to the assembly, critical appraisal, and synthesis of all relevant studies that address a specific clinical question" (p. 5). The specific clinical question referenced here by these authors is often quite narrow and defined explicitly in terms of such factors as population and setting, patient/client condition of interest, exposure to an intervention, and/or one or more particular outcomes. The control of researcher bias is advanced via an exhaustive search of all pertinent studies using explicit and known inclusion/exclusion criteria as the bases for selection decisions. The primary studies' designs, characteristics, data analyses, and results are critiqued and interpreted—all with a view toward synthesizing the literature and, thereby, informing clinical practice as well as suggesting areas of needed research.

A subtle yet important distinction needs to be made at this point regarding two types of systematic reviews: the *critical systematic review* and the *meta-analytic systematic review*. Although the focus of this section is obviously on the critical systematic review, its nature cannot be completely understood unless briefly contrasted here with the meta-analytic systematic review (to be developed more fully in the next section).

BARE BONES BOX 9-1

Essential Features of the Traditional Narrative Review Research Method

- Conducted with a view toward identifying, categorizing, analyzing, and synthesizing efforts of earlier researchers who completed independent studies.
- Intent is to characterize the current state of knowledge in a given research area by giving a broad-based perspective on a topic.
- Provides a selective — though not necessarily exhaustive — coverage of previous independent studies on a given research problem.
- Most appropriate for portraying the history or development of a problem area, describing encouraging developments if available research is sparse or limited by faulty methodologies, and conceptually integrating two or more previously unrelated areas of research.
- Focus may be on either (a) original data-based studies wherein numerical and/or verbal data were analyzed or (b) studies primarily conceptual or theoretical in nature that inform a chosen research problem area.
- As implied, relies on a narrative summary of the procedures and results of various studies addressing a focused problem area.
- Attempts to formulate conclusions across various studies so as to inform the theory surrounding the problem area.
- Potential to provide insight on those mechanisms underlying the results of the individual studies reviewed.
- Potential to form theory-based categories of studies and compare their findings, thus resulting in conclusions not possible via any one earlier study.
- Potential to summarize the current state of research in a problem area and suggest needed avenues of future research.
- Limitations include the following: seldom exhaustive in coverage of studies in a research area, possible research bias in selection of studies to review, frequent absence of specific inclusion/exclusion criteria for study selection, typical absence of systematic weighting of different study features, inconsistency in identifying which studies constitute the bulk of research evidence, and questionable value in providing detailed quantitative insight on specific clinical issues.

- Integrative Research Category
  - Synthesis-Oriented Research Strategy
    - Traditional Narrative Review Method
    - **Critical Systematic Review Method**
    - Meta-Analytic Systematic Review Method
    - Best-Evidence Synthesis Method
    - Qualitative Systematic Review Methods
      - Qualitative Meta-Synthesis Method
      - Qualitative Meta-Summary Method

FIGURE 9-3 ■ Spotlight on the critical systematic review method in affiliation with the synthesis-oriented research strategy (bold emphasis designates coverage in this section).

As characterized by Cook et al. (1998), then, "a meta-analysis is a type of systematic review that uses statistical methods to combine and summarize the results of several primary studies" (p. 5). Furthermore, Onyskiw (1996) noted that meta-analysis serves (a) to systematically aggregate and integrate empirical findings derived from individual yet similar studies, (b) to analyze statistically the outcomes from these earlier research efforts and, thereby, (c) to enhance the precision of our estimates of the effects of treatments or interventions.

Systematic reviews that include this statistical component known as meta-analysis are referred to as meta-analytic systematic reviews. By contrast, however, systematic reviews that *do not* include meta-analysis but *do* encompass all of the other features of a systematic review as detailed earlier are labeled critical systematic reviews.

Though not permitting quantitative analyses of results across the primary studies, critical systematic reviews do improve our understanding of inconsistent/inconclusive findings across diverse types of studies. This occurs largely because of the objective critical appraisal of primary studies that is the essence of this form of systematic review. In turn, problem solving by clinicians is facilitated more readily than is typically the case when one must rely on the outcomes of a single study. Be that as it may, this type of systematic review is obviously not a substitute for appropriate clinical reasoning.

Illustrations of the critical systematic review method exemplifying the essential features of this approach to research synthesis include investigations by Moraska (in press), Ernst and Fialka (1994), and Koes, Assendelft, van der Heijden, Bouter, and Knipschild (1991). These studies focused on sports massage, the clinical effectiveness of massage therapy, and spinal manipulation/mobilization for back and neck pain, respectively. Each of these investigations addressed such defining research procedures as focused research questions along with explicitly defined populations, conditions of interest, exposures to treatment, and one or more

BARE BONES BOX 9-2

Essential Features of the Critical Systematic Review Research Method

- Conducted with a view toward applying scientific strategies in an unbiased way to collect, critique, and synthesize all relevant primary studies that address a specific clinical question.
- Research question is narrow, falls in the clinical realm, and is defined explicitly regarding the following areas: population and setting, condition of interest, exposure to a treatment, and/or one or more specific outcomes.
- Potential researcher bias is controlled via the use of explicit inclusion and exclusion criteria for study selection.
- Exhaustive search of all relevant primary studies is conducted using the explicit inclusion/exclusion criteria.
- Primary studies' designs, characteristics, data analyses, and results are critiqued and interpreted.
- Resulting critique and interpretation of primary studies lead to an objective synthesis of pertinent literature useful for informing clinical practice and suggesting needed research.
- Absence of meta-analytic technique precludes the systematic aggregating and integrating of empirical data across the several primary studies for purpose of better estimating effects of treatments.
- Improves one's understanding of inconsistencies and inconclusiveness across diverse types of research by critically appraising primary studies.
- Facilitates problem solving by clinicians more readily than is typical with results from a single study only.
- Enhances clinical decision making, yet does not substitute for appropriate clinical reasoning.

specific outcomes. Furthermore, explicit inclusion/exclusion criteria were used to assemble an exhaustive collection of relevant studies. Study designs, characteristics, analyses, and results were then appraised and interpreted. In each of these three critical reviews, the systematic procedures led to a synthesis of the acquired studies' implications that in turn informed both clinical practice and the direction of future research.

Additional examples of critical systematic reviews consistent with our discussion thus far include the several following studies: Ernst (1998, 1999a, 1999b); Furlan, Brosseau, Imamura, and Irvin (2002); van der Heijden, van der Windt, and de Winter (1997); and Weldon and Hill (2003). Box 9-2 lists those essential features that define the critical systematic review method and also acknowledges the absence of meta-analysis as a statistical technique for combining quantitative data across studies.

It may be of value to mention one final point. The presence of all of the defining features of a systematic review—but with the absence of meta-analysis for examining results across primary studies—is labeled by some authors as a *qualitative systematic review* or simply as *qualitative*. Examples of this usage are found in the works of Cook et al. (1998) and Furlan et al. (2002). Obviously, this is not the usage adopted in this book for the following principal reasons: (a) the use of the term *qualitative* in this particular context—as demonstrated by the two sources just cited—is quite infrequent; (b) our earlier use of the term *qualitative* as

specified in Chapter 8 on qualitative research category is considerably more prevalent; and (c) the fifth and sixth research methods still to be covered in the current chapter are designated as qualitative systematic reviews quite consistent with the prevailing literature in the qualitative tradition (cf. Patterson, Thorne, Canam, & Jillings, 2001).

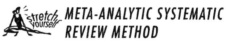 ## META-ANALYTIC SYSTEMATIC REVIEW METHOD

The third of six research methods that make possible the synthesis-oriented research strategy is the **meta-analytic systematic review research method**, which is spotlighted in Figure 9-4.

One of the most significant advances in quantitative methodology and analyses during the final quarter of the 20th century was that of meta-analysis (Glass, 1976). In his seminal article, Gene Glass

- Integrative Research Category
  - • Synthesis-Oriented Research Strategy
    - • • Traditional Narrative Review Method
    - • • Critical Systematic Review Method
    - • • **Meta-Analytic Systematic Review Method**
    - • • Best-Evidence Synthesis Method
    - • • Qualitative Systematic Review Methods
      - • • • Qualitative Meta-Synthesis Method
      - • • • Qualitative Meta-Summary Method

FIGURE 9-4 ■ Spotlight on the meta-analytic systematic review method in affiliation with the synthesis-oriented research strategy (bold emphasis designates coverage in this section).

distinguished among primary, secondary, and meta-analyses of research as follows:

> **Primary analysis** *is the original analysis of data in a research study. It is what one typically imagines as the application of statistical methods.* ... **Secondary analysis** *is the re-analysis of data for the purpose of answering the original research question with better statistical techniques, or answering new questions with old data.* ... **Meta-analysis** *refers to the analysis of analyses. I use it to refer to the statistical analysis of a large collection of analysis results from individual studies for the purpose of integrating the findings. It connotes a rigorous alternative to the casual, narrative discussions of research studies which typify our attempts to make sense of the rapidly expanding research literature. (p. 3)*

Some features of the terminology here deserve further emphasis. Onyskiw (1996) correctly noted that the prefix **meta** derives from the Greek meaning "transcending." What is "transcended" here are the results of several primary studies in that meta-analysis views as "subjects" the results from the various primary studies that have been systematically selected for scrutiny by use of explicitly declared inclusion/exclusion criteria. Meta-analysis then analyzes the already existing analyses across the several primary studies (hence, Glass's original reference to "analysis of analyses").

To accomplish this analysis of analyses in performing a meta-analytic systematic review, several measurement and statistical realities come into play as prerequisites of sorts. Although it is beyond the scope of this book to delve deeply into the computational intricacies of meta-analysis, we will at least consider some of these principal features and steps from a predominantly conceptual viewpoint. Box 9-3 provides a summary of these meta-analytic sequential steps as succinctly presented by Onyskiw (1996, pp. 71–78), followed by a discussion of these steps.

Steps 1 and 2 are fairly generic and actually apply to either of the two types of systematic reviews that we are considering. Defining the *research problem* area via a specific formulation of the research question of necessity requires the researcher to stipulate such things as the target population, treatment or intervention of interest, and outcome measure. *Inclusion/exclusion criteria* likewise need to be specifically identified as well as justified as the bases for designating only certain studies as admissible to the analysis. Regarding the *retrieval of relevant studies*, both published and unpublished studies need to be considered in the context of the various means available for locating studies in the first place.

Box 9-3	SUMMARY OF SEQUENTIAL STEPS ESSENTIAL TO PERFORMING A META-ANALYSIS

1. Defining the problem and establishing inclusion criteria for admissible studies.
2. Retrieving relevant studies.
3. Classifying and coding study characteristics.
4. Converting the outcome measure to a common scale or metric.
5. Aggregating the study findings.
   a. Estimating a summary measure of effect size.
   b. Calculating the variance of the summary measure.
   c. Testing for homogeneity.
   d. Calculating confidence intervals.
6. Interpreting the study findings.

Modified from Onyskiw, J. E. (1996). The meta-analytic approach to research integration. *Canadian Journal of Nursing Research, 28*(3), 69–85.

The locating of studies task naturally brings into play such resources as computer searches, abstract and indexing services, reference lists in published studies, and informal professional networks (cf. Cooper, 1982, on this latter point of search guidelines).

Step 3 involves the **classification and coding** tasks pertaining to the characteristics of the primary studies assembled. These primary study characteristics in a sense represent the independent variables of the meta-analytic effort. Study characteristics include both methodological and substantive features of the primary studies. Methodological characteristics or features (e.g., research design, sampling method, rating of study quality, to name but a few) and substantive characteristics (e.g., including but not limited to research question, theoretical framework, and intervention administered) are classified and then coded. The coding form used for this task must be developed and employed in such a way as to protect its validity and reliability. Procedures are well established for ensuring these technical features of the coding effort (cf. McCain, Smith, & Abraham, 1986).

Step 4 technically involves converting the outcome measure to a **common scale or metric**. This step focuses mainly on what is considered to be the dependent variable in the meta-analysis, or the effect size. Conceptually, **effect size** is so named because it indicates the effectiveness of the experimental treatment in a study. It provides valuable information about the magnitude and direction of the treatment's effect on the outcome measure of interest. In its most basic form, effect size is indexed as a measure of the mean difference between the experimental group and the control group measured in standard deviation unit. Translated, this means that the effect size—designated by either Cohen's *d* statistic or Hedges's *g* statistic—is calculated as the difference between the mean of the treatment group and the mean of the control group divided by the standard deviation. (The standard deviation used here can be either the control-group standard deviation or the pooled within-group standard deviation; cf. Glass, McGaw, & Smith, 1981.) The interpretation here is in terms of the number of standard deviation units by which the control group could have benefited or failed to benefit—depending on the sign of the effect size index—had that group received the experimental intervention. Again, Onyskiw's (1996) discussion of these matters is highly recommended in that it is very lucid and well founded on the seminal writings related to meta-analysis (e.g., Cohen, 1988; Devine, 1990; Glass, 1976; Glass et al., 1981; Hedges & Olkin, 1985; and Rosenthal, 1984).

Step 5 in the meta-analytic study may seem to be the most intricate because it involves four substeps; however, this part of the meta-analysis only builds on and extends what we have already seen. This step is designated as *aggregating the study findings* and serves the function of statistically combining the data present in each of the primary studies that have been assembled.

The series of four substeps starts with *estimating a summary measure of effect size* that descriptively indexes the summarized value for the effect of the independent variable on the dependent variable across the entire accumulation of primary studies. The second substep involves *calculating the variance of the summary measure of effect size* that indexes the variability associated with the summary measure. The importance of this substep is that the degree of variability may provide insight regarding the presence of confounding variables among the primary studies analyzed. More specifically, for example, a large variance may indicate a problematic presence of confounding variables. The third substep *tests for the homogeneity of effect sizes* across the several primary studies assembled. Confirmation of homogeneity allows the meta-analyst to interpret with confidence the summary measure of effect size because existing variation in effect sizes across the studies is presumed to be driven by sampling error. The fourth and final substep involves *calculating*

a confidence interval that estimates the possible range of summary effect size values that *captures* the true summary effect size. This is done at a given probability (conventionally 95%), thereby resulting in a 95% confidence interval.

The sixth and final step in the meta-analysis is that of *interpreting the study findings*. The interpretation intended here is that of relating the findings to those study characteristics classified and coded at the outset. You may recall that (a) the study characteristics are the independent variables in the meta-analysis and (b) they are typically classified as representing methodological and substantive features of the primary studies assembled. An assumption here is that the meta-analyst has a comprehensive enough grasp of the research domain investigated to allow making sense of the meta-analytic results and deriving appropriate conclusions.

Having reviewed the six steps necessary for conducting a meta-analysis, let us now consider several of the advantages that have been associated with doing a meta-analytic systematic review. Slavin (1995) has cited these advantages as relating most directly to such areas as the following: the *inclusiveness* of primary studies, assembled as a way to control somewhat researcher bias that might otherwise infiltrate the selection process; the use of *systematic quantitative techniques* to standardize and aggregate the outcomes of the several assembled studies; and the *systematic investigation of patterns* across the primary studies by *classifying and coding study characteristics* and then *aggregating* the study findings. Onyskiw (1996), likewise, has weighed in on meta-analytic advantages found in such features as the following: *improved quality of research integration*; *explicitly documented study protocol* allowing other researchers to evaluate the adequacy of the methodology and encouraging replication; *greater statistical power than primary studies*, thus making the detection of a treatment effect more likely and a Type II error less likely; provides a *thorough and objective description of current status in a research domain*, thereby identifying gaps in knowledge and giving direction to future research.

In the interest of a balanced assessment of meta-analysis, certain limitations as cited by Slavin (1995) should be acknowledged. One limitation is the rarity with which even one study is described in detail, even exemplary and important studies whose contrast with the meta-analytic findings may be of interest. Also, biases inherent in one or more of the primary studies assembled frequently go undetected

BARE BONES BOX 9-4

Essential Features of the Meta-analytic Systematic Review Research Method

- Meta-analysis is an "analysis of analyses" in that it is the quantitative analysis of a large collection of results from earlier primary studies for the purpose of integrating the findings.
- Meta-analysis views as "subjects" the results from various primary studies that have been systematically selected for scrutiny by way of explicitly declared inclusion/exclusion criteria.
- Already existing analyses across the assembled primary studies are analyzed.
- Sequential steps to performing a meta-analysis are as follows:
  Research problem area or domain is defined.
  Inclusion/exclusion criteria for admissible studies are identified.
  Relevant primary studies meeting the inclusion criteria are identified and retrieved.
  Study characteristics are classified and coded; these represent the independent variables.
  Outcome measures from primary studies are converted to a common scale or metric mainly via reliance on effect size calculations; the converted common metric is the dependent variable.
  Findings across the primary studies are aggregated mainly via reliance on estimating a summary measure of effect size, calculating the variance of the summary measure, testing for homogeneity, and calculating confidence intervals.
  Study findings are interpreted.
- Advantages of meta-analysis include the following: improved quality of research integration; explicitly documented study protocol; inclusiveness of primary studies assembled; systematic investigation of patterns across primary studies via the classifying, coding, and aggregating procedures; use of systematic quantitative techniques; greater statistical power than primary studies; and thorough and objective description of current status in a research domain.
- Limitations of meta-analysis include the following: rarity of exemplary primary studies being described in detail; biases inherent in one or more primary studies potentially undetected and, hence, present in meta-analysis; mechanistic procedures at times due to heightened concern over researcher bias; and potential loss of focus on better comprehending the research domain under study.

and, therefore, are often included in the meta-analysis. Finally, because of heightened concerns regarding researcher bias, meta-analyses are typically mechanistic. This feature is more often the consequence of attention to reliability and replicability issues rather than a preferred focus on better comprehending the research domain being studied.

In summation, Box 9-4 displays those essential features of the meta-analytic systematic review method. In doing so, this summary highlights those major characteristics, procedures, advantages, and limitations discussed earlier.

In addition to the sources already cited throughout this section, additional important references that may elaborate on our discussion of meta-analysis include the following: Assendelft, Morton, Yu, Suttorp, and Shekelle (2003); Chalmers, Berrier, Sacks, Levin, Reitman, and Nagalingam (1987); Conn, Valentine, Cooper, and Rantz (2003); Greenhalgh (1998, 2001); Griffin (1998); L'Abbe, Detsky, and O'Rourke (1987); Moher and Olkin (1995); Moher, Cook, Eastwood, Olkin, Rennie, and Stroup (1999); Mosteller and Colditz (1996);

Moyer, Rounds, and Hannum (2004); and van Tulder, Ostelo, Vlaeyen, Linton, Morley, and Assendelft (2000).

The Moher et al. (1999) citation is particularly helpful in that it identifies a standard format for meta-analyses. This is the result of an effort by an international advisory board that met in conjunction with the Quality of Reporting of Meta-analyses (QUOROM) conference.

Before concluding this section, please note that toward the latter part of this chapter we provide an illustration of the meta-analytic systematic review method. This illustration is in the form of a complete research article by Moyer et al. (2004). The full text of this meta-analytic study is accompanied by a critique consistent with the meta-analytic procedures suggested by Onyskiw (1996). Also, the critique follows the evaluative criteria discussed throughout this section and summarized in Box 9-5 through a critical appraisal checklist.

BEST-EVIDENCE SYNTHESIS METHOD

Moving right along, the fourth of six research methods included in the synthesis-oriented strategy

---

BOX 9-5   CRITICAL APPRAISAL CHECKLIST FOR CRITIQUING A META-ANALYTIC SYSTEMATIC REVIEW RESEARCH ARTICLE

Question 1. Is the research problem or domain identified via a specific research question that reflects the target population, treatment of interest, and outcome measure?

Question 2. Are clearly specified inclusion/exclusion criteria identified for determining which primary studies are to be included in the meta-analysis?

Question 3. Is the strategy for identifying and retrieving relevant primary studies specified in terms of computer searches, abstract and indexing services, reference lists in published studies, and informal professional networks?

Question 4. Are the independent variables of the meta-analysis (i.e., the characteristics of the assembled primary studies) classified and coded in terms of both methodological and substantive features?

Question 5. Are the validity and reliability of the coding form established?

Question 6. What technique is used to convert the outcome measure in the study to a common scale or metric (realizing that the common scale or metric is the dependent variable in the meta-analysis)?

Question 7. With respect to aggregating the study findings, what analyses are reported regarding (a) estimating a summary measure of effect size, (b) calculating the variance of the summary measure, (c) testing for homogeneity, and (d) calculating confidence intervals?

Question 8. Are the meta-analytic findings interpreted in reference to those characteristics of the assembled primary studies that were classified and coded at the outset?

Question 9. What are the implications of the study, and are there any recommendations regarding additional primary studies or meta-analyses that are needed?

Question 10. Is the overall study protocol explicitly documented enough to allow other researchers (a) to evaluate the methodology used and (b) to replicate the study?

---

is known as the **best-evidence synthesis research method** and is spotlighted in Figure 9-5.

Our journey so far through the integrative research category has taken us across the traditional narrative review, the critical systematic review, and the meta-analytic systematic review methods. In the traditional narrative review, we have an approach that provides a selective–though not necessarily exhaustive–coverage of previous independent studies in a given research domain or problem area. The researcher

- Integrative Research Category
  - • Synthesis-Oriented Research Strategy
    - • • Traditional Narrative Review Method
    - • • Critical Systematic Review Method
    - • • Meta-Analytic Systematic Review Method
    - • • **Best-Evidence Synthesis Method**
    - • • Qualitative Systematic Review Methods
      - • • • Qualitative Meta-Synthesis Method
      - • • • Qualitative Meta-Summary Method

FIGURE 9-5 ■ Spotlight on the best-evidence synthesis method in affiliation with the synthesis-oriented research strategy (bold emphasis designates coverage in this section).

here attends to methodological and substantive issues with the latitude to elaborate at length on individual studies. The selection of studies, though, is typically not based on explicit inclusion/exclusion criteria. This fact invites the criticism that researcher bias is not being controlled and, consequently, the data-based and conceptual/theoretical studies reviewed may lead to incomplete and questionable conclusions. Finally, there is the drawback of this type of review typically not involving any type of quantitative insight as a basis for its findings.

The critical systematic review speaks to many of the deficiencies associated with the narrative review method just mentioned. Perhaps most important is the reliance here on explicit inclusion/exclusion criteria that systematically and objectively drive the selection of primary studies for review. The assembled collection of studies is intended to be exhaustive, to focus on a clinically based research problem quite narrow in scope, and to facilitate problem solving by clinicians. Although meta-analytic techniques are not involved, the researcher here does provide a detailed yet synthesizing critique of the primary studies' designs, characteristics, data analyses, and results.

The meta-analytic systematic review includes all of the procedural features of the critical systematic review; however, as the name indicates, meta-analytic techniques are invoked. This allows the researcher to transcend the results of whatever an individual study can denote in terms of its own quantitative findings. This is accomplished by an "analysis of analyses" that standardizes the results of individual studies and then aggregates them across the assembled collection of several studies. In completing all of the tasks just mentioned, the researcher is committed to being as exhaustive and inclusive as possible to ensure a thoroughly comprehensive coverage of studies. Once assembled, the methodological and substantive characteristics of the individual studies are classified and coded. These characteristics are the independent variables of the meta-analysis; the standardized common metric (e.g., Cohen's d statistic) to which a study's outcome measure is converted is the dependent variable.

This quick review of the ground covered in this chapter provides a context in which we can now consider the best-evidence synthesis research method. The preceding review was critical because this best-evidence method builds on all of the advantages of the three earlier methods. It chooses, however, to be selectively exhaustive in its identification and assemblage of those primary studies that are eventually meta-analyzed.

This method for synthesizing research literature was introduced in a seminal paper by Slavin in 1986. It is largely an effort to improve on the positive features of the three review methods summarized earlier, but with an adjustment made for what Slavin perceives to be a drawback to conventional meta-analyses. Specifically, Slavin argued that meta-analyses must include in their assemblage of primary studies only those that represent the "best evidence" available at the time in a particular research domain. More to the point, Slavin (1986) claimed that his paper

proposes an alternative to both meta-analytic and traditional reviews. This method, "best-evidence synthesis," combines the quantification of effect sizes and systematic study selection procedures of quantitative syntheses with the attention to individual studies and methodological and substantive issues typical of the best narrative reviews. Best-evidence syntheses focus on the "best evidence" in a field, the studies highest in internal and external validity, using well-specified and defended a priori inclusion criteria, and use effect

size data as an adjunct to a full discussion of the literature being reviewed. (p. 5)

In a subsequent paper as well (Slavin, 1995, p. 11), the defining feature of the best-evidence synthesis is explained by way of a legal analogy: "In law, there is a principle that the same evidence that would be essential in one case might be disregarded in another because in the second case there is better evidence available." Slavin went on to illustrate this legal principle in terms of a disputed authorship case wherein a word-processed document might represent important evidence if indeed no handwritten version were available. If a handwritten copy were available, however, the word-processed version would no longer be admissible for the obvious reason that it no longer represents the best available evidence.

This principle, then, is extended to the tasks of literature reviews where best-evidence syntheses are concerned. The **best-evidence principle** functions well in legal matters because there are certain types of cases for which a priori (beforehand) criteria exist for judging the adequacy of evidence. Although Slavin hastened to admit that such **a priori criteria** are not necessarily available for all areas of research, he acknowledges that such criteria could conceivably be proposed for individual research subfields as they are reviewed. This process of generating appropriate a priori criteria could take the form of examining earlier narrative and meta-analytic reviews.

From an operational standpoint, the best-evidence synthesis method replaces the all-inclusive and exhaustive identification and retrieval of studies prevalent in a conventional meta-analytic study. Instead, the researcher relies on open and explicit procedures that are visible to the reader regarding (a) the details of each study reviewed and (b) the nature of the evidence that each study provides.

Specifying the a priori criteria for use in determining which studies are to be included in the review is a defining task in the best-evidence approach. This task is driven mainly by the reasons underlying the review in the first place. There are, however, certain themes that give direction to formulating the criteria that will drive the inclusion of particular studies, and they include the following (cf. Slavin, 1995): (a) relevance or germaneness of the study to the research domain investigated; (b) methodological adequacy of the study, particularly as it relates to minimizing bias; (c) equally high external as well as internal validity in a study; (d) sample size of the study, with caution exercised

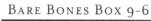

BARE BONES BOX 9-6

Essential Features of the Best-Evidence Synthesis Research Method

- Best-evidence synthesis builds on the principal advantages of the traditional narrative review, critical systematic review, and meta-analytic review methods.
- Represents an alternative to traditional narrative reviews, critical systematic reviews, and conventional meta-analyses.
- Combines the attention to (a) individual studies and methodological and substantive issues of traditional reviews and (b) the quantification of effect sizes and systematic study selection procedures of conventional meta-analyses.
- Corrects for a drawback in conventional meta-analyses wherein the all-inclusive and exhaustive collection of primary studies may include studies not representing the best available evidence in a given research domain.
- Is "selectively exhaustive" in its identification and collection of primary studies that are eventually meta-analyzed.
- Focuses on the best evidence available in a research domain, that is, studies highest in internal and external validity, using well-specified and defended a priori inclusion/exclusion criteria, and using effect size indices as an adjunct to a full discussion of the literature being reviewed.
- Appeals to a legal analogy whereby the same evidence that would be essential in one case might be disregarded in another because in the second case there is better evidence available.
- Predicated, therefore, on the principle of best evidence and the corresponding a priori criteria used for identifying episodes of best evidence.
- A priori criteria for best evidence determinations could be proposed for individual research subfields via examining earlier narrative, critical systematic, and meta-analytic reviews.
- Principal themes helping to formulate a priori criteria for best evidence selections include relevance to the research domain investigated, methodological adequacy, equally high external and internal validity, sample size of study, relevant studies with diverse methods having compensating flaws, justification for exclusion of certain well-designed studies, and justification for retention of quality studies meriting discussion.

for those studies with very small samples; (e) germane studies using diverse methods that have compensating flaws; (f) explanations of why certain well-designed studies were excluded, thus making the inclusion criteria clearer; and (g) retention of certain studies that do not yield effect sizes, yet are of appropriate quality meriting discussion.

A best-evidence synthesis incorporates the advantages of each of the other review methods. The principle of best evidence, though, is invoked as the basis for refining and determining exactly which studies eventually appear in the exhaustive collection. We do arrive at an exhaustive collection of primary studies, yet qualified in that the inclusion/exclusion criteria reflecting what is considered "admissible evidence" govern the selection process.

Box 9-6 displays the essential features of the best-evidence synthesis method in its attempt to augment the advantageous characteristics already affiliated with the other three literature review methods.

As an example of this research review method, Spitzer et al. (1990) used the best-evidence synthesis method in a study of the links between passive smoking and disease. Further illustrations of the best-synthesis method being applied in efforts to integrate the literature in certain research domains

include Gutierrez and Slavin (1992) and Slavin (1987a, 1987b, 1990).

QUALITATIVE SYSTEMATIC REVIEW METHODS

The final two of our six research methods for implementing a synthesis-oriented research strategy involve systematic reviews from the perspective of the qualitative tradition. Our coverage of the qualitative tradition in Chapter 8 established the context within which we now consider the following two methods: the *qualitative meta-synthesis research method* and the *qualitative meta-summary research method*. These methods and their positioning in the context of a synthesis-oriented strategy are spotlighted in Figure 9-6.

The relatively recent emergence of qualitative research studies in the health and behavioral science professions has created a need for qualitative researchers to address the integrative research category. Finfgeld (2003) urged researchers in this tradition to synthesize findings from related studies so as to render those qualitative results more accessible to clinicians, researchers, and policymakers. Accordingly, qualitative research proponents are initiating efforts to translate the integrative features of the research process into approaches consistent with the constructivist perspective and

- Integrative Research Category
  - • Synthesis-Oriented Research Strategy
    - • • Traditional Narrative Review Method
    - • • Critical Systematic Review Method
    - • • Meta-Analytic Systematic Review Method
    - • • Best-Evidence Synthesis Method
    - • • **Qualitative Systematic Review Methods**
      - • • • **Qualitative Meta-Synthesis Method**
      - • • • **Qualitative Meta-Summary Method**

FIGURE 9-6 ■ Spotlight on the qualitative systematic review methods in affiliation with the synthesis-oriented research strategy (bold emphasis designates coverage in this section).

its corresponding research methods (see, for example: Finfgeld, 2003; Patterson, Thorne, Canam, & Jillings, 2001; and Sandelowski & Barroso, 2003).

One result of this trend is a multitude of suggested approaches that appear in the professional literature under such headings as meta-study, meta-synthesis, meta-analysis, meta-data analysis, meta-method, meta-theory, and meta-summary. The seemingly never-ending references to "meta-this" or "meta-that" can indeed be confusing to even the veteran researcher. To make this situation somewhat manageable for purposes of this chapter, our coverage in this section is restricted to a discussion of the qualitative meta-synthesis and the qualitative meta-summary methods. Part of the reasoning here is to address the qualitative systematic review function from both a global/general vantage point (i.e., the meta-synthesis) and a particular/specific view (i.e., the meta-summary). Understanding the qualitative meta-synthesis method initially sets the stage for then understanding the meaning of the qualitative meta-summary method.

Qualitative Meta-Synthesis Method

Working in the context of the qualitative tradition, Finfgeld (2003) characterized *meta-synthesis* as a broad, global, encompassing, or umbrella term designating the synthesis of research findings (not simply raw data) across several qualitative studies for the expressed purpose of rendering a new interpretation. The synthesizing function here is interpretive, given the qualitative research focus as opposed to the more aggregative or collective emphasis as found, for example, in a quantitative meta-analysis. Certain quantitative researchers may understandably take issue with this apparent distancing of the interpretive function from their work. The close affiliation of the interpretive function with the

qualitative tradition, however, is the principal point intended here rather than an attempt to dislodge the importance of interpretation from the quantitative *researcher's activities*.

As you can gather from this brief description, the major goal or objective of meta-synthesis is to generate "a new and integrative interpretation of findings that is more substantive than those resulting from individual investigations. This methodology allows for the clarification of concepts and patterns, and results in refinement of existing states of knowledge and emergent operational models and theories" (Finfgeld, 2003, p. 894).

A particularly pertinent illustration of the **qualitative meta-synthesis research method** is a study by Jensen and Allen (1994). These researchers have provided a synthesis of qualitative research on the concepts of wellness and illness. In so doing, they have derived substantive interpretations about health, disease, wellness, and illness from a total of 112 qualitative studies representing primarily the grounded theory, phenomenological, and ethnographic perspectives. A theoretical explanation of the health-disease experience resulted inductively and reflected a synthesis of common perceptions of health and disease across individuals. The synthesizing interpretations made possible in this qualitative systematic review are thought to be more informative and insightful of the phenomenon studied than would be possible from any one of the studies reviewed.

Another example of the qualitative meta-synthesis method is a study by Arman and Rehnsfeldt (2003). These researchers investigated suffering as a lived phenomenon in the context of women with breast cancer. The findings of 14 qualitative studies were synthesized regarding (a) the experience of the disease from the patient's perspective and (b) the interpretation of that experience from the perspective of suffering. Other valuable illustrations of the qualitative meta-synthesis method—as well as the research domains studied—include the following: Barroso and Powell-Cope (2000), living with HIV; Beck (2001), postpartum depression; and Frederickson (1999), understandings of presence, touch, and listening in a caring conversation.

Qualitative Meta-Summary Method

As shown in the previous section, the qualitative meta-synthesis method integrates the research findings and interpretations of several previously completed qualitative studies so as to formulate a more comprehensive interpretation of the phenomenon studied. Sandelowski and Barroso (2003, p. 227) characterized the qualitative *meta-synthesis* as "a form of systematic review or integration of qualitative research findings in a target domain that are themselves **interpretive syntheses of data** [emphasis added], including phenomenologies, ethnographies, grounded theories, and other integrated and coherent descriptions or explanations of phenomena, events, or cases."

In the case of the **qualitative meta-summary research method**, however, the effort here is on qualitative reports whose findings are summarized as opposed to synthesized; therefore, these reports do not lend themselves to a meta-synthesis. The summarized findings of these reports are more reminiscent of features of a survey. They typically assume the form of lists and frequency counts of topics and themes, and they rely more on the naming of concepts as opposed to interpreting concepts. In this regard, Sandelowski and Barroso (2003, p. 227) characterized the qualitative meta-summary as "a form of systematic review or integration of qualitative findings in a target domain that are themselves **topical or thematic summaries or surveys of data** [emphasis added]." These authors also go on to explain the three essential techniques associated with performing a meta-summary: (a) extraction of findings, (b) abstraction of findings, and (c) calculation of effect sizes.

The *extraction of findings* task refers to formulating interpretations, judgments, or conclusions based on study data generated in the form of lists and frequencies of topics, themes, and concepts. These interpretations of the study data constitute the findings in a meta-summary effort and must literally be extracted from the data accumulated. The *abstraction of findings* step entails reducing the earlier extracted findings to a smaller subset of interpretive statements that parsimoniously and accurately represent the principal meanings inherent in all the findings. The third and final step of *calculating manifest effect sizes* involves quantitatively transforming the qualitative data (represented by the abstracted findings) into variations of frequency counts labeled frequency effect size and intensity effect size. These two effect sizes are called manifest effect sizes because each reflects the content manifested in the abstracted findings. The frequency and intensity effect sizes here can be viewed as the qualitative researcher's analogs or counterparts to the quantitative researcher's summary measure of effect size used in meta-analyses.

Further elaboration on these three steps constituting the meta-summary methodology is available

in the Sandelowski and Barroso (2003) source already acknowledged. This source, furthermore, illustrates this method in the context of qualitative research on HIV-positive women with findings pertaining to motherhood.

Box 9-7 presents the essential features of the **qualitative systematic review research methods** involving meta-syntheses and meta-summaries.

ILLUSTRATION OF THE META-ANALYTIC SYSTEMATIC REVIEW METHOD: AN ANALYSIS OF A COMPLETE RESEARCH ARTICLE (MOYER, ROUNDS, & HANNUM, 2004)

Box 9-8 contains the complete research report by Moyer, Rounds, and Hannum (2004) that illustrates the meta-analytic systematic review research method. As indicated in the title and abstract, this meta-analysis is of the massage therapy (MT) research literature, spans 37 studies, and focuses on nine dependent variables.

As a follow-up to your reading of the Moyer et al. (2004) article, let us now critique this research study based on our discussions in this chapter of the meta-analytic review method. More specifically, we will use the 10 questions that constitute the critical appraisal checklist displayed in Box 9-5 and repeated in this section.

FOCUS OF CRITIQUE QUESTION 1: RESEARCH PROBLEM AND TARGETED POPULATION, TREATMENT, AND OUTCOME

Is the research problem or domain identified via a specific research question that reflects the target population, treatment of interest, and outcome measure?

The introductory section is extensively developed in that it speaks to the history of MT, an overview of MT in terms of definitions and various forms, MT theories, possible effects of MT, and predictions for MT in the context of the several studies meta-analyzed. The purpose statement for the study implies the study's research question. In so doing, the authors identify the target population as that set of MT primary studies involving human participants other than infants that also accommodate the several inclusion/exclusion criteria established (and to be addressed in critique question 2). As we will examine shortly, the procedures used by the

Text continued on p. 210

BARE BONES BOX 9-7

Essential Features of the Qualitative Systematic Review Research Methods Involving Meta-syntheses and Meta-summaries (cf. Finfgeld, 2003; Sandelowski & Barroso, 2003)

Need for qualitative researchers to translate the integrative function of the research process into approaches consistent with the constructivist perspective and its corresponding research methods.

Qualitative systematic reviews can be viewed from two polar perspectives, namely, the global/general vantage point (i.e., the meta-synthesis method) and the particular/specific view (i.e., the meta-summary method).

Meta-Synthesis Method

- Broad, global, encompassing, umbrella term designating the synthesis of research findings (not simply data) across several qualitative studies so as to render a new interpretation.
- Form of systematic review or integration of qualitative research findings in a target domain that are themselves interpretive syntheses of data, including phenomenologies, ethnographies, grounded theories, and other integrated and coherent descriptions of phenomena or events.
- Synthesizing function is interpretive given the qualitative research focus as opposed to the more aggregative emphasis found (e.g., in a quantitative meta-analysis).
- Major goal is to generate a new and integrative interpretation of findings that is more substantive than those resulting from individual investigations.

Meta-Summary Method

- Focus on qualitative reports whose findings are summarized rather than synthesized; hence, these reports do not lend themselves to a meta-synthesis.
- Summarized findings of these qualitative studies are reminiscent of survey features, typically assume the form of lists and frequency counts of topics and themes, and rely more on naming concepts rather than interpreting them.
- Form of systematic review or integration of qualitative research findings in a target domain that are themselves topical or thematic summaries or surveys of data.
- Three techniques or procedures involved in performing a meta-summary are (a) extraction of findings, (b) abstraction of findings, and (c) calculation of manifest effect sizes.

BOX 9-8   A META-ANALYSIS OF MASSAGE THERAPY RESEARCH

Christopher A. Moyer, James Rounds, and James W. Hannum
University of Illinois at Urbana-Champaign

Massage therapy (MT) is an ancient form of treatment that is now gaining popularity as part of the complementary and alternative medical therapy movement. A meta-analysis was conducted of studies that used random assignment to test the effectiveness of MT. Mean effect sizes were calculated from 37 studies for 9 dependent variables. Single applications of MT reduced state anxiety, blood pressure, and heart rate but not negative mood, immediate assessment of pain, and cortisol level. Multiple applications reduced delayed assessment of pain. Reductions of trait anxiety and depression were MT's largest effects, with a course of treatment providing benefits similar in magnitude to those of psychotherapy. No moderators were statistically significant, though continued testing is needed. The limitations of a medical model of MT are discussed, and it is proposed that new MT theories and research use a psychotherapy perspective.

Massage therapy (MT), the manual manipulation of soft tissue intended to promote health and well-being, has a history extending back several thousand years. Recorded in writing as far back as 2000 B.C. (Fritz, 2000, p. 13), massage was a part of many ancient cultures including that of the Chinese, Egyptians, Greeks, Hindus, Japanese, and Romans, and was often considered to be a medicinal practice (Elton, Stanley, & Burrows, 1983, p. 275). The Greek physician Hippocrates (460–377 B.C.) advocated rubbing as a treatment for stiffness; later, the physicians Celsus (25 B.C.–A.D. 50) and Galen (A.D. 129–199) wrote extensively on the medicinal and therapeutic value of massage and related techniques such as anointing, bathing, and exercise. However, in Western cultures, the association between massage and medicine eventually diminished as Greco-Roman traditions were abandoned. Although the practice of massage continued as a folk medicine treatment during the Middle Ages, its adoption by the common people served to separate it from the scientific and medical milieu, and in this way, massage fell out of favor with the medical establishment (Fritz, 2000; Salvo, 1999).

BOX 9-8   A META-ANALYSIS OF MASSAGE THERAPY RESEARCH — CONT'D

This schism continued during the early part of the 19th century, during which time Per Henrik Ling developed Swedish massage, the basis of many modern forms of MT. Ling, who was not trained in medicine, applied his ideas and techniques to the treatment of disease, a practice that met opposition from the Swedish medical community. Despite this resistance, Ling gained support from his influential clients and was eventually able to teach his system to physicians, who adopted his techniques and shared them with like-minded colleagues. Soon after, in the later part of the century, the Dutch physician Johann Mezger was successful in reintroducing massage to the scientific community, presenting it to his colleagues as a medical treatment, and codifying some of its elements with terms that are still in use today (Fritz, 2000, pp. 16–17; Salvo, 1999, pp. 9–11).

Interest in MT has continued to grow among the scientific community and consumers alike. Currently, in the United States, MT is one of the fastest growing sectors of the expanding complementary and alternative medical therapy movement. Visits to massage therapists increased 36% between 1990 and 1997, with consumers now spending between $4 and $6 billion annually for MT (Eisenberg et al., 1998), in pursuit of benefits such as improved circulation, relaxation, feelings of well-being, and reductions in anxiety and pain, all of which are endorsed as benefits of MT by the American Massage Therapy Association (AMTA, 1999b). At the same time, numerous studies across several fields including psychology, medicine, nursing, and kinesiology support MT's therapeutic value. Field (1998) reviewed the effectiveness of MT in treating symptoms associated with a host of clinical conditions, including pregnancy, labor, burn treatment, postoperative pain, juvenile rheumatoid arthritis, fibromyalgia, back pain, migraine headache, multiple sclerosis, spinal cord injury, autism, attention-deficit/hyperactivity disorder, posttraumatic stress disorder, eating disorders, chronic fatigue, depression, diabetes, asthma, HIV, and breast cancer. In addition to the beneficial outcomes that were unique to these specific conditions, Field proposed a set of common findings by indicating that "across studies, decreases were noted in anxiety, depression, [and] stress hormones (cortisol)" (p. 1278).

Even the popular press has picked up on the increase in MT practice and research. A feature in *Time* suggested that MT is on the rise, in part, because of "people's greater awareness of the effect stress has on health" (Luscombe, 2002, p. 49). It is also reported that the National Institutes of Health have begun funding MT research, and that the White House Commission on Complementary and Alternative Medicine Policy (2002) has called for more research and public education on MT. The *Time* article concludes by noting that the Commission's chairman, physician James Gordon, indicates that MT is known to be effective in decreasing anxiety, reducing pain, and improving mood (Luscombe, 2002, p. 50).

If MT can be effective in the ways indicated by the AMTA, Field, and Gordon, it would represent a therapy of interest to a variety of fields. One can imagine its use expanding beyond the private practices of massage therapists, and extending to places such as hospitals, nursing homes, psychological treatment centers, sports performance clinics, and workplaces. In addition, MT could establish itself as a treatment supported by insurance carriers and health maintenance organizations. These are, in fact, trends that are already occurring in a limited way. Nevertheless, for these trends to continue (indeed, to determine if they even should continue), what is needed is a more rigorous and quantitative examination of MT's effectiveness than that which currently exists.

There are three meta-analyses of MT research, but each is very limited in scope. Ottenbacher et al. (1987) quantified 19 studies that examined the effects of tactile stimulation on infants and young children, and found statistically significant beneficial outcomes for five of the six categories examined: motor–reflex, cognitive–language, social–personal, physiological, and overall development. Labyak and Metzger (1997) examined nine studies that sought to measure the effect of effleurage back massage on physiological indicators of relaxation, and concluded that this form of MT was effective in promoting relaxation. However, interpretation of this finding is made problematic by their decision to include within-groups designs in the analysis, leaving open the possibility that the observed effects could be attributable to spontaneous recovery, placebo effect, or statistical regression (Field, 1998, p. 1270), and by the fact that only limited information is provided on the individual studies and their effect sizes. Ernst (1998) reviewed seven studies that assessed the effect of postexercise MT as a treatment for delayed-onset muscle soreness, reaching the tentative conclusion that MT may be a promising treatment, a conclusion that is hampered, like that of Labyak and Metzger, by a lack of sufficient statistics reported in the review itself.

No study to date has quantitatively reviewed the range of commonly reported MT effects in physically mature individuals. The present study is intended to address this problem. By means of a more exhaustive literature search than those conducted in previous reviews, we seek to unite the spectrum of MT studies that appear in a range of scientific disciplines including psychology, medicine, nursing, and kinesiology. In addition, by limiting inclusion to studies that use a between-groups design with random assignment of participants, the present study more accurately measures MT's true effects than reviews that have included other designs that are open to bias and do not permit strong causal claims.

Overview of MT

In modern practice, MT is not a single technique, or even a single set of techniques. Rather, it is a broad heading for a range of approaches that share common characteristics, a fact that is evident in definitions provided by the AMTA. The AMTA defines *massage* as "manual soft tissue manipulation [that] includes holding, causing movement, and/or applying pressure to the body," and *massage therapy* as "a profession in which the practitioner applies manual techniques, and may apply adjunctive therapies, with the intention of positively affecting the health and well-being of the client" (AMTA, 1999a). Clearly, these definitions provide latitude for a variety of approaches to exist under the rubric of MT. In one instance, MT may consist of a treatment lasting an hour or more, with long, firm strokes applied to numerous sites of the client's body, while that client lies

Continued

Box 9-8 A META-ANALYSIS OF MASSAGE THERAPY RESEARCH — CONT'D

partially disrobed on a specially designed table in a private clinic. In another instance, an MT client may receive a 10-min treatment of kneading focused on the shoulders while seated fully clothed in a specially designed chair, in a public space such as a shopping mall or workplace. Duration of treatment, types of touch and strokes administered, the sites of the body where treatment is applied, the apparatus used to facilitate treatment, and where that treatment takes place can all vary considerably. In addition, there is also considerable variability in the explanatory mechanisms that massage therapists (and recipients) subscribe to. Finally, the outcomes being pursued may vary widely; whereas one client may undergo MT in the hopes of obtaining relief from backache, another may receive MT to reduce emotional tension. In the present study, we define MT as the manual manipulation of soft tissue intended to promote health and well-being, a definition that encompasses the diverse nature of this form of treatment.

Though MT can take a variety of forms, the common element that allows these forms to be grouped together is their use of interpersonal touch in the form of soft tissue manipulation. This element forms the basis for the predominant theories encountered in MT research that are concerned with how it may provide the benefits of reductions in anxiety, depression, stress hormones, and pain. In several of these theories, the pressure applied to the body by means of MT is thought to trigger certain physiological responses that ultimately result in beneficial outcomes. It should be noted, however, that the pressure required by these theories has not been quantified, nor do existing clinical studies of MT routinely report on the amount of pressure administered in a way that would permit precise replication. Although at least one study utilizing infants as subjects observed differential effects in terms of weight gain for firm versus light strokes (Scafidi et al., 1986), no study to date has examined pressure as an independent variable with a sample of physically mature participants.

MT Theories

Unfortunately, there has been little emphasis on theory in the MT literature, with many researchers choosing to emphasize their predictions and results without testing, or in some cases even discussing, possible explanatory mechanisms. In other instances, theories are offered, but important details are omitted. Researchers have rarely specified such things as whether a theory explains immediate versus lasting effects, or if activation of a theoretical mechanism requires a course of treatment as opposed to a single application. For the theories that follow, we suggest that only the first one, the gate control theory of pain reduction, is logically limited to providing an immediate effect. Each of the remaining theories, to various degrees, could potentially offer immediate or lasting effects, or provide benefits that accumulate over a course of treatment. However, it must be noted that these are strictly suppositions and have not yet been tested.

The order in which these theories are presented reflects their frequency in the literature. Those that appear first are most frequently cited.

Gate Control Theory of Pain Reduction

Melzack and Wall (1965) theorized that the experience of pain can be reduced by competing stimuli such as pressure or cold, because of the fact that these stimuli travel along faster nervous system pathways than pain. In this way, MT performed with sufficient pressure would create a stimulus that interferes with the transmission of the pain stimuli to the brain, effectively "closing the gate" to the reception of pain before it can be processed (e.g., Barbour, McGuire, & Kirchhoff, 1986; Field, 1998; Malkin, 1994). This notion, that MT may have an analgesic effect consistent with gate control theory, appears in the literature more than any other theory pertaining to MT.

Promotion of Parasympathetic Activity

MT may provide its benefits by shifting the autonomic nervous system (ANS) from a state of sympathetic response to a state of parasympathetic response. A sympathetic response of the ANS occurs as an individual's body prepares to mobilize or defend itself when faced with a threat or challenge, and is associated with increased cardiovascular activity, an increase in stress hormones, and feelings of tension. Conversely, the parasympathetic response occurs when an individual's body is at rest and not faced with a threat, or is recovering from a threat that has since passed, and is associated with decreased cardiovascular activity, a decrease in stress hormones, and feelings of calmness and well-being (Sarafino, 2002, p. 40).

The pressure applied during MT may stimulate vagal activity (Field, 1998, pp. 1273, 1276–1277), which in turn leads to a reduction of stress hormones and physiological arousal, and a subsequent parasympathetic response of the ANS (e.g., Ferrell-Torry & Glick, 1993; Hulme, Waterman, & Hillier, 1999; Schachner, Field, Hernandez-Reif, Duarte, & Krasnegor, 1998). By stimulating a parasympathetic response through physiological means, MT may promote reductions in anxiety, depression, and pain that are consistent with a state of calmness. This same mechanism may also be responsible for several condition-specific benefits resulting from MT, such as increased immune system response in HIV-positive individuals (Diego et al., 2001), or improved functioning during a test of mental performance, in which study participants receiving MT also displayed changes in electro-encephalograph pattern consistent with increased relaxation and alertness (Field, Ironson, et al., 1996). However, support for this theory is not universal, and it has even been suggested that MT may promote a sympathetic response of the ANS (e.g., Barr & Taslitz, 1970).

Box 9-8 A META-ANALYSIS OF MASSAGE THERAPY RESEARCH — CONT'D

Influence on Body Chemistry

Two studies have linked MT with increased levels of serotonin (Field, Grizzle, Scafidi, & Schanberg, 1996: Ironson et al., 1996), which "may inhibit the transmission of noxious nerve signals to the brain" (Field, 1998, p. 1274). Others have suggested that manipulations such as rubbing, or applying pressure, may stimulate a release of endorphins into the bloodstream (Andersson & Lundeberg, 1995; Oumeish, 1998). In these ways, MT may provide pain relief or feelings of well-being by influencing the body chemistry of the recipient.

Mechanical Effects

Articles concerned with sports performance, exercise recovery, and injury management highlight the possibility that MT may speed healing and reduce pain by mechanical means. The manipulations and pressure of MT may break down subcutaneous adhesions and prevent fibrosis (Donnelly & Wilton, 2002, p. 5) and promote circulation of blood and lymph (Fritz, 2000, pp. 475–478), processes that may lead to reductions in pain associated with injury or strenuous exercise. However, as a group, studies concerned with measuring MT's effect on circulation have generated inconsistent results (Tidus, 1999).

Promotion of Restorative Sleep

Individuals deprived of deep sleep may experience changes in body chemistry that lead to increases in pain. In the absence of deep sleep, levels of substance P increase and levels of somatostatin decrease, and both of these changes have been linked with the experience of pain (Sunshine et al., 1996). Sunshine et al. (1996) concluded that MT may have promoted deeper, less disturbed sleep in a sample of fibromyalgia sufferers who experienced a reduction in pain during the course of treatment. Chen, Lin, Wu, and Lin (1999) reached the conclusion that acupressure treatment may have been effective in improving sleep quality in a sample of elderly residents at an assisted-living facility. In this way, MT may reduce pain indirectly by promoting restorative sleep.

Interpersonal Attention

The five theories previously described, the majority of which attempt to explain the role MT may play in reducing pain, are the only ones that appear consistently in the scientific literature. However, the element of interpersonal attention that may be present in MT must also be considered. It is occasionally noted that some portion of MT effects may result from the interpersonal attention that the recipient experiences, as opposed to resulting entirely from the activation of physiological mechanisms (Field, 1998, p. 1270; Malkin, 1994). However, although this possible effect of interpersonal attention is acknowledged in the research literature, it is almost universally treated as a nuisance variable, and comparison treatments are selected in such a way that different groups receive the same amount of attention. In this way it is believed that any benefits demonstrated by the MT group that exceed those of the comparison group can be attributed to a specific ingredient of MT, specifically interpersonal touch in the form of soft tissue manipulation. Although many studies, including all of those in the present analysis, attempt to control for interpersonal attention, no study to date has examined it as an independent variable. As such, the role that interpersonal attention may play in MT effects is not well understood.

Effects

The present study examines both psychological and physiological effects resulting from MT. The psychological effects correspond with those suggested by Field and Gordon and endorsed by the AMTA, and are also of interest because MT can be considered a novel way of treating these conditions, which are more routinely addressed by means of psychotherapy or pharmaceuticals. The physiological effects nominate themselves because MT is a physical therapy.

We contend that MT effects can also be divided into single-dose effects and multiple-dose effects. Single-dose effects include MT's influence on states, either psychological or physiological, that are transient in nature and that might reasonably be expected to be influenced by a single session of MT. These include state anxiety, negative mood, pain assessed immediately following treatment, heart rate, blood pressure, and cortisol level. Multiple-dose effects are restricted to MT's influence on variables that are typically considered to be more enduring, or that would likely be influenced only by a series of MT sessions performed over a period of time, as opposed to a single dose. These variables include trait anxiety and depression, as well as pain when it is assessed at a time considerably after treatment has ended.

Frequently, researchers elect to examine both single-dose effects and multiple-dose effects within the same study. Diego et al. (2001) is one such study, in which treatment group participants received MT twice weekly for a period of 12 weeks, and comparison group participants engaged in progressive muscle relaxation (PMR) according to the same schedule. Assessments of state anxiety were made immediately prior to, and immediately following, both the first and last sessions of MT or PMR in the study. Depression, a condition expected to be more resistant to change, was assessed prior to the first session of MT or PMR, and not again until after the 24th and last sessions of either treatment. Many studies, particularly those conducted by the Touch Research Institute, use such a design in order to examine both single- and multiple-dose effects.

It must be noted that the terms single-dose effect and multiple-dose effect are not yet in common usage. Research into MT generated by the Touch Research Institute typically uses the terms short-term effect and long-term effect to make a similar distinction, but no consistent terminology

Continued

BOX 9-8   A META-ANALYSIS OF MASSAGE THERAPY RESEARCH—CONT'D

has been used among other MT researchers. The decision to use this terminology is motivated by the desire to prevent any confusion that may arise with regard to how long an effect may last following the termination of treatment. Very few studies have attempted to examine whether any MT effects may last beyond the final day on which a participant receives treatment, making the use of the term *long-term effect* potentially confusing. All effects in the present study, with the exception of one outcome variable, were assessed on the same day that a treatment took place. The exception is MT's effect on delayed assessment of pain, for which assessments took place at various time periods significantly after treatment had been discontinued. Presently, pain appears to be the only variable in the MT literature that has been assessed in this way; the possibility that MT may have enduring effects on other variables has gone essentially unaddressed.

Single-Dose Effects

State anxiety. State anxiety is a momentary emotional reaction consisting of apprehension, tension, worry, and heightened ANS activity. Because state anxiety can be understood as a reaction to one's condition or environment, the intensity and duration of such a state is determined by an individual's perception of a situation as threatening (Spielberger, 19722, p. 489). Many of the samples used in MT research are drawn from populations experiencing serious and chronic health problems that can lead to feelings of anxiety (Hughes, 1987; Popkin, Callies, Lentz, Cohen & Sutherland, 1988). If MT is effective in reducing state anxiety, it may be doubly valuable to such patient populations, in that it could both improve subjective well-being and promote physical health. In physically healthy populations, the improvement in subjective well-being and promote physical health. In physically healthy populations, the improvement in subjective well-being alone may be the primary benefit of a reduction in state anxiety.

Negative mood. Some studies have examined the effect of MT on mood, which may be defined as "transient episodes of feeling or affect" (Watson, 2000, p. 4). Although the primary studies do not specify a model for mood, virtually all the studies appear to be concerned with MT's ability to bring about a reduction of negative affect rather than an increase in positive affect.

Pain. Several studies have examined MT's immediate effect on pain, the unpleasant emotional and sensory experience that is associated with actual or potential tissue damage (Merkskey et al., 1979). The sources of pain in the primary studies are diverse, and include conditions such as headache (Hernandez-Reif, Dieter, Field, Swerdlow, & Diego, 1998), backache (Hernandez-Reif, Field, Krasnegor, & Theakston, 2001), and labor pain (Hemenway, 1993) among others.

Cortisol. Some MT studies have attempted to measure a change in participants' cortisol levels. Cortisol is a stress hormone associated with the sympathetic response of the ANS (Field, 1998). MT, a therapy commonly thought of as relaxing, it expected to reduce cortisol levels, a finding that would be consistent with facilitating a parasympathetic response of the ANS (e.g., Field et al., 1992; Ironson et al., 1996).

Blood pressure. A handful of studies have examined MT's effect on blood pressure. Although predictions are not always offered, most commonly MT is expected to reduce blood pressure consistent with a parasympathetic response of the ANS (Hernandez-Reif, Field, et al., 2000; Okvat, Oz, Ting, & Namerow, 2002).

Heart rate. A few studies examining MT have attempted to measure its physiological effects in terms of heart rate. Researchers have not always offered clear predictions for this variable (Barr & Taslitz, 1970), but in cases where a prediction is evident, most often a decrease in heart rate is predicted, consistent with a parasympathetic response of the ANS (Cottingham, Porges, & Richmond, 1988; Okvat et al., 2002). Nevertheless, some researchers have noted that the opposite effect could be observed in cases in which MT was a novel experience for research participants (Reed & Held, 1988, p. 1232).

Multiple-Dose Effects

Trait anxiety. Several studies have examined MT's potential to reduce *trait anxiety*, the "relatively stable individual differences in anxiety proneness as a personality trait" (Spielberger, 1972, p. 482). In contrast with the transient and situation-specific nature of state anxiety, trait anxiety is a dispositional, internalized proneness to be anxious (Phillips, Martin, & Meyers, 1972, p. 412). Persons with high levels of trait anxiety tend to perceive the world as more dangerous or threatening, and experience anxiety states more frequently and with greater intensity than those with lower levels of trait anxiety (Spielberger, 1972, p. 482).

Depression. Ingram and Siegle (2002) noted that, in the course of research, the concept of depression has been defined many different ways, including as a mood state, a symptom, a syndrome, a mood disorder, and a disease. In the current meta-analysis, studies included in this category have been chosen on the basis of their utilization of a measure believed to capture something beyond "ordinary unhappiness" or a "sad mood," symptoms that would more accurately belong to the previously discussed category of negative mood. Subclinical depression, likely the best description of the type of depression most often assessed in MT research, consists of the aforementioned symptoms combined with symptoms such as mild to moderate levels of motivational and cognitive deficits, vegetative signs, and disruptions in interpersonal relationships (Ingram & Siegle, 2002, p. 90).

Delayed assessment of pain. A few studies have assessed participants' experience of pain at one or more time points significantly after a course of treatment has ended. The majority of these studies have done so at intervals that range from a few days to 6 weeks (Cen, 2000;

BOX 9-8   A META-ANALYSIS OF MASSAGE THERAPY RESEARCH — CONT'D

Dyson-Hudson, Shiflett, Kirshblum, Bowen, & Druin, 2001; Preyde, 2000; Shulman & Jones, 1996), although one study included an assessment that took place 42 weeks after treatment ended (Cherkin et al., 2001). Because of the small number of studies, and the range of times at which delayed assessments were made, it is not expected that the present study will be able to determine precisely how long an analgesic effect resulting from MT lasts, or the rate at which such an effect decays; rather, the aim is simply to examine whether or not MT may have a lasting analgesic effect.

Moderators

A number of potentially interesting moderator variables have gone unexamined in MT research. Primary studies, for instance, have neglected to examine whether the length of MT sessions, or characteristics of the therapist and the recipient, influence the magnitude of MT effects. Similarly, only a few studies have used more than one comparison group, making it difficult to determine whether the type of treatment to which MT is compared may moderate its effects. Although within-study examinations of such moderators would permit stronger inferences to be made, their importance can be explored in the present study by means of between-study comparisons. In addition, the present study also examines a potential moderator that cannot be examined within an individual study, that of a laboratory effect.

Minutes of MT per session. It is common for treatment studies in medicine (e.g., Bollini, Pampallona, Tibaldi, Kupelnick, & Munizza, 1999; Yyldyz & Sachs, 2001) and in psychotherapy (e.g., Bierenbaum, Nichols, & Schwartz, 1976; Turner, Valtierra, Talken, Miller, & DeAnda, 1996) to examine dosage as an independent variable. However, no studies concerned with MT have done so. It is not known whether there is a minimal amount, in terms of minutes of MT administered per session, required to produce benefits, nor it is known whether there is an optimal amount of MT that produces benefits most efficiently. Fortunately, the studies that exist vary considerably in the amount of MT administered to participants in each session, from as little as 5 min (Fraser & Kerr, 1993; Wendler, 1999) to as much as an hour (Levin, 1990). By examining the relationship between the magnitude of effects generated and the amount of MT administered per session, the present study aims to determine whether there are minimum or optimum dosages of MT.

Mean age of participants. Although MT research has been performed on samples with a variety of age ranges, no study has sought to determine whether MT offers effects of differing magnitude to participants who differ in age. The present study examines whether there is a relationship between the mean age of the participants in a study and the magnitude of effects.

Gender of participants. Only one study to date, using a very small sample, has examined whether MT effects might vary according to the gender or the recipients (Weinrich & Weinrich, 1990). The present study more powerfully examines the possibility that the gender of the recipient might moderate MT effects by examining whether study outcomes vary according to gender.

Type of comparison treatment. In discussing the research findings for a different treatment modality (psychotherapy), Wampold (2001) noted that there is a distinction that must be made between absolute and relative efficacy. *Absolute efficacy* "refers to the effects of treatment vis-à-vis no treatment and accordingly is best addressed by a research design where treated participants are contrasted with untreated participants" (Wampold, 2001, p. 59). By contrast, *relative efficacy* "is typically investigated by comparing the outcomes of two treatments" when one wishes to determine which, if either, is superior (Wampold, 2001, p. 73). Clearly, the type of efficacy one wishes to measure plays an important part in determining what will be an appropriate choice for a comparison, as a study designed to measure one does not necessarily measure the other. This issue of distinguishing absolute efficacy (does MT work better than no treatment at all?) from relative efficacy (does MT work better than a specific alternative treatment, such as PMR?) has not been made explicit enough in MT research. However, a wide variety of comparison treatments have been used in MT research, some of which resemble a wait-list (no treatment) condition, whereas others use active treatments (such as the aforementioned PMR, or chiropractic care) as a point of comparison, or placebo-type comparison treatments that are meant to account for the effect of receiving attention (such as transcutaneous electrical stimulation performed with a machine that is not delivering any current to the participant). Logically, if MT has any effect whatsoever, we expect the MT effects that result from comparison with a no-treatment condition would be larger than those that result from comparing MT to any treatment condition, including so-called placebo conditions in which the participants receive no viable treatment. Combining the results of such different studies without attempting to account for these different comparison points could be problematic. For this reason, we have divided the comparison treatments in the primary studies, when possible, as belonging to either wait-list equivalent or active/placebo categories.

The wait-list equivalent category consists of comparison treatments that most closely resemble having received no treatment, and includes wait-list controls, standard care (in studies where all participants had a medical condition and continued to receive care for the condition regardless of group assignment), rest, reading, or a work break. The active/placebo category consists of all other comparison treatments, which are grouped according to the expectation that each could reasonably be expected to have some effect, including the possibility of a placebo effect. These include treatments such as PMR, acupuncture, chiropractic care, and various forms of attention, among others. Studies that used multiple comparison groups that could not be included together within a single category were not included in either category.

Therapist training. Treatment research in fields such as psychology (Pinquart & Soerensen, 2001; Weisz, Weiss, Alicke, & Klotz, 1987) and medicine (Lin et al., 1997; Tiemens et al., 1999) sometimes examines the existence of training effects to determine whether practitioners with

Continued

BOX 9-8 A META-ANALYSIS OF MASSAGE THERAPY RESEARCH — CONT'D

greater amounts of training provide greater benefit to those being treated. No MT research, however, has examined the training of the massage therapist as an independent variable. However, the studies that do exist vary in regard to who performs MT on participants. The majority of studies use one or more fully trained and licensed massage therapists. Others utilize a layperson with only minimal training in providing massage, usually just enough to facilitate the study (e.g., Fischer, Bianculli, Sehdev, & Hediger, 2000; Weinrich & Weinrich, 1990; Wendler, 1999). By contrasting the results of studies that used a fully trained massage therapist with those that used a layperson to provide treatment, the present meta-analysis may be able to determine whether a therapist's training plays an important role in providing MT benefits.

Laboratory effect. Much of the research in this area, and especially the most recent research, is the product of a single laboratory, the Touch Research Institute (Field, 1998). Because this one source is responsible for a large proportion of MT studies, it is important to determine whether the results coming from this research group differ in a significant way from those of other researchers. If a difference is found, it would be important to examine more closely what factors contribute to that difference.

Predictions

MT is expected to promote significant and desirable reductions for each of the following variables, consistent with the existing explanatory theories outlined above: state anxiety, negative mood, pain (immediate and delayed assessment), cortisol, heart rate, blood pressure, trait anxiety, and depression. It is expected that greater reductions in these variables will be associated with higher doses of MT, in the form of minutes of MT administered per session, a relationship one would expect to observe if MT is a viable treatment. MT effects are not expected to vary according to the age or gender of participants. It is expected that MT effects generated from studies using wait-list equivalent comparison treatments will be larger than those generated from studies with active/placebo comparison treatments. Finally, no prediction is made concerning therapist training, or the existence of a laboratory effect.

Method

Literature Search and Criteria for Inclusion

A literature search was performed by Christopher A. Moyer and a graduate student in library and information sciences hired-as a research assistant. The PsycINFO, MEDLINE, CINAHL, SPORT Discus, and *Dissertation Abstracts International* databases were searched using the following key words: *massage, massotherapy, acupressure* (and *acupressure*), *applied kinesiology, bodywork musculoskeletal manipulation, reflexology, relaxation techniques, Rolfing, Touch Research Institute,* and *Trager.* Author searches were conducted within the same databases for the following authors associated with MT research: Burman, I.; Field, T.; Hart, S.; Hernandez-Reif, M.; Kuhn, C.; Peck, M.; Quintino, O.; Schanberg, S.; Taylor, S.; Theakston, H.; Weinrich, M.; and Weinrich, S. The Internet Web sites of the AMTA (www.amtamassage.org), the AMTA Foundation (www.amta-foundation.org), and the Touch Research Institute (http://www.miami.edu/touch-research/) were inspected for references, and the Touch Research Institute was also contacted directly to request unpublished data. The reference lists of all studies located by these means were then manually searched to yield additional studies.

All studies were inspected to ensure that they examined a form of MT consistent with the present study's operational definition, in which MT is defined as the manual manipulation of soft tissue intended to promote health and well-being. Studies were limited to those that administered MT to human participants other than infants, and that reported results in English. Studies concerned with chiropractic, heat therapy, hydrotherapy, passive motion, or progressive relaxation treatments were not included, unless the study also included an MT group. Studies examining therapeutic touch, a nursing intervention distinct from MT (in that it does not actually require physical contact to occur), were also excluded unless they also had an MT group. Several studies used more than two groups; in these cases, study results were combined in order to yield a between-groups comparison of all subjects receiving MT versus all subjects receiving non-MT treatments. Studies concerned with ice massage, participants performing self-massage, or massage performed with the aid of mechanical devices were excluded, as were studies that only included MT as part of a combination treatment (e.g., MT combined with exercise and movement therapy). MT administered with scented oil or MT administered with background music were not considered to be combination treatments, as these are common elements of MT in clinical practice, and studies using such treatment were included. Studies that did not explicitly label a treatment as "massage" or as "massage therapy," but used a treatment that fit the authors' operational definition of MT, were included.

These criteria yielded 144 studies concerned with outcomes of MT. Each study was reviewed independently by Christopher A. Moyer and James Rounds for possible inclusion in the meta-analysis. Studies were examined to ensure that they (a) compared an MT group with one or more non-MT control groups, (b) used random assignment to groups, and (c) reported sufficient data for a between-groups effect size to be generated on at least one dependent variable of interest. These three criteria accounted for approximately equal proportions of excluded studies.

BOX 9-8 A META-ANALYSIS OF MASSAGE THERAPY RESEARCH — CONT'D

The first two inclusion criteria were necessary to ensure that effects where a result of treatment. When participants in MT research serve as their own controls (e.g., Bauer & Dracup, 1987; Fakouri & Jones, 1987) there is no way to know whether effects are attributable to treatment or are instead the result of spontaneous recovery, placebo effect, or statistical regression (Field, 1998, p. 1270). Similarly, random assignment of participants to groups is necessary to control for the possibility of selection effects. Glaser (1990) is an example of a study that is threatened in this way. Because treatment participants were previously enrolled in an MT program, and were compared with a group of participants who were not enrolled, it is likely that these groups differed in their predisposition toward MT in a way that could affect results.

When studies met all criteria apart from reporting sufficient data for calculating between-groups effects, and contact information was available, study authors were contacted in an attempt to obtain the necessary data. Specifically, there were seven studies from the Touch Research Institute for which this was the case (Field et al., 1999; Field et al., 2000; Field, Peck, et al., 1998; Field, Quintino, Henteleff, Wells-Keife, & Delvecchio-Feinberg, 1997; Field, Schanberg, et al., 1998; Field, Sunshine, et al., 1997; Sunshine et al., 1996). Upon our request, we were informed that the data needed from these studies (standard deviations) were no longer available. For this reason, these studies could not be included in the meta-analysis.

Interrater agreement for the inclusion process was 93%. The 10 studies for which there was initial disagreement, which occurred most frequently as a result of uncertainty regarding random assignment, were then reviewed jointly, with the subsequent decision made to exclude 8 of these. This resulted in a total of 37 studies meeting the inclusion criteria.

Variables and Measures

The nine variables for which effect sizes were calculated, and the instruments used to assess them, are as follows:

State anxiety. Fifteen of the 21 studies examining MT's effect on anxiety used the state anxiety portion of the State-Trait Anxiety Inventory (Spielberger, 1983). Five studies used a visual analogue scale, and one study used an investigator-constructed measure.

Negative mood. Seven of eight studies assessing negative mood used the Profile of Mood States (McNair, Lorr, & Droppleman, 1971). The remaining study used a visual analogue scale.

Immediate assessment of pain. Eight of the 15 studies assessing pain immediately following treatment used visual analogue scales alone. Two studies used a visual analogue scale in conjunction with either the Short-Form McGill Pain Questionnaire (Melzack, 1987) or the Menstrual Distress Questionnaire (Moos, 1968). Two studies used investigator-constructed measures, and the remaining studies relied on the Neck Pain Questionnaire (Leack et al., 1994), the revised Oswestry Low Back Pain Questionnaire (Hudson-Cook, Tomes-Nicholson, & Breen, 1989), or behavioral observation.

Cortisol. Of the seven studies that assessed cortisol levels, four relied on salivary samples, two on urinary samples, and one on a blood sample. In each case, samples were collected 20 min after the application of MT, to account for the fact that bodily cortisol levels are indicative of responses occurring 20 min prior to sampling (Field, Hernandez-Reif, Quintino, Schanberg, & Kuhn, 1998, p. 233).

Blood pressure. Five studies offer data pertaining to participants' blood pressure, assessed by means of a sphygmomanometer. Measures of diastolic and systolic blood pressure were combined into one effect size, because only a few studies report on this variable, and differ in regard to which values they report.

Heart rate. Of the six studies that assessed the effect of MT on heart rate, four used some type of automatic monitoring device, and one study indicated that pulse was assessed manually. One study did not specify the means by which heart rate was assessed.

Trait anxiety. Three studies of the seven assessing trait anxiety used the Symptom Checklist-90-Revised (SCL-90-R; Derogatis, 1983). One study combined the Conners Teacher Rating Scale (Conners, 1969) and the Revised Children's Manifest Anxiety Scale (Reynolds & Richmond, 1985). The three remaining studies used either the Beck Anxiety Inventory (Beck, Brown, Epstein, & Steer, 1988), the trait portion of the State-Trait Anxiety Inventory (Spielberger, 1983), or an investigator-constructed measure.

Depression. Five of the 10 studies assessing depression utilized the Center for Epidemiological Studies — Depression Scale (CES-D; Radloff, 1977). Two used the SCL-90-R, and one combined the CES-D and the SCL-90-R. The remaining studies used either the Children's Depression Inventory — Short Form (Kovacs, 1992) or an investigator-constructed measure.

Delayed assessment of pain. The five studies assessing pain at a time significantly after treatment ended relied on five different instruments. These were the Neck Pain Questionnaire (Leak et al., 1994), the Wheelchair User's Shoulder Pain Index (Curtis et al., 1995), the McGill Pain Questionnaire (Melzack, 1975), a visual analogue scale, and an investigator-constructed measure.

Statistical Analysis

Effect sizes. Between-groups comparisons on variables of interest were converted to Hedges's g effect size. Hedges's g, calculated as (Group Mean 1 − Group Mean 2) ÷ pooled standard deviation, estimates the number of standard deviations by which the average member of a treatment group differs from the average number of a comparison group for a given outcome. In cases where a study used more than one measure to examine the same outcome variable, results of multiple measures were standardized and then averaged in order to result in one effect size per variable for any study. Similarly, if a study examined the immediate effects of more than one application of treatment, or examined the treatment effect on

Continued

Box 9-8   A META-ANALYSIS OF MASSAGE THERAPY RESEARCH — CONT'D

delayed assessments of pain at more than one time point, the results of the multiple applications or assessments were standardized and then averaged in order to calculate a single effect size for that study. Effect sizes were coded such that positive values, for any variable, indicate a more desirable outcome (e.g., a reduction in anxiety) for the participants who received MT.

This process was done independently by both the first and second authors for the entire set of effect sizes; these initial results were then compared in order to determine agreement and eliminate errors. Agreement rate (AR) of initial calculations for the entire set of 84 effect sizes was 88%. Within outcome categories, the initial rates of agreement were as follows: state anxiety, $AR = 86\%$ ($n = 21$); negative mood, $AR = 88\%$ ($n = 8$); immediate assessment of pain, $AR = 87\%$ ($n = 15$); cortisol, $AR = 86\%$ ($n = 7$); blood pressure, $AR = 60\%$) ($n = 5$); heart rate, $AR = 100\%$ ($n = 6$); trait anxiety, $AR = 86\%$ ($n = 7$); depression, $AR = 90\%$ ($n = 10$); and delayed assessment of pain, $AR = 60\%$ ($n = 5$). When discrepancies were observed, calculations were reviewed jointly to correct errors, and a consensus was reached.

Individual study effect sizes were then subjected to a correction for small sample bias, then weighted by their inverse variance and averaged to generate a mean effect size for each outcome variable (Lipsey & Wilson, 2001). An overall, nonspecific effect size was also calculated by averaging all effects within each study, and then calculating a weighted overall effect from these effect sizes. All effect sizes were calculated according to a random effects model of error estimation.

Statistical significance of the mean effect sizes was assessed by calculating the 95% confidence interval (CI) for the population parameter. A significance level of .05 or better is inferred when zero is not contained within the CI. For effect sizes reaching statistical significance, the likelihood and possible influence of publication bias — the possibility that studies retrieved for the meta-analysis may not be a random sample of all studies actually conducted (Rosenthal, 1998) — was assessed by means of a trim and fill procedure (Duval & Tweedie, 2000), a nonparametric statistical technique of examining the symmetry and distribution of effect sizes plotted by inverse variance. This technique first estimates the number of studies that may be missing as a result of publication bias, and then allows a new, attenuated effect size to be calculated on the basis of the influence such studies would have if they were included in the analysis. The trim and fill procedure was performed with the Division of Vector-Borne Infectious Diseases library using the statistical computing program S-PLUS (Bigger-staff, 2000), which generates results for the three estimators of missing studies (L_0, R_0, and Q_0) described by Duval and Tweedie (2000). Per the suggestion of these authors, the number of missing studies resulting from each estimator was considered before the eventual decision was made to report results according to the L_0 and R_0 estimators, which are considered preferable for most situations (Duval & Tweedie, 2000).

Moderators.   As with effect sizes, moderator variable data were also coded independently by both the first and second authors. Agreement rate for initial coding of all moderator data across categories was 97% ($n = 158$). Within moderator variable categories, initial agreement rates were as follows: minutes per session, $AR = 100\%$ ($n = 34$); mean age, $AR = 100\%$ ($n = 25$); comparison type, $AR = 97\%$ ($n = 31$); training, $AR = 87\%$ ($n = 31$); and laboratory effect, $AR = 100\%$ ($n = 34$); proportion of female participants was coded only by the first author. The influence of moderator variables was assessed by performing a weighted regression analysis (Lipsey & Wilson, 2001) on the set of overall, nonspecific effect sizes for all studies.

Results

Table 1 lists the effect sizes (Hedges's g) for each study by outcome variable, as well as important study characteristics. The 37 studies included in the meta-analysis used a total of 1,802 participants, including 795 who received MT. Of the 1,007 participants who received a comparison treatment, 49% received one of the five treatments categorized as wait-list equivalent, and the remaining 51% received a treatment categorized as active/placebo. The mean number of participants for a study was 48.7 ($SD = 49.0$), and mean age of all participants was 40.6 years ($SD = 13.9$). Participants received an average of 21.7 min ($SD = 14.0$) of MT per application of treatment. Sixty-five percent of studies reported using a trained massage therapist (or therapists), 22% reported using a minimally trained person (or persons) to deliver treatment, and 14% did not indicate the level of training of the person (or persons) administering MT. Thirty-two percent of studies were conducted by the Touch Research Institute.

Table 2 graphically represents the distribution of overall study effect sizes by means of a stem and leaf plot. Table 3 lists the mean effect size for each outcome variable, as well as the number of studies contributing to the effect size, its 95% CI, and the results of trim and fill procedures applied to statistically significant effects. The nonspecific, overall mean effect was statistically significant ($g = 0.34$, $p < 0.01$). Among the nine specific outcome variables examined, six displayed statistically significant effect sizes. For the single-dose effects category, these included state anxiety ($g = 0.37$, $p < 0.01$), blood pressure ($g = 0.25$, $p < 0.02$), and heart rate ($g = 0.41$, $p < 0.01$). Negative mood ($g = 0.34$), immediate assessment of pain ($g = 0.28$) and cortisol ($g = 0.14$) were nonsignificant. All outcome variables examined within the multiple-dose effects category, including trait anxiety ($g = 0.75$, $p < 0.01$), depression ($g = 0.62$, $p < 0.01$), and delayed assessment of pain ($g = 0.31$, $p < 0.01$), were statistically significant.

The results of trim and fill analyses conducted on the statistically significant outcome variables indicated that the results are fairly robust to the threat of publication bias. For overall effects, an analysis based on the L_0 estimator yielded 10 studies missing as a result of publication bias, which

BOX 9-8   A META-ANALYSIS OF MASSAGE THERAPY RESEARCH—CONT'D

TABLE I   INDIVIDUAL STUDY CHARACTERISTICS AND EFFECT SIZES(g) BY OUTCOME VARIABLE

STUDY	PARTICIPANTS	N	% FEMALE	MEAN AGE	MIN/SESSION	COMP. TYPE	TRAINED THERAPIST?	TRI STUDY?	g
State anxiety									
Chang et al. (2002)	Pregnant women	60	100	28	30	WL	No	No	0.45
Chin (1999)	Surgery patients	85	100	42	10	WL	No	No	−0.50
Delaney et al. (2002)	Health adults	30	53	31	20	WL	Yes	No	0.20
Diego et al. (2002)	Spinal cord patients	20	25	39	40	A/P	Yes	Yes	0.57
Diego et al. (2001)	HIV + adolescents	24	92	17	20	A/P	Yes	Yes	0.87
Field et al. (2002)	Fibromyalgia patients	20	—	51	30	A/P	Yes	Yes	0.11
Field, Ironson, et al. (1996)	Medical staff	50	80	26	15	A/P	Yes	Yes	0.48
Fischer et al. (2000)	Amniocentesis patients	200	100	34	—	WL	No	No	0.00
Fraser & Kerr (1993)	Institutionalized elderly	21	—	—	5	C	—	No	1.20
Groer et al. (1994)	Healthy adults	32	69	64	10	WL	No	No	−0.21
Hernandez-Reif, Field, et al. (1998)	Multiple sclerosis patients	24	75	48	45	WL	Yes	Yes	1.33
Hernandez-Reif, et al. (2001)	Back pain patients	24	54	40	30	A/P	Yes	Yes	0.07
Hernandez-Reif, Field, et al. (2000)	Hypertensive adults	30	53	52	30	A/P	Yes	Yes	0.24
Hernandez-Reif, Martinez, et al. (2000)	PDD patients	22	100	33	30	A/P	Yes	Yes	0.84
Leivadi et al. (1999)	University dance students	30	100	20	30	A/P	Yes	Yes	0.21
Levin (1990)	Healthy adults	36	—	27	60	WL	Yes	No	1.30
Menard (1995)	Surgery patients	30	100	52	45	WL	Yes	No	1.12
Mueller Hinze (1988)	Healthy women	48	100	27	10	C	—	No	0.50
Okvat et al. (2002)	Cardiac catheter patients	78	24	61	10	A/P	Yes	No	−0.06
Richards (1993)	Hospitalized elderly men	69	0	66	6	C	No	No	0.80
Wendler (1999)	Soldiers	93	10	30	5	A/P	No	No	0.54
Negative mood									
Abrams (1999)	Children/adolescents with ADHD	30	17	13	20	WL	Yes	Yes	0.09
Field et al. (2002)	Fibromyalgia patients	20	—	51	30	A/P	Yes	Yes	0.00
Field, Ironson, et al. (1996)	Medical staff	50	80	26	15	A/P	Yes	Yes	1.09
Hernandez-Reif, Field, et al. (1998)	Multiple sclerosis patients	24	75	48	45	WL	Yes	Yes	0.32

Continued

BOX 9-8   A META-ANALYSIS OF MASSAGE THERAPY RESEARCH —CONT'D

TABLE I   INDIVIDUAL STUDY CHARACTERISTICS AND EFFECT SIZES(g) BY OUTCOME VARIABLE —CONT'D

STUDY	PARTICIPANTS	N	% FEMALE	MEAN AGE	MIN/SESSION	COMP. TYPE	TRAINED THERAPIST?	TRI STUDY?	g
Hernandez-Reif et al. (2001)	Back pain patients	24	54	40	30	A/P	Yes	Yes	−0.07
Hernandez-Reif, Martinez, et al. (2000)	PDD patients	24	400	33	30	A/P	—	Yes	1.27
Leivadi et al. (1999)	University dance students	30	100	20	30	A/P	Yes	Yes	−0.49
Levin (1990)	Healthy adults	36	—	27	60	WL	Yes	No	0.46
Immediate assessment of pain									
Cen (2000)	Neck pain patients	31	75	48	30	C	Yes	No	1.21
Chang et al. (2002)	Pregnant women	60	100	28	30	WL	No	No	0.99
Chin (1999)	Surgery patients	85	100	42	10	WL	No	No	−0.30
Field et al. (2002)	Fibromyalgia patients	20	—	51	30	A/P	Yes	Yes	0.85
Fischer et al. (2000)	Amniocentesis patients	200	100	34	—	WL	No	No	−0.13
Hemenway (1993)	Labor pain patients	32	100	23	10	A/P	No	No	0.38
Hernandez-Reif, Dieter, et al. (1998)	Headache patients	26	—	40	30	WL	Yes	Yes	0.52
Hernandez-Reif, et al. (2001)	Back pain patients	24	54	40	30	A/P	Yes	Yes	0.35
Hernandez-Reif, Martinez, et al. (2000)	PDD patients	24	100	33	30	A/P	Yes	Yes	0.81
Hsieh et al. (1992)	Back pain patients	63	—	34	—	A/P	Yes	No	−0.94
Leivadi et al. (1999)	University dance students	30	100	20	30	A/P	Yes	Yes	0.21
Mueller Hinze (1988)	Healthy women	48	100	27	10	C	—	No	0.81
Okvat et al. (2002)	Cardiac catheter patients	78	24	61	10	A/P	Yes	No	0.16
Weinrich & Weinrich (1990)	Cancer patients	28	36	62	10	A/P	No	No	−0.04
Wilkie et al. (2000)	Hospice care center patients	29	31	63	30	WL	Yes	No	−0.14
Cortisol									
Abrams (1999)	Children/adolescents with ADHD	30	17	13	20	WL	Yes	Yes	0.07
Chin (1999)	Surgery patients	85	100	42	10	WL	No	No	0.07
Field, Ironson, et al. (1996)	Medical staff	50	80	26	15	A/P	Yes	Yes	0.45
Hernandez-Reif et al. (2001)	Back pain patients	24	54	40	30	A/P	Yes	Yes	−0.39
Hernandez-Reif, Field, et al. (2000)	Hypertensive adults	30	53	52	30	A/P	Yes	Yes	0.18
Hernandez-Reif et al. (2002)	Parkinson's disease patients	16	50	58	30	A/P	Yes	Yes	0.41
Leivadi et al. (1999)	University dance students	30	100	20	30	A/P	Yes	Yes	0.13

Continued

Blood pressure

Delaney et al. (2002)	Healthy adults	30	53	31	20	WL	Yes	No	−0.06
Hernandez-Reif, Field, et al. (2000)	Hypertensive adults	30	53	52	30	A/P	Yes	Yes	0.29
Mueller Hinze (1988)	Healthy women	48	100	27	10	C	—	No	0.49
Okvat et al. (2002)	Cardiac catheter patients	78	24	61	10	A/P	Yes	No	0.16
Wendler (1999)	Soldiers	93	10	30	5	A/P	No	No	0.34

Heart rate

Cottingham et al. (1988)	Healthy men	32	0	27	45	WL	Yes	No	0.22
Delaney et al. (2002)	Healthy adults	30	53	31	20	WL	Yes	No	0.53
Mueller Hinze (1988)	Healthy women	48	100	27	10	C	—	No	0.82
Okvat et al. (2002)	Cardiac catheter patients	78	24	61	10	A/P	Yes	No	0.16
Richards (1993)	Hospitalized elderly men	69	0	66	6	C	No	No	0.35
Wendler (1999)	Soldiers	93	10	30	5	A/P	No	No	0.52

Trait anxiety

Abrams (1999)	Children/adolescents with ADHD	30	17	13	20	WL	Yes	Yes	0.94
Hernandez-Reif, Dieter, et al. (1998)	Headache patients	26	—	40	30	A/P	Yes	Yes	0.52
Hernandez-Reif et al. (2001)	Back pain patients	24	54	40	30	A/P	Yes	Yes	0.98
Hernandez-Reif, Field, et al. (2000)	Hypertensive adults	30	53	52	30	A/P	Yes	Yes	2.11
Rexilius et al. (2002)	Patient caregivers	35	72	52	30	C	Yes	No	0.31
Scherder et al. (1998)	Alzheimer's patients	16	—	86	30	A/P	—	No	0.68
Shulman & Jones (1996)	Employees	33	61	40	15	WL	Yes	No	0.06

Depression

Abrams (1999)	Children/adolescents with ADHD	30	17	13	20	WL	Yes	Yes	0.29
Diego et al. (2002)	Spinal cord patients	20	25	39	40	A/P	Yes	Yes	0.32
Diego et al. (2001)	HIV + adolescents	24	92	17	20	A/P	Yes	Yes	0.74
Field et al. (2002)	Fibromyalgia patients	20	—	51	30	A/P	Yes	Yes	0.63
Hernandez-Reif, Dieter, et al. (1998)	Headache patients	26	—	40	30	WL	Yes	Yes	0.38
Hernandez-Reif et al. (2001)	Back pain patients	24	54	40	30	A/P	Yes	Yes	0.80
Hernandez-Reif, Field, et al. (2000)	Hypertensive adults	30	53	52	30	A/P	Yes	Yes	0.82
Hernandez-Reif, Martinez, et al. (2000)	PDD patients	24	100	33	30	A/P	—	Yes	0.28
Rexilius et al. (2002)	Patient caregivers	35	72	52	30	C	Yes	No	0.91
Scherder et al. (1998)	Alzheimer's patients	16	—	86	30	A/P	—	No	1.50

BOX 9-8 A META-ANALYSIS OF MASSAGE THERAPY RESEARCH—CONT'D

TABLE I INDIVIDUAL STUDY CHARACTERISTICS AND EFFECT SIZES (g) BY OUTCOME VARIABLE—CONT'D

STUDY	PARTICIPANTS	N	% FEMALE	MEAN AGE	MIN/SESSION	COMP. TYPE	TRAINED THERAPIST?	TRI STUDY?	g
Delayed assessment of pain									
Cen (2000)	Neck pain patients	31	75	48	30	C	Yes	No	0.36
Cherkin et al. (2001)	Back pain patients	262	58	45	—	C	Yes	No	0.25
Dyson-Hudson et al. (2001)	Wheelchair users	18	22	45	45	A/P	Yes	No	0.35
Preyde (2000)	Back pain patients	73	51	45	30	C	Yes	No	0.49
Stratford et al. (1989)	Tendinitis patients	40	50	43	10	WL	—	No	0.30

Note: Dashes indicate that data were not reported. Comp. = comparison; TRI = Touch Research Institute; A/P = active/placebo; C = combination; WL = wait-list equivalent; PDD = premenstrual dysphoric disorder; ADHD = attention-deficit/hyperactivity disorder.

BOX 9-8 A META-ANALYSIS OF MASSAGE THERAPY RESEARCH — CONT'D

TABLE 2 STEM AND LEAF PLOT OF 37 OVERALL STUDY EFFECT SIZES

STEM	LEAF
−0.9	4
−0.8	
−0.7	
−0.6	
−0.5	
−0.4	
−0.3	
−0.2	14
−0.1	4
−0.0	47
0.0	26
0.1	1
0.2	2259
0.3	0558
0.4	0114579
0.5	8
0.6	17
0.7	2389
0.8	013
0.9	
1.0	9
1.1	2
1.2	0

result in an attenuated but still significant effect ($g = 0.20$, 95% CI $= 0.06, 0.34$); the funnel plot of actual and filled study effect sizes for this analysis is represented in Figure 1. The same analysis performed with the R_0 estimator indicates no missing studies. Of the six specific outcome variables that generated significant effects, results of trim and fill analyses indicated that only state anxiety and delayed assessment of pain effects were likely overestimated due to publication bias. A trim and fill analysis performed on the state anxiety effect using the L_0 estimator yielded an estimate of four studies likely missing as a result of publication bias. When the influence such studies would have on state anxiety is calculated, the adjusted effect is nonsignificant ($g = 0.22$, 95% CI $= -0.01, 0.45$). A trim and fill analysis performed on the delayed assessment of pain outcome variable using the L_0 estimator yielded a slightly smaller but still significant effect ($g = 0.26$, 95% CI $= 0.07, 0.44$). When the same analyses were performed with the R_0 estimator, no missing studies were indicated in either case.

An analysis of potential moderator variables for the set of overall effect sizes was not statistically significant, $Q_R(6) = 5.80$. Despite the nonsignificance of the regression model, the decision was made to inspect the significance of the individual moderator variables. Minutes of MT administered per session ($z = 155$, $p = 0.06$, one-tailed) was the only moderator that approached the predetermined alpha for statistical significance ($p < 0.05$). To examine this variable a bit further, we calculated separate weighted effect sizes for two categories of studies. Studies that administered ≥ 30 min of MT per session generated an effect that was substantially larger than that resulting from the entire set of studies ($g = 0.54$, 95% CI $= 0.32, 0.76$). Studies that administered < 30 min of MT per session demonstrated an effect that was slightly smaller than that of the entire set of studies, but still significant ($g = 0.30$, 95% CI $= 0.08, 0.52$).

Discussion

This meta-analysis supports the general conclusion that MT is effective. Thirty-seven studies yielded a statistically significant overall effect as well as six specific effects out of nine that were examined. Significant results were found within the single-dose and multiple-dose categories, and for

Continued

BOX 9–8 A META-ANALYSIS OF MASSAGE THERAPY RESEARCH—CONT'D

TABLE 3 MEAN EFFECT SIZES (g) AND RESULTS OF TRIM AND FILL ANALYSES BY OUTOME VARIABLE

OUTOME VARIABLE	k	g	95% CI	L_0	ADJUSTED g BASED ON $k + L_0$	ADJUSTED 95% CI
Overall	37	0.34**	0.21, 0.48	10	0.20**	0.06, 0.34
Single-dose effects						
State anxiety	21	0.37**	0.14, 0.59	4	0.22	−0.01, 0.45
Negative mood	8	0.34	−0.08, 0.76	—		
Immediate pain	15	0.28	−0.01, 0.57	—		
Cortisol	7	0.14	−0.10, 0.38	—		
Blood pressure	5	0.25*	0.03, 0.48	0		
Heart rate	6	0.41**	0.19, 0.62	0		
Multiple-dose effects						
Trait anxiety	7	0.75**	0.27, 1.22	0		
Depression	10	0.62**	0.37, 0.88	0		
Delayed pain	5	0.31**	0.10, 0.52	3	0.26**	0.07, 0.44

Note: A positive g indicates a reduction for any outcome variable. Dashes indicate data not calculated because of nonsignificance of effect size. CI = confidence interval; L_0 = estimate of missing studies resulting from trim and fill procedure.
* $p < .05.$ ** $p < .01.$

BOX 9-8   A META-ANALYSIS OF MASSAGE THERAPY RESEARCH — CONT'D

both physiological and psychological outcome variables. Confidence in these findings is bolstered by the results of trim and fill analyses, which indicate that the results are not unduly threatened by publication bias.

Single-Dose Effects

Three of the six single-dose effects examined were statistically significant. The magnitude of MT's effect on state anxiety means that the average participant receiving MT experienced a reduction of state anxiety that was greater than 64% of participants receiving a comparison treatment. MT was also more effective than comparison treatments in reducing blood pressure and heart rate. The average MT participant experienced a reduction in blood pressure that was greater than 6% of comparison group participants, whereas for heart rate, the reduction resulting from MT was greater than 60% of comparison group participants, findings that are consistent with the theory that MT may promote a parasympathetic response of the ANS. Cortisol, however, another outcome variable that would be expected to decrease if MT promotes a parasympathetic response, was not significantly reduced, a finding that contrasts with the conclusion previously reached by Field (1998). Despite this inconsistent support for MT promoting a parasympathetic response, the significant finding for the cardiovascular variables suggests that future research should examine whether MT might have an enduring effect on blood pressure such that it could be used in treating hypertension.

   MT did not exhibit an effect on immediate assessment of pain. This finding contrasts with the commonly offered notion that MT may provide analgesia by competing with painful stimuli in a way consistent with the gate control theory of pain. MT's effect on negative mood was also nonsignificant.

Multiple-Dose Effects

Some of MT's largest and most interesting effects belong to the multiple-dose effects category. Despite the fact that MT did not demonstrate an effect on immediate assessment of pain, a significant effect was found for delayed assessment of pain. MT participants who received a course of

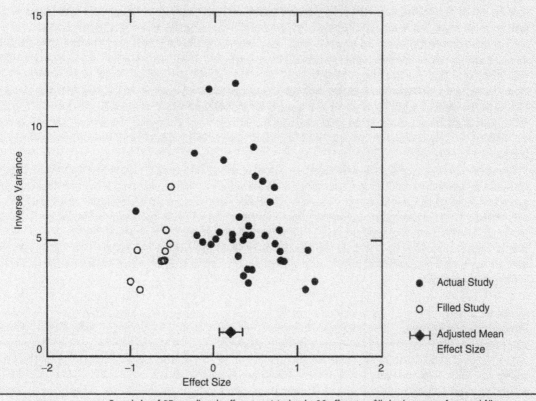

FIGURE 1 ■ Funnel plot of 37 overall study effect sizes (*g*) plus the 10 effect sizes filled in by means of trim and fill procedure using the L_0 estimator; no filled studies are indicated using the R_0 estimator.

Continued

BOX 9-8 A META-ANALYSIS OF MASSAGE THERAPY RESEARCH — CONT'D

treatment and were assessed several days or weeks after treatment ended exhibited levels of pain that were lower, on average, than 62% of comparison group participants. This finding is consistent with the theory that MT may promote pain reduction by facilitating restorative sleep, but without data on sleep patterns, this possibility is only conjecture.

Reductions of trait anxiety and depression following a course of treatment were MT's largest effects. The average MT participant experienced a reduction of trait anxiety that was greater than 77% of comparison group participants, and a reduction of depression that was greater than 73% of comparison group participants. These effects are similar in magnitude to those found in meta-analyses examining the absolute efficacy of psychotherapy, a more traditional treatment for either condition, in which it is estimated that the average psychotherapy client fares better than 79% of untreated clients (Wampold, 2001, p. 70). Considered together, these results indicate that MT may have an effect similar to that of psychotherapy.

Moderators

All six moderators that were examined were nonsignificant. In most cases, this was not surprising, given that we did not expect effects to vary according to recipient characteristics and made no predictions concerning therapist training or laboratory effect. However, it was unexpected that neither the minutes of MT administered per session nor type of comparison treatment moderated effects in a way that was statistically significant.

Minutes of MT administered per session was the only moderator that approached the predetermined alpha for statistical significance. This, combined with the logic that if MT has an effect, longer doses should likely be more potent, leads us to suspect that our analysis failed to find a relationship because of insufficient statistical power rather than the true absence of any moderating effect. Nevertheless, it must be concluded that this moderator may not be as important as we predicted, and that even short sessions of MT can be effective. Future studies could more powerfully examine the role of session length by including two levels of this variable, something that does not appear to have been done in any study to date.

Whether studies used a wait-list equivalent or active/placebo comparison group was not significant for overall effects. This finding does not support the prediction of studies using wait-list equivalent comparison treatments would yield larger effects. Because stronger inferences can be made from within-study comparisons, we decided to compare this result with those from studies that included both an active/placebo and a wait-list equivalent comparison group within the design. Three studies fitting this criterion examined state anxiety as an outcome. Richards (1993), in a study that involved 69 participants, found that wait-list participants improved significantly less than those who received a combination of muscle relaxation, mental imagery, and relaxing music. By contrast, Fraser and Kerr (1993), in a study that involved 21 participants, found no statistically significant difference in outcome between two comparison groups, one of which received attention in the form of conversation (active/placebo), the other of which received no intervention (wait-list equivalent). Similarly, Mueller Hinze (1988), in a study with 48 participants, found no differences in outcome for three comparison groups including therapeutic touch (active/placebo), transcutaneous electrical stimulation without current (active/placebo), and a no-treatment control (wait-list equivalent). As a group, these contrasting results seem to agree with the nonsignificant finding in the meta-analysis in suggesting that whether MT is compared with an active/placebo or wait-list equivalent treatment does not substantially influence effects. However, no primary studies that examined MT's largest effects — on depression and trait anxiety — used such a design; the influence of such a moderator may be more evident in relation to these more robust effects, and could be examined in future studies by using both types of comparison groups.

The prediction that effects would not vary according to the age or gender of participants was supported. Neither of these recipient characteristics was significantly associated with overall effects. Therapist training did not have a significant effect on outcome. This finding, however, should not be used to conclude that training is of no consequence. In the present meta-analysis, this variable could only be dummy coded according to whether a study involved a trained massage therapist, or a layperson trained by a massage therapist for the purposes of conducting the study. It was not possible to differentiate the levels of experience various massage therapists may have had, nor was it possible to know how much training laypersons involved in the studies had received. The only conclusion that can be definitively reached from this result is that laypersons provided with some training can provide beneficial MT, information that may be valuable to researchers working with limited resources. No evidence of a laboratory effect was found.

MT Theories

Mixed support for existing theories. It is interesting to note that, among the theories that are commonly offered to explain MT effects, the most popular theories are the ones least supported by the present results. The failure to find a significant effect for immediate assessment of pain contradicts the theory that MT provides stimuli that interfere with pain consistent with gate control theory. Reductions in blood pressure and heart rate resulting from MT do support the theory that MT promotes a parasympathetic response, although, if this theory is true, it would also be expected that a significant reduction in cortisol levels would have occurred, which did not. By contrast, the remaining theories are not inconsistent with he current results. MT's effects on state anxiety, trait anxiety, and depression may come about as a result of MT's influence on body chemistry,

BOX 9-8 A META-ANALYSIS OF MASSAGE THERAPY RESEARCH — CONT'D

whereas the ability of a course of MT treatment to provide lasting pain relief may result from the mechanical promotion of circulation and breakdown of adhesions, or from improved sleep promoted by the treatment.

MT from a psychotherapy perspective. Another theory that has not previously been put forth may also account for MT effects. MT may provide benefit in a way that parallels the common-factors model of psychotherapy. Substantial evidence suggests that the considerable efficaciousness of psychotherapy results not from any specific ingredient of treatment, but rather from the factors that all forms of psychotherapy share (Wampold, 2001). In this model, factors such as a client who has positive expectations for treatment, a therapist who is warm and has positive regard for the client, and the development of an alliance between the therapist and client are considered to be more important than adherence to a specific modality of psychotherapy. The same model can be extended to MT, given the possibility that benefits arising from it may come about more from factors such as the recipient's attitude toward MT, the therapist's personal characteristics and expectations, and the interpersonal contact and communication that take place during treatment, as opposed to the specific form of MT used or the site to which it is applied.

Several of the findings in the present study are consistent with such a model applied to MT. The finding that MT has an effect on trait anxiety and depression that is similar in magnitude to what would be expected to result from psychotherapy suggests the possibility that these different treatments may be more similar than previously considered. Further support comes from the fact that MT training was not predictive of effects. Possibly, MT effects are more closely linked with characteristics of the massage provider that are independent of skill or experience in performing soft tissue manipulation.

In addition to having similar effects, MT parallel psychotherapy in structure. Both forms of therapy routinely rely on repeated, private interpersonal contact between two persons. Studies contributing effects to the trait anxiety and depression outcome categories used treatment protocols similar to those that might be maintained in short-term psychotherapy, with twice-weekly meetings over a span of 5 weeks being most common; other studies used similar protocols. Interestingly, the length of individual sessions in these studies ranged from 15 to 40 min, with 30 min being the most common session length. Had these studies used a session length equivalent to he "50-minute hour" that is routine in psychotherapy, it is possible that MT's effect for these variables would have matched or exceeded that expected of psychotherapy.

Application of such a psychotherapeutic, common-factors model to MT has important ramifications for future research. Different questions need to be asked, different moderators tested, and different comparisons made. Foremost among the questions is whether MT is as effective as psychotherapy. No study has directly compared these treatments, a comparison that would be justified given the finding that some MT effects may be very similar to those of psychotherapy. Similarly, it could be interesting to determine whether a combination of MT and psychotherapy could be significantly more effective than either alone. Another critical issue that needs to be examined is whether these specific MT effects are enduring. Current studies contributing to these effects all performed assessments on the final day of treatment, making it impossible to know if the effects last. Studies that administer a course of MT treatment should make assessments not only immediately after treatment has ended, but also several weeks or months later, to determine whether reductions of anxiety, depression, or other conditions are maintained.

Despite the fact that MT is a treatment that relies on interpersonal contact, no research has attempted to manipulate, or even measure, the kind of psychological interactions that undoubtedly take place between the provider and recipient of MT. Details worth examining include (a) the amount and types of communication, both verbal and nonverbal, that take place between massage therapist and recipient; (b) the recipient's and therapist's expectations for whether treatment will be beneficial; (c) the amount of empathy perceived by the recipient on behalf of the therapist; (d) whether the psychological state of the therapist is of importance; and (e) whether personally traits of the therapist, of the recipient, or any interaction between those personality traits influence outcomes. An examination of such personally, process, and therapeutic relationship variables may reveal that benefiting from MT is just as much about feeling valued as it is about being kneaded.

Finally, the possibility that MT may provide a significant portion of its benefit in a way that parallels psychotherapy has a bearing on the selection of comparison treatments used in future research. Viewed from a medical perspective, comparison treatments in MT research are thought to function as placebo treatments, in that they control for incidental aspects of the treatment (most notably attention in MT research) while withholding what is thought to be the specific effective ingredient (soft tissue manipulation). However, the same logic cannot be applied if the treatment being examined is thought to be beneficial because of incidental aspects, because the double-blind condition favored in medicine trials, where neither the participants nor the researchers involved in the study are aware of who is receiving viable treatment and who is receiving the placebo, is logically impossible (Wampold, 2001, p. 129). Those supervising and administering treatment in MT research, as in psychotherapy research, are aware of the treatment being delivered and know if it is intended to be therapeutic. This is critical factor to consider if the treatment being studied relies on the therapist's beliefs and intentions in order to be effective. The placebo treatment, derived from medical trials intended to examine the effectiveness of specific ingredients, cannot control for the incidental aspects of a treatment such as MT. When a common-factors model is applied to MT, the notion that a comparison treatment such as progressive muscle relaxation controls for attention is incorrect. The attention provided to comparison group participants is identical in quantity but not in quality, and cannot be expected to function as a control for the attention received by participants in the MT treatment group.

Continued

BOX 9-8   A META-ANALYSIS OF MASSAGE THERAPY RESEARCH — CONT'D

The idea that MT has significant parallels with psychotherapy, and that perspectives gained from psychotherapeutic research should be applied to future research, is not meant to suggest that MT delivers effects entirely by psychological means. Clearly MT is at least partially a physical therapy, and some of its benefits almost certainly occur through physiological mechanisms. In fact, one of the most interesting aspects of MT is that it may deliver benefit in multiple ways; specific ingredients and common factors may each play a role, with each being differentially important depending on the desired effect. However, whether researchers wish to study MT as a physical therapy, as a psychological one, or as both, new research should examine not merely the effects resulting from MT, but also the ways in which these effects come about. It is only by testing MT theories that a better understanding of this ancient practice will result.

References

References marked with an asterisk indicate studies included in the meta-analysis.

*Abrams, S. M. (1999). Attention-deficit/hyperactivity disordered children and adolescents benefit from massage therapy (Doctoral dissertation, University of Miami, 1999). *Dissertation Abstracts International, 60,* 5218.

American Massage Therapy Association. (1999a). AMTA definition of massage therapy. Retrieved April 6, 2003, from http://www.amtamassage.org/about/definition.html

American Massage Therapy Association (1999b). Enhancing your health with therapeutic massage. Retrieved April 6, 2003, from http://www.amtamassage.org/publications/enhancing-health.htm

Andersson, S., & Ludeberg, T. (1995). Acupuncture — From empiricism to science: Functional background to acupuncture effects in pain and disease. *Medical Hypotheses, 45,* 271–281.

Barbour, L. A., McGuire, D. B., & Kirchhoff, K. T. (1986). Nonanalgesic methods of pain control used by cancer outpatients. *Oncology Nursing Forum, 13,* 56–60.

Barr, J. S., & Taslitz, N. (1970). The influence of back massage on autonomic functions. *Physical Therapy, 50,* 1679–1691.

Bauer, W. C., & Dracup, K. A. (1987). Physiologic effect of back massage in patients with acute myocardial infarction. *Focus on Critical Care, 14,* 42–46.

Beck, A., Brown, G., Epstein, N., & Steer, R. (1988). An inventory for measuring clinical anxiety: Psychometric properties. *Journal of Consulting and Clinical Psychology, 56,* 893–897.

Bierenbaum, H., Nichols, M. P., & Schwartz, A. J. (1976). Effects of varying session length and frequency in brief emotive psychotherapy. *Journal of Consulting and Clinical Psychology, 44,* 790–798.

Bigerstaff, B. (2000). S-Plus library DVBID (dvbidlib.exe) [Computer software]. Retrieved from http://www.stat.colostate.edu/~bradb/files/

Bollini, P., Pampallona, S., Tibaldi, G., Kupelnick, B., & Munizza, C. (1999). Meta-analysis of dose-effect relationships in randomized clinical trials. *British Journal of Psychiatry, 174,* 297–303.

*Cen, S. Y. (2000). *The effect of traditional Chinese therapeutic massage on individuals with neck pain.* Unpublished master's thesis, California State University, Northridge.

*Chang, M. Y., Wang, S. Y., & Chen, C. H. (2002). Effects of massage on pain and anxiety during labour: A randomized controlled trial in Taiwan. *Journal of Advanced Nursing, 38,* 68–73.

Chen, M. L., Lin, L. C., Wu, S. C., & Lin, J. G. (1999). The effectiveness of acupressure in improving the quality of sleep of institutionalized residents. *Journals of Gerontology: Series A: Medical Sciences, 54,* M389–M394.

*Cherkin, D. C., Eisenberg, D., Sherman, K. J., Barlow, W., Kaptchuk, T. J., Street, J., et al. (2001). Randomized trial comparing traditional Chinese medical acupuncture, therapeutic massage, and self-care education for chronic low back pain. *Archives of Internal Medicine, 161,* 1081–1088.

*Chin, C. C. (1999). The effects of back massage on surgical stress responses and postoperative pain (Doctoral dissertation, Case Western Reserve University, 1999). *Dissertation Abstracts International, 61,* 776.

Conners, C. K. (1969). A teacher rating scale for use in drug studies with children. *American Journal of Psychiatry, 126,* 884–889.

*Cottingham, J. T., Porges, S. W., & Richmond, K. (1988). Shifts in pelvic inclination angle and parasympathetic tone produced by Rolfing soft tissue manipulation. *Physical Therapy, 68,* 1364–1370.

Curtis, K. A., Roach, K. E., Applegate, E. B., Amar, T., Benbow, C. S., Genecco, T. D., et al. (1995). Development of the Wheelchair User's Shoulder Pain Index. *Paraplegia, 33,* 290–293.

*Delaney, J. P., Leong, K. S., Watkins, A., & Brodie, D. (2002). The short-term effects of myofascial trigger point massage therapy on cardiac autonomic tone in healthy subjects. *Journal of Advanced Nursing 37,* 364–371.

Box 9-8   A META-ANALYSIS OF MASSAGE THERAPY RESEARCH — CONT'D

Derogatis, L. R. (1983). *SCL-90-R administration, scoring and procedures manual.* Towson, MD: Clinical Psychometric Research.

*Diego, M. A., Field, T., Hernandez-Reif, M., Hart, S., Brucker, B., Field, T., et al. (2002). Spinal cord patients benefits from massage therapy. *International Journal of Neuroscience, 112,* 133–142.

*Diego, M. A., Field, T., Hernandez-Reif, M., Shaw, K., Firedman, L., & Ironson, G. (2001). HIV adolescents show improved immune function following massage therapy. *International Journal of Neuroscience, 106,* 35–45.

Donnelly, C. J., & Wilton, J. (2002). The effect of massage to scars on active range of motion and skin mobility. *British Journal of Hand Therapy, 7,* 5–11.

Duval, S., & Tweedie, R. (2000). A nonparametric "trim and fill" method of accounting for publication bias in meta-analysis. *Journal of the American Statistical Association, 95,* 89–98.

*Dyson-Hudson, T. A., Shiflett, S. C., Kirshblum, S. C., Bowen, J. E., & Druin, E. L. (2001). Acupuncture and Trager psychophysical integration in the treatment of wheelchair user's shoulder pain in individuals with spinal cord injury. *Archives of Physical Medicine and Rehabilitation, 82,* 1038–1046.

Eisenberg, D. M., Davis, R. B., Ettner, S. L., Appel, S., Wilkey, S., Van Rompay, M., et al. (1998). Trends in alternative medicine use in the United States, 1990–1997: Results of a follow-up national survey. *Journal of the American Medical Association, 280,* 1569–1575.

Elton, D., Stanley, G., & Burrows, G. (1983). *Psychological control of pain.* New York: Grune & Stratton.

Ernst, E. (1998). Does post-exercise massage treatment reduce delayed onset muscle soreness? A systematic review. *British Journal of Sports Medicine, 32,* 212–214.

Fakouri, C., & Jones, P. (1987). Relaxation Rx: Slow stroke back rub. *Journal of Gerontological Nursing, 13,* 32–35.

Ferrell-Torry, A. T., & Glick, O. J. (1993). The use of therapeutic massage as a nursing intervention to modify anxiety and the perception of cancer pain. *Cancer Nursing, 16,* 93–101.

Field, T. M. (1998). Massage therapy effects. *American Psychologist 53,* 1270–1281.

*Field, T., Diego, M., Cullen, C., Hernandez-Reif, M., Sunshine, W., & Douglas, S. (2002). Fibromyalgia pain and substance p decrease and sleep improves after massage therapy. *Journal of Clinical Rheumatology, 8,* 72–76.

Field, T., Grizzle, N., Scafidi, F., & Schanberg, S. (1996). Massage and relaxation therapies' effects on depressed adolescent mothers. *Adolescence, 31,* 903–911.

Field, T., Hernandez-Reif, M., Hart, S., Theakston, H., Schanberg, S., & Kuhn, C. (1999). Pregnant women benefit from massage therapy. *Journal of Psychosomatic Obstetrics and Gynaecology, 20,* 31–38.

Field, T. M., Hernandez-Reif, M., Quintino, O., Schanberg, S., & Kuhn, C. (1998). Elder retired volunteers benefit from giving massage therapy to infants. *Journal of Applied Gerontology, 17,* 229–239.

*Field, T., Ironson, G., Scafidi, F., & Nawrocki, T., Goncalves, A., & Burman, I. (1996). Massage therapy reduces anxiety and enhances EEG pattern of alertness and math computations. *International Journal of Neuroscience, 86,* 197–206.

Field, T., Morrow, C., Valdeon, C., Larson, S., Kuhn, C., & Schanberg, S. (1992). Massage reduces anxiety in child and adolescent psychiatric patients. *Journal of the American Academy of Child & Adolescent Psychiatry, 31,* 124–131.

Field, T., Peck, M., Hernandez-Reif, M., Krugman, S., Burman, I., & Ozment-Schenck, L. (2000). Postburn itching pain, and psychological symptoms are reduced with massage therapy. *Journal of Burn Care Rehabilitation, 21,* 189–193.

Field, T., Peck, M., Krugman, S., Tuchel, T., Schanberg, S., Kuhn, C., et al. (1998). Burn injuries benefit from massage therapy. *Journal of Burn Care and Rehabilitation, 19,* 241–244.

Field, T., Quintino, O., Henteleff, T., Wells-Keife, L., & Delvecchio-Feinberg, G. (1997). Job stress reduction therapies. *Alternative Therapies, 3,* 54–56.

Field, T., Schanberg, S., Kuhn, C., Field, T., Fierro, K., Henteleff, T., et al. (1998). Bulimic adolescents benefit from massage therapy. *Adolescence, 33,* 555–563.

Field, T. M., Sunshine, W., Hernandez-Reif, M., Quintino, O., Schanberg, S., Kuhn, C., et al. (1997). Massage therapy effects on depression and somatic symptoms in chronic fatigue syndrome. *Journal of Chronic Fatigue Syndrome, 3,* 43–51.

*Fischer, R. L., Bianculli, K. W., Sehdev, H., & Hediger, M. L. (2000). Does light pressure effleurage reduce pain and anxiety associated with genetic amniocentesis? A randomized clinical trial. *Journal of Maternal-Fetal Medicine, 9,* 294–297.

*Fraser, J., & Kerr, J. R. (1993). Psychophysiological effects of back massage on elderly institutionalized patients. *Journal of Advanced Nursing, 18,* 238–245.

Fritz, S. (2000). *Mosby's fundamentals of therapeutic massage.* St. Louis, MO: Mosby.

Glaser, D. (1990). The effects of a massage program on reducing the anxiety of college students (Master's thesis, San Jose State University, 1990). *Masters Abstracts International, 29,* 263.

Continued

Box 9-8　A META-ANALYSIS OF MASSAGE THERAPY RESEARCH — CONT'D

*Groer, M., Mozingo, J., Droppleman, P., Davis, M., Jolly, M. L., Boynton, M., et al. (1994). Measures of salivary secretory immunoglobulin A and state anxiety after a nursing back rub. *Applied Nursing Research, 7*, 2–6.

*Hemenway, C. B. (1993). The effects of massage on pain in labor (Master's thesis, University of Florida, 1993). *Masters Abstracts International, 33*, 515.

*Hernandez-Reif, M., Dieter, J., Field, T., Swerdlow, B., & Diego, M. (1998). Migraine headaches are reduced by massage therapy. *International Journal of Neuroscience, 96*, 1–11.

*Hernandez-Reif, M., Field, T., Field, T., & Theakston, H. (1998). Multiple sclerosis patients benefit from massage therapy. *Journal of Bodywork and Movement Therapies, 2*, 168–174.

*Hernandez-Reif, M., Field, T., Krasnegor, J., & Theakston, H. (2001). Lower back pain is reduced and range of motion increased after massage therapy. *International Journal of Neuroscience, 106*, 131–145.

*Hernandez-Reif, M., Field, T., Krasnegor, J., Theakston, H., Hossain, Z., & Burman, I. (2000). High blood pressure and associated symptoms were reduced by massage therapy. *Journal of Bodywork and Movement Therapies, 4*, 31–38.

*Hernandez-Reif, M., Field, T., Largie, S., Cullen, C., Beutler, J., Sanders, C., et al. (2002). Parkinson's disease symptoms are differentially affected by massage therapy vs. progressive muscle relaxation: A pilot study. *Journal of Bodywork and Movement Therapies, 6*, 177–182.

*Hernandez-Reif, M., Martinez, A., Field, T., Quintero, O., Hart, S., & Burman, I. (2000). Premenstrual symptoms are relieved by massage therapy. *Journal of Psychosomatic Obstetrics and Gynecology, 21*, 9–15.

*Hsieh, C. Y., Phillips, R. B., Adams, A. H., & Pope, M. H. (1992). Functional outcomes of low back pain: Comparison of four treatment groups in a randomized controlled trial. *Journal of Manipulative and Physiological/Therapeutics, 15*, 4–9.

Hudson-Cook, N., Tomes-Nicholson, K., & Breen, A. (1989). A revised Oswestry disability Questionnaire. In M. O. Roland & J. R. Jennifer (Eds.), *Back pain: New approaches to rehabilitation and education* (pp. 197–204). New York: Manchester University Press.

Hughes, J. E. (1987). Psychological and social consequences of cancer. *Cancer Surveys, 6*, 455–475.

Hulme, J., Waterman, H., & Hillier, V. F. (1999). The effect of foot massage on patients' perception of care following laparoscopic sterilization as day case patients. *Journal of Advanced Nursing, 30*, 460–468.

Ingram, R. E., & Siegle, G. J. (2002). Contemporary methodological issues in the study of depression: Not your father's Oldsmobile. In I. H. Gotlib & C. L. Hammen (Eds.), *Handbook of depression* (pp. 86–114). New York: Guilford Press.

Ironson, G., Field, T., Scafidi, F., Kumar, M. Patarca, R., Price, A., et al. (1996). Massage therapy is associated with enhancement of the immune system's cytotoxic capacity. *International Journal of Neuroscience, 84*, 205–218.

Kovacs, M. (1992). *The Children's Depression Inventory: A self-rated depression scale for school-aged youngsters.* Unpublished manuscript.

Labyak, S. E., & Metzger, B. L (1997). The effects of effleurage backrub on the physiological components of relaxation: A meta-analysis. *Nursing Research, 46*, 59–62.

Leak, A. M., Cooper, J., Dyer, S., Williams, K. A., Turner-Stokes, L., & Frank, A. O. (1994). The Northwick Park Neck Pain Questionnaire devised to measure neck pain and disability. *British Journal of Rheumatology, 33*, 469–474.

*Leivadi, S., Hernandez-Reif, M. H., Field, T., O'Rourke, M., D'Arienzo, S., Lewis, D., et al. (1999). Massage therapy and relaxation effects on university dance students. *Journal of Dance Medicine and Science, 3*, 108–112.

*Levin, S. R. (1990). *Acute effects of massage on the stress response.* Unpublished master's thesis, University of North Carolina, Greensboro.

Lin, E. H., Katon, W. J., Simon, G. E., Von Korff, M., Bush, T. M., Rutter, C. M., et al. (1997). Achieving guidelines for the treatment of depression in primary care: Is physician education enough? *Medical Care, 35*, 831–842.

Lipsey, M. W., & Wilson, D. B. (2001). *Practical meta-analysis.* Thousand Oaks, CA: Sage.

Luscombe, B. (2002, July 29). Massage goes mainstream. *Time, 160*, 48–50.

Malkin, K. (1994). Use of massage in clinical practice. *British Journal of Nursing, 3*, 292–294.

McNair, D. M., Lorr, M., & Droppleman, L. F. (1971). *Profile of Mood States.* San Diego, CA: Educational and Industrial Testing Service.

Melzack, R. (1975). The McGill Pain Questionnaire: Major properties and scoring methods. *Pain, 1*, 277–299.

Melzack, R. (1987). The short-form McGill Pain Questionnaire. *Pain, 30*, 191–197.

Melzack, R., & Wall,. P. D. (1965, November 19), Pain mechanisms: A new theory. *Science, 150*, 971–979.

*Menard, M. B. (1995). The effect of therapeutic massage on post surgical outcomes (Doctoral dissertation, University of Virginia, 1995). *Dissertation Abstracts International, 57*, 276.

Merskey, H., Albe-Fessard, D. G., Bonica, J. J., Carmen, A., Dubner, R., Kerr, F. W. L., et al. (1979). IASP sub-committee on taxonomy. *Pain, 6*, 249–252.

BOX 9-8   A META-ANALYSIS OF MASSAGE THERAPY RESEARCH—CONT'D

Moos, R. H. (1968). The development of a menstrual distress questionnaire. *Psychosomatic Medicine, 30,* 853–867.

*Mueller Hinze, M. L. (1988). The effects of therapeutic touch and acupressure on experimentally-induced pain (Doctoral dissertation, University of Texas at Austin, 1988). *Dissertation Abstracts International, 49,* 4755.

*Okvat, H. A., Oz, M. C., Ting, W., & Namerow, P. B. (2002). Massage therapy for patients undergoing cardiac catheterization. *Alternative Therapies in Health and Medicine, 8,* 68–75.

Ottenbacher, K. J., Muller, L., Brandt, D., Heintzelman, A., Hojem, P., & Sharpe, P. (1987). The effectiveness of tactile stimulation as a form of early intervention: A quantitative evaluation. *Development and Behavioral Pediatrics, 8,* 68–76.

Oumeish, O. Y. (1998). The philosophical, cultural, and historical aspects of complementary, alternative, unconventional, and integrative medicine in the Old World. *Archives of Dermatology, 134,* 1373–1386.

Phillips, B. N., Martin, R. P., & Meyers, J. (1972). Interventions in relation to anxiety in school. In C. D. Spielberger (Ed.), *Anxiety: Vol. 2. Current trends in theory and research* (pp. 409–464). New York: Academic Press.

Pinquart, M., & Soerensen, S. (2001). How effective are psychotherapeutic and other psychosocial interventions with older adults? A meta-analysis. *Journal of Mental Health and Aging, 7,* 207–243.

Popkin, M. M., Callies, A. L., Lentz, R. D., Cohen, E. A., & Sutherland, D. E. (1988). Prevalence of major depression, simple phobia, and other psychiatric disorders in patients with long-standing Type-I diabetes mellitus. *Archives of General Psychiatry, 45,* 64–68.

*Preyde, M. (2000). Effectiveness of massage therapy for subacute low-back pain: A randomized controlled trial. *Canadian Medical Association Journal, 162,* 1815–1820.

Radloff, L. (1977). The CES-D Scale: A self-report depression scale for research in the general population. *Applied Psychological Measurement, 1,* 385–401.

Reed, B. V., & Held, J. (1988). Effects of sequential connective tissue massage on autonomic nervous system of middle-aged and elderly adults. *Physical therapy, 68,* 1231–1234.

*Rexilius, S. J., Mundt, C. A., Megel, M. E., & Agrawal, S. (2002). Therapeutic effects of massage therapy and healing touch on caregivers of patients undergoing autologous hematopoietic stem cell transplant. *Oncology Nursing Forum, 29,* E35–E44.

Reynolds, C. R., & Richmond, B. O. (1985). *Revised Children's Manifest Anxiety Scale (RCMAS) manual.* Los Angeles: Western Psychological Services.

*Richards, K. C. (1993). The effect of a muscle relaxation, imagery, and relaxing music intervention and a back massage on the sleep and psychophysiological arousal of elderly males hospitalized in the critical care environment (Doctoral dissertation, University of Texas at Austin, 1993). *Dissertation Abstracts International, 54,* 2443.

Rosenthal, R. (1998). Writing meta-analytic reviews. In A. E. Kazdin (Ed.), *Methodological issues and strategies in clinical research* (2nd ed., pp. 767–790). Washington, DC: American Psychological Association.

Salvo, S. G. (1999). *Massage therapy: Principles and practice.* Philadelphia: Saunders.

Sarafino, E. P. (2002). *Health psychology: Biopsychosocial interactions.* New York: Wiley.

Scafidi, F., Field, T., Schanberg, S., Bauer, C., Vega-Lahr, N., Garcia, R., et al. (1986). Effects of tactile/kinesthetic stimulation on the clinical course and sleep/wake behavior of preterm neonates. *Infant Behavior and Development, 13,* 91–105.

Schachner, L., Field, T., Hernandez-Reif, M., Duarte, A. M., & Krasnegor, J. (1998). Atopic dermatitis symptoms decreased in children following massage therapy. *Pediatric Dermatology, 15,* 390–395.

*Scherder, E., Bouma, A., & Steen, L. (1998). Effects of peripheral tactile nerve stimulation on affective behavior of patients with probable Alzheimer's disease. *American Journal of Alzheimer's Disease, 13,* 61–69.

*Shulman, K. R., & Jones, G. E. (1996). The effectiveness of massage therapy intervention on reducing anxiety in the workplace. *Journal of Applied Behavioral Science, 32,* 160–173.

Spielberger, C. D. (1972). Conceptual and methodological issues in anxiety research. In C. D. Spielberger (Ed.), *Anxiety: Vol. 2. Current trends in theory and research* (pp. 481–493). New York: Academic Press.

Spielberger, C. D. (1983). *Manual for the State-Trait Anxiety Inventory.* Palo Alto, CA: Consulting Psychologists Press.

*Stratford, P. W., Levy, D. R., Gauldie, S., Miseferi, D., & Levy, K. (1989). The evaluation of phonophoresis and friction massage as treatments for extensor carpi radialis tendonitis: A randomized controlled trial. *Physiotherapy Canada, 41,* 93–99.

Sunshine, W., Field, T. M., Quintino, O., Fierro, K., Kuhn, C., Burman, I., et al. (1996). Fibromyalgia benefits from massage therapy and transcutaneous electrical stimulation. *Journal of Clinical Rheumatology, 2,* 18–22.

Tiemens, B. G., Ormel, J., Jenner, J. A., van der Meer, K., Van Os, T. W., van den Brink, R. H., et al. (1999). Training primary-care physicians to recognize, diagnose and manage depression: Does it improve patient outcomes? *Psychological Medicine, 29,* 833–845.

Continued

Box 9-8   A META-ANALYSIS OF MASSAGE THERAPY RESEARCH—CONT'D

Tiidus, P. M. (1999). Massage and ultrasound as therapeutic modalities in exercise-induced muscle damage. *Canadian Journal of Applied Physiology, 24*, 267–278.

Turner, P. R., Valtierra, M., Talken, T. R., Miller, V. I., & DeAnda, J. R. (1996). Effect of session length on treatment outcome for college students in brief therapy. *Journal of Counseling Psychology, 43*, 228–232.

Wampold, B. E. (2001). *The great psychotherapy debate.* Mahwah, NJ: Erlbaum.

Watson, D. (2000). *Mood and temperament.* New York: Guilford Press.

*Weinrich, S. P., & Weinrich, M. C. (1990). The effect of massage on pain in cancer patients. *Applied Nursing Research, 3,* 140–145.

Weisz, J. R., Weiss, B., Alicke, M. D., & Klotz, M. L. (1987). Effectiveness of psychotherapy with children and adolescents: A meta-analysis for clinicians. *Journal of Consulting and Clinical Psychology, 55,* 542–549.

*Wendler, M. C. (1999). An investigation of selected outcomes of Tellington touch in healthy soldiers (Doctoral dissertation, University of Colorado, 1999). *Dissertation Abstracts International, 60,* 5439.

White House Commission on Complementary and Alternative Medicine Policy. (2002, March). *White House Commission on Complementary and Alternative Medicine Policy: Final report.* Retrieved May 4, 2003, from http://govinfo.library.unt.edu/whccamp/finalreport.html

*Wilkie, D. J., Kampbell, J., Cutshall, S., Halabisky, H., Harmon, H., Johnson, L. P., et al. (2000). Effects of massage on pain intensity, analgesics and quality of life in patients with cancer pain: A pilot study of a randomized clinical trial conducted within hospice care delivery. *Hospice Journal, 15,* 31–53.

Yyldyz, A., & Sachs, G. S. (2001). Administration of antidepressants: Single versus split dosing: A meta-analysis. *Journal of Affective Disorders, 66,* 199–206.

Christopher A. Moyer, James Rounds, and James W. Hannum, Department of Educational Psychology, University of Illinois at Urbana-Champaign.

We wish to thank Sue Duval, Carol Webber, and the Interlibrary Borrowing Staff at the Illinois Research and Reference Center, University of Illinois at Urbana-Champaign, for their invaluable contributions to this project. Patrick Armstrong and James Wardrop also contributed.

Correspondence concerning this article should be addressed to James Rounds, Department of Educational Psychology, University of Illinois at Urbana-Champaign, 1310 South Sixth Street, Champaign, IL 61820-6990. E-mail: jrounds@uiuc.edu

From Moyer, C. A., Rounds, J., & Hannum, J. W. (2004). A meta-analysis of massage therapy research. *Psychological Bulletin, 130*(1), 3–18.

researchers actually identified 37 studies that represented this investigation's sample of primary studies meeting the inclusion/exclusion criteria. The treatment is obviously MT intervention that is contrasted with wait-list or active/placebo controls. The study's principal outcomes focus on nine dependent variables (DVs) considered in two categories: (a) single-dose effects that might reasonably be thought of as being influenced by a single session of MT and (b) multiple-dose effects that might necessitate a series of MT sessions. The single-dose effects or outcomes investigated are state anxiety, negative mood, pain immediately assessed, cortisol, blood pressure, and heart rate. The multiple-dose effects include trait anxiety, depression, and delayed assessment of pain.

In addition to these nine principal outcomes, effects, or DVs, this study also examines six moderator variables. As indicated by Kendall, Flannery-Schroeder, and Ford (1999, p. 352), "a *moderator* is a variable that influences either the direction or the strength of the relationship between an independent . . . variable and a dependent . . . variable." In other words, the independent variables (IV) and DVs are related in such a way that their relationship is being influenced by another variable, the moderator variable that is exerting what might be called a "moderating effect." Viewed another way, the moderator variable influences when certain outcomes will occur as a consequence of a treatment. The six moderator variables in this study include the minutes of MT per session, mean age of participants, gender of participants, type of comparison treatment, therapist training, and laboratory effect.

FOCUS OF CRITIQUE QUESTION 2: INCLUSION/EXCLUSION CRITERIA

Are clearly specified inclusion/exclusion criteria identified for determining which primary studies are to be included in the meta-analysis?

Yes, the authors communicate the inclusion/exclusion criteria in explicit and operational ways in the first part of the methods section labeled "Literature Search and Criteria for Inclusion." As noted in the article itself, these criteria address predominantly—though not exclusively—the research design and data reporting features of the individual studies themselves. The application of these criteria resulted in 37 primary studies being included in the meta-analysis.

FOCUS OF CRITIQUE QUESTION 3: SEARCH AND RETRIEVAL STRATEGY

Is the strategy for identifying and retrieving relevant primary studies specified in terms of computer searches, abstract and indexing services, reference lists in published studies, and informal professional networks?

Yes, the first paragraph in the method section details extensively the search strategy used and the various sources of primary studies accessed at the outset of the process. Enough information is given in these areas to permit a reader to evaluate the comprehensiveness of the effort or to replicate the effort in this research domain or a related one. In later parts of the method section, the authors indicate additional strategies used to obtain data from those authors of certain reports that did not contain the requisite data needed for meta-analysis purposes.

FOCUS OF CRITIQUE QUESTION 4: CLASSIFICATION AND CODING OF CHARACTERISTICS OF THE ASSEMBLED PRIMARY STUDIES

Are the independent variables of the meta-analysis (i.e., the characteristics of the assembled primary studies) classified and coded in terms of both methodological and substantive features?

The research domain of interest is clearly the type of manual intervention aimed at positively affecting the health and well-being of the client. More specifically, one level of intervention—or one level of the IV—is that of MT. The second level of the IV contrasted with MT is any one of three possibilities: a wait-list comparison "treatment," an active comparison treatment (e.g., progressive muscle relaxation), or a placebo comparison treatment.

Additionally, this study identifies six other factors or variables, each of which could indeed function as an IV in another study. In this meta-analysis, however, each of these six variables serves as a moderator variable as explained earlier. And because of their status as moderator variables, each one can potentially influence the relationship between the type of manual intervention (i.e., the IV) and any one of the nine effects measured (i.e., the DV).

The classification and coding schemes used in this study, therefore, are discussed and then displayed in terms of the aforementioned characteristics for each of the 37 assembled primary studies. Specifically, for each study there is a mean effect size index (to be discussed later in this critique) as well as descriptive data pertaining to the six moderator variables. Furthermore, these characteristics of each study are discussed and displayed for *each* of the nine effects (outcomes or DVs) investigated. The principal display giving form to what has just been described is Table 1, with Tables 2 and 3 complementing the more comprehensive data presented in Table 1.

FOCUS OF CRITIQUE QUESTION 5: VALIDITY AND RELIABILITY OF CODING FORM

Are the validity and reliability of the coding form established?

The validity of the implied coding form used to document and classify the several study characteristics cited previously appears to be established. Specifically, the researchers based their classification of study characteristics on the MT literature available in the following areas: (a) accepted operational definition and common element of MT, (b) MT theories that give a context for investigating MT as an intervention and its effects, (c) nine recognized categories of MT effects, and (d) six recognized categories of possible moderating influences.

Regarding the issue of reliability, the authors discuss in the method section the degree of inter-rater agreement or consistency. The data provided here suggest a high degree of reliability in using the interface of the inclusion/exclusion criteria and study characteristics. The bases for, and approaches to, the decisions made regarding primary studies assembled and examined appear to be objective, valid, and consistent.

FOCUS OF CRITIQUE QUESTION 6: BASIS FOR CONVERTING PRIMARY STUDY OUTCOME MEASURE TO A COMMON METRIC

What technique is used to convert the outcome measure in the study to a common scale or metric (realizing that the common scale or metric is the dependent variable in the meta-analysis)?

The technique used is that of Hedges's *g* statistic, which, along with Cohen's *d* statistic, is one of the two prevalent effect size indices. The *g effect size* metric/statistic is provided for each study per each of the nine effects, or DVs, measured (see Table 1).

Furthermore, an *overall g effect size* metric is provided for each study in the collection of 37 (see Table 2).

FOCUS OF CRITIQUE QUESTION 7: AGGREGATED STUDY FINDINGS

With respect to aggregating the study findings, what analyses are reported regarding (a) estimating a summary measure of effect size, (b) calculating the variance of the summary measure, (c) testing for homogeneity, and (d) calculating confidence intervals?

The principal summary measure in the meta-analysis is that of the *mean effect size (g)* provided not only *for each of the nine outcome variables but also overall* (see Table 3). Furthermore, a *95% confidence interval (CI)* was calculated to assess which of the mean effect sizes were statistically significant. Adjusted mean effects sizes (g) and adjusted 95% CIs were provided to reflect possible publication bias; however, these analyses are beyond the scope of our current discussion.

FOCUS OF CRITIQUE QUESTION 8: INTERPRETATION OF FINDINGS RELATIVE TO CHARACTERISTICS OF PRIMARY STUDIES ASSEMBLED

Are the meta-analytic findings interpreted in reference to those characteristics of the assembled primary studies that were classified and coded at the outset?

Most definitely, the authors do a commendable job of discussing the multitude of findings in this study in specific reference to both the methodological and substantive features of the primary studies. In particular, the authors interpret their findings in the context of the introductory section's extensive coverage of topics such as single-dose versus multiple-dose effects, moderator variables, and the several MT theories. Of particular note is the interpretation of this study's findings relative to MT as viewed from a psychotherapeutic perspective.

FOCUS OF CRITIQUE QUESTION 9: IMPLICATIONS AND RECOMMENDED FUTURE RESEARCH

What are the implications of the study, and are there any recommendations regarding additional primary studies or meta-analyses that are needed?

Building on the response to critique question 8, this study's implications are most directly related to the following areas: (a) the nature of MT intervention in terms of both specific ingredients and common factors, (b) its likely underlying mechanisms in both physiological and psychological realms, (c) the distinction between single- and multiple-dose effects, (d) the potential role of moderators, and (e) the common factors feature of MT that should distinguish research in this area from the conventional medical model of reliance on double-blind studies and extensive use of placebo comparisons.

The recommendations for further research are totally in terms of future primary studies that speak to the five areas of implications cited in the preceding paragraph. Of particular emphasis, however, is the call for future research that (a) expands the search for underlying mechanisms beyond the physiological to include the psychological as well and (b) considers the common factors theme in addition to the specific ingredients focus in MT interventions.

FOCUS OF CRITIQUE QUESTION 10: EXTENT AND VALUE OF STUDY PROTOCOL DOCUMENTATION

Is the overall study protocol explicitly documented enough to allow other researchers (a) to evaluate the methodology used and (b) to replicate the study?

The study's protocol is meticulously laid out for the reader. This allows one to reflect from an informed position on the extent to which the findings of this study are objective, unbiased, and credible. The extensive degree of specificity with which the protocol is explained also permits an interested party to engage in either a full or partial replication of the study either in this research domain or in a related one.

WHERE DO WE GO FROM HERE?

In Part Four of this book, we considered two research categories that may be viewed as either alternatives or complements to quantitative research, the qualitative research and integrative research categories. Chapters 2 through 9, therefore, provide a survey of various options available to researchers in the health and behavioral sciences.

Part Five comprises one chapter in the form of two reprinted documents. The first document (AMTA Foundation & Kahn, 2002) provides somewhat of a historical context from which to consider the current emphasis on massage therapy research competencies (MTRCs). This report details the insights of the Massage Research Agenda Workgroup (MRAW) that was commissioned by the then AMTA Foundation (re-named the Massage Therapy

Foundation in September 2004), which convened for a three-day conference in March 1999. The second document (Hymel, 2003) presents several ideas that researchers, practitioners, and policymakers may want to consider with a view toward advancing research competencies in the massage therapy profession.

Although the forthcoming Chapter 10 is couched in terms of massage therapy, the majority of themes addressed in the two reprints apply as well to related health science professions that share an interest in advancing research competencies.

REFERENCES

AMTA Foundation, & Kahn, J. (2002). *Massage therapy research agenda*. Evanston, IL: AMTA Foundation. Retrieved July 29, 2004, from www.amtafoundation. org/massageagenda.html.

Arman, M., & Rehnsfeldt, A. (2003). The hidden suffering among breast cancer patients: A qualitative metasynthesis. *Qualitative Health Research, 13*(4), 510–527.

Assendelft, W. J. J., Morton, S. C., Yu, E. I., Suttorp, M. J., & Shekelle, P. G. (2003). Spinal manipulative therapy for low back pain. *Annals of Internal Medicine, 138*, 871–881.

Bangert-Downs, R. L. (1995). Misunderstanding meta-analysis. *Evaluation & the Health Professions, 18*(3), 304–314.

Barroso, J., & Powell-Cope, G. M. (2000). Metasynthesis of qualitative research on living with HIV infection. *Qualitative Health Research, 10*, 340–353.

Beck, C. T. (2001). Caring within nursing education: A metasynthesis. *Journal of Nursing Education, 40*, 101–109.

Callaghan, M. J. (1993). The role of massage in the management of the athlete: A review. *British Journal of Sports Medicine, 27*(1), 28–33.

Chalmers, T. C., Berrier, J., Sacks, H. S., Levin, H., Reitman, D., & Nagalingam, R. (1987). Meta-analysis of clinical trials as a scientific discipline. II: Replicate variability and comparison of studies that agree and disagree. *Statistics in Medicine, 6*, 733–744.

Cohen, J. (1988). *Statistical power for the behavioral sciences* (2nd ed.). Hillsdale, NJ: Lawrence Erlbaum.

Conn, V. S., Valentine, J. C., Cooper, H. M., & Rantz, M. J. (2003). Grey literature in meta-analyses. *Nursing Research, 52*(4), 256–261.

Cook, D. J., Mulrow, C. D., & Haynes, B. (1998). Synthesis of best evidence for clinical decisions. In C. Mulrow & D. Cook (Eds.), *Systematic reviews: Synthesis of best evidence for health care decisions* (pp. 5–12). Philadelphia: American College of Physicians.

Cooper, H. M. (1982). Scientific guidelines for conducting integrative research reviews. *Review of Educational Research, 52*(2), 291–302.

Davis, G. C. (2003). Improved sleep may reduce arthritis pain. *Holistic Nursing Practice, 17*(3), 128–135.

Devine, E. C. (1990). Meta-analysis: A new approach for reviewing research. In N. L. Chaska (Ed.), *The nursing profession: Turning points* (pp. 180–185). St. Louis: Mosby.

Ernst, E. (1998). Does post-exercise massage treatment reduce delayed onset muscle soreness? A systematic review. *British Journal of Sports Medicine, 32*, 212–214.

Ernst, E. (1999a). Abdominal massage therapy for chronic constipation: A systematic review of controlled clinical trials. *Forsch Komplementarmed (Research in Complemenatry Medicine), 6*, 149–151.

Ernst, E. (1999b). Massage therapy for low back pain: A systematic review. *Journal of Pain Symptom Management, 17*(1), 65–69.

Ernst, E., & Fialka, V. (1994). The clinical effectiveness of massage therapy—A critical review. *Forsch Komplementarmed, 1*, 226–232.

Field, T. (1998). Massage therapy effects. *American Psychologist, 53*(12), 1270–1281.

Finfgeld, D. L., (2003). Metasynthesis: The state of the art—so far. *Qualitative Health Research, 13*(7), 893–904.

Fredriksson, L. (1999). Modes of relating in a caring conversation: A research synthesis on presence, touch and listening. *Journal of Advanced Nursing, 30*, 1167–1176.

Furlan, A. D., Brosseau, L., Imamura, M., & Irvin, E. (2002). Massage for low-back pain: A systematic review within the framework of the Cochrane Collaboration Back Review Group. *Spine, 27*(17), 1896–1910.

Glass, G. (1976). Primary, secondary, and meta-analysis of research. *Educational Researcher, 5*, 3–8.

Glass, G., McGaw, B., & Smith, M. L. (1981). *Meta-analysis in social research*. Beverly Hills, CA: Sage.

Greenhalgh, T. (1998). Commentary: Meta-analysis is a blunt and potentially misleading instrument for analyzing models of service delivery. *BMJ, 317*, 395–396.

Greenhalgh, T. (2001). *How to read a paper: The basics of evidence based medicine* (2nd ed.). London: BMJ.

Griffin, S. (1998). Diabetes care in general practice: Meta-analysis of randomised control trials. *BMJ, 317*, 390–394.

Gutierrez, R., & Slavin, R. E. (1992). Achievement effects of the nongraded elementary school: A best-evidence synthesis. *Review of Educational Research, 62*, 333–376.

Harris, S. (2004). *Einstein simplified: Cartoons on science by Sidney Harris* (Rev. ed.). New Brunswick, NJ: Rutgers University Press.

Hedges, L. V., & Olkin, I. (1985). *Statistical methods for meta-analysis*. Toronto: Academic Press.

Hymel, G. M. (2003). Advancing massage therapy research competencies: Dimensions for thought and action. *Journal of Bodywork and Movement Therapies, 7*(3), 194–199.

Jensen, L. A., & Allen, M. N. (1994). A synthesis of qualitative research on wellness-illness. *Qualitative Health Research, 4*(4), 349–369.

Kendall, P. C., Flannery-Schroeder, E. C., & Ford, J. D. (1999). Therapy outcome research methods. In P. C. Kendall, J. N. Butcher, & G. N. Holmbeck (Eds.),

Handbook of research methods in clinical psychology (2nd ed.) (pp. 330–363). New York: John Wiley & Sons.

Koes, B. W., Assendelft, W. J. J., van der Heijden, G. J. M. G., Bouter, L. M., & Knipschild, P. G. (1991). Spinal manipulation and mobilisation for back and neck pain: A blinded review. *BMJ, 303*, 1298–1303.

L'Abbe, K. A., Detsky, A. S., & O'Rourke, K. (1987). Meta-analysis in clinical research. *Annals of Internal Medicine, 107*, 224–233.

McCain, N. L., Smith, M. C., & Abraham, I. L. (1986). Meta-analyses of nursing interventions: The codebook as a research instrument. *Western Journal of Nursing Research, 8*(2), 155–167.

Moher, D., Cook, D. J., Eastwood, S., Olkin, I., Rennie, D., & Stroup, D. F. (1999). Improving the quality of reports of meta-analyses of randomised controlled trials: The QUOROM statement. *The Lancet, 354*, 1896–1900.

Moher, D., & Olkin, I. (1995). Meta-analysis of randomized controlled trials: A concern for standards. *Journal of the American Medical Association, 274*(24), 1962–1964.

Moraska, A. (in press). Sports massage–A critical review. *Journal of Sports Medicine and Physical Fitness.*

Mosteller, F., & Colditz, G. A. (1996). Understanding research synthesis (meta-analysis). *Annual Review of Public Health, 17*, 1 – 23.

Moyer, C. A., Rounds, J., & Hannum, J. W. (2004). A meta-analysis of massage therapy research. *Psychological Bulletin, 130*(1), 3–18.

Onyskiw, J. E. (1996). The meta-analytic approach to research integration. *Canadian Journal of Nursing Research, 28*(3), 69–85.

Patterson, B. L., Thorne, S. E., Canam, C., & Jillings, C. (2001). *Meta-study of qualitative health research: A practical guide to meta-analysis and meta-synthesis.* Thousand Oaks, CA: Sage.

Rosenthal, R. (1984). *Meta-analytic procedures for social research: Applied social research methods series.* London: Sage.

Sandelowski, M., & Barroso, J. (2003). Creating metasummaries of qualitative findings. *Nursing Research, 52*(4), 226–233.

Schaefer, K. M. (2003). Sleep disturbances linked to fibromyalgia. *Holistic Nursing Practice, 17*(3), 120–127.

Slavin, R. E. (1986). Best-evidence synthesis: An alternative to meta-analytic and traditional reviews. *Educational Researcher, 15*(9), 5–11.

Slavin, R. E. (1987a). Ability grouping and student achievement in elementary schools: A best-evidence synthesis. *Review of Educational Research, 57*, 347–350.

Slavin, R. E. (1987b). Mastery learning reconsidered. *Review of Educational Research, 57*, 175–213.

Slavin, R. E. (1990). Ability grouping and student achievement in secondary schools: A best-evidence synthesis. *Review of Educational Research, 60*, 471–499.

Slavin, R. E. (1995). Best evidence synthesis: An intelligent alternative to meta-analysis. *Journal of Clinical Epidemiology, 48*(1), 9–18.

Spitzer, W. O., Lawrence, V., Dales, R., Hill, G., Archer, M. C., Clark, P., et al. (1990). Links between passive smoking and disease: A best-evidence synthesis. *Clinical and Investigative Medicine, 13*(1), 17–42.

Tiidus, P. M. (1997). Manual massage and recovery of muscle function following exercise: A literature review. *Journal of Orthopaedic and Sports Physical Fitness, 25*(2), 107–112.

van der Heijden, G. J. M. G., van der Windt, D. A. W. M., & de Winter, A. F. (1997). Physiotherapy for patients with soft tissue shoulder disorders: A systematic review of randomized clinical trials. *BMJ, 315*, 25–30.

van Tulder, M. W., Ostelo, R., Vlaeyen, J. W. S., Linton, S. J., Morley, S. J., & Assendelft, W. J. J. (2000). Behavioral treatment for chronic low back pain: A systematic review within the framework of the Cochrane Back Review Group. *Spine, 25*(20), 2688–2699.

Weldon, S. M., & Hill, R. H. (2003). The efficacy of stretching for prevention of exercise-related injury: A systematic review of the literature. *Manual Therapy, 8*(3), 141–150.

ADDITIONAL RECOMMENDED RESOURCES

Cooper, H. M. (1984). *The integrative research review: A systematic approach.* Beverly Hills, CA: Sage.

Cooper, H., & Hedges, L. V. (Eds.). *The handbook of research synthesis.* New York: The Russell Sage Foundation.

Egger, M., & Smith, G. D. (1997). Meta-analysis: Potentials and promise. *BMJ, 315*, 1371–1374.

Egger, M., & Smith, G. D. (1998). Meta-analysis: Bias in location and selection of studies. *BMJ, 316*, 61–66.

Egger, M., Smith, G. D., & Phillips, A. N. (1997). Meta-analysis: Principles and procedures. *BMJ, 315*, 1533–1537.

Egger, M., Schneider, M., & Smith, G. D. (1998). Meta-analysis: Spurious precision? Meta-analysis of observational studies. *BMJ, 316*, 140–144.

Glasziou, P., Irwig, L., Bain, C., & Colditz, G. (2001). *Systematic reviews in health care: A practical guide.* New York: Cambridge University Press.

Hedges, L. V. (1982). Estimation of effect size from a series of independent experiments. *Psychological Bulletin, 92*(2), 490–499.

Kazdin, A. E. (Ed.). (2003). *Methodological issues & strategies in clinical research* (3rd ed.). Washington, DC: American Psychological Association.

Kendall, P. C., Butcher, J. N., & Holmbeck, G. N. (Eds.). (1999). *Handbook of research methods in clinical psychology* (2nd ed.). New York: John Wiley & Sons.

Lipsey, M. W., & Wilson, D. B. (2001). *Practical meta-analysis.* Thousand Oaks, CA: Sage.

Mulrow, C., & Cook, D. (Eds.). (1998). *Systematic reviews: Synthesis of best evidence for health care decisions.* Philadelphia: American College of Physicians.

Rosenthal, R., & Rubin, D. B. (1982). Comparing effect sizes of independent studies. *Psychological Bulletin, 92*(2), 500–504.

Smith, G. D., & Egger, M. (1998). Meta-analysis: Unresolved issues and future developments. *BMJ, 316*, 221–225.

Smith, G. D., Egger, M., & Phillips, A. N. (1997). Meta-analysis: Beyond the grand mean? *BMJ, 315*, 1610–1615.

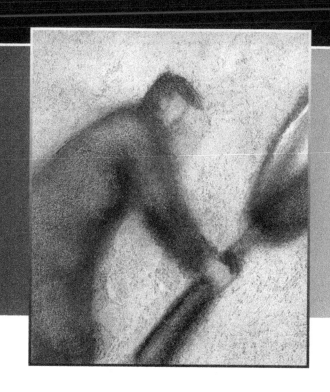

PART FIVE

ADVANCING THE MASSAGE THERAPY RESEARCH AGENDA

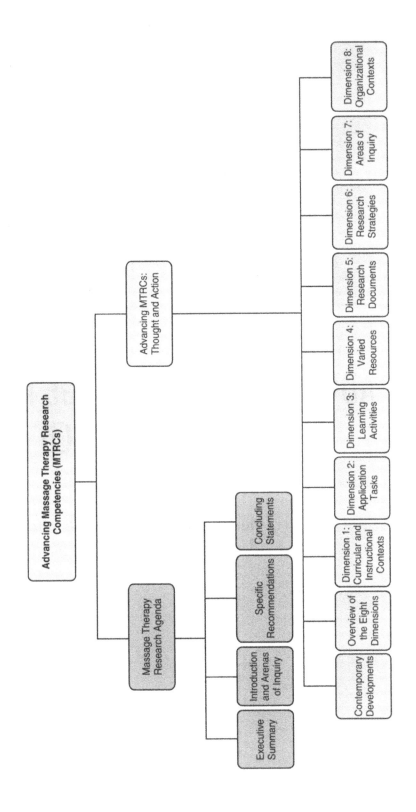

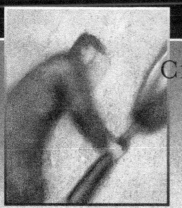

10

ADVANCING MASSAGE THERAPY RESEARCH COMPETENCIES: RECENT CONTEXTS AND PROJECTED DIRECTIONS

OUTLINE

OBJECTIVES

Upon completion of this chapter, the reader will have the information necessary to perform the following tasks:

1 Regarding the outcomes document generated by the Massage Research Agenda Workgroup (MRAW),
   a. discuss the major factors leading to the MRAW's three-day conference in March 1999;
   b. identify the two distinct categories into which the general arena of clinical research on safety and efficacy may be divided;
   c. identify and discuss at least five activities associated with the group's recommendation to build a massage research infrastructure;
   d. identify and discuss at least five considerations regarding the group's recommendation to fund research into the safety and efficacy of massage therapy;
   e. identify and discuss the following three areas in which the MRAW suggests that studies be conducted: primary prevention studies, secondary prevention studies, and replication studies;
   f. characterize the group's recommendation to fund studies of the physiological (and other) mechanisms by which massage therapy achieves its effects;
   g. discuss the group's recommendation to fund studies stemming from a wellness paradigm;
   h. identify and discuss at least three suggestions regarding the MRAW's recommendation to fund studies of the profession of therapeutic massage.

KEY TERMS

COMTA
Massage Research Agenda Workgroup
 (MRAW)
Massage research infrastructure

Massage Therapy Foundation
Massage therapy research competency
 dimensions
Massage therapy safety and efficacy

Profession of massage therapy
Underlying mechanisms
Wellness paradigm

2 Regarding the reprinted article on advancing massage therapy research competencies,
  a. cite and discuss at least three contemporary developments leading to the current emphasis on research competency;
  b. discuss each of the following eight dimensions in which possibilities exist for advancing massage therapy research competencies (MTRCs): curricular and instructional contexts; application tasks for demonstrating MTRCs; learning activities for enhancing MTRCs; print, electronic, and personnel resources; varieties of research documents; potential research strategies; potential areas of inquiry in massage therapy research; and organizational contexts for supporting massage therapy research.

WHERE HAVE WE BEEN AND WHERE ARE WE NOW? THE CONNECTION

Chapters 2 through 9 surveyed the complete range of research categories inclusive of quantitative, qualitative, and integrative research. Also, research strategies affiliated with the three categories have been examined with a particular focus on those research methods, designs, and procedures that come into play. Our coverage of this material has been sequential and linear with realistic illustrations built in at appropriate stages.

This type of introductory exposure to the research process should convey the broad range of several possibilities that one may encounter when studying what earlier investigators have uncovered. Also, it should indicate the several possible options available if one wants to become actively engaged in the research process as a member of a research team.

From these perspectives of research consumer or active researcher, it should be helpful to learn of the recent historical context for much of the current attention to massage therapy research. Furthermore, in building on that context, it should prove beneficial for one to learn of directions in which the profession needs to travel in order to position its work on a more scientific base. The two reprinted documents constituting this chapter provide that historical context as well as those needed dimensions giving direction to how we think and act professionally (cf. AMTA Foundation & Kahn, 2002; and Hymel, 2003).

MASSAGE THERAPY RESEARCH AGENDA: OUTCOMES DOCUMENT OF THE MASSAGE RESEARCH AGENDA WORKGROUP (MRAW)

The first document considered here provides some of the recent background to the current attention being given to research in the **profession of**

massage therapy (AMTA Foundation & Kahn, 2002). It reflects the deliberations, insight, recommendations, and conclusions of the **Massage Research Agenda Workgroup (MRAW)** commissioned by the then AMTA Foundation (now the **Massage Therapy Foundation**) when it convened for a three-day conference in March 1999.

This effort by the MRAW identifies two distinct categories within the general arena of clinical research on **massage therapy safety and efficacy**: studies that compare the relative effectiveness of specific massage modalities to one another and studies that examine massage in comparison with other treatments. In the realm of specific recommendations, the outcomes document lists the following five: (a) build a **massage research infrastructure,** (b) fund research into the safety and efficacy of massage therapy, (c) fund studies of physiological mechanisms (or other **underlying mechanisms**) by which massage therapy achieves its effects, (d) fund studies stemming from a **wellness paradigm,** and (e) fund studies of the profession of therapeutic massage.

Against this backdrop, then, Box 10-1 presents the MRAW's outcomes document in its entirety.

BOX 10-1 MASSAGE THERAPY RESEARCH AGENDA*

Executive Summary

1. **Build a research infrastructure within the massage therapy profession.** Encourage development of a research literate massage therapy profession through several means. Work with the Commission on Massage Therapy Accreditation (COMTA), the AMTA Council of Schools (COS) and the National Certification Board for Therapeutic Massage and Bodywork (NCBTMB) to establish research as a core competency in the professional education of massage therapists. Fund the education of massage therapy researchers. Foster collaborations, create pathways and establish linkages which encourage interactions of massage therapists with physicians; clinical and experimental researchers; and with social scientists.

2. **Fund research into the safety and efficacy of massage therapy.** Begin by funding studies which compare the relative effectiveness of different massage modalities for a given condition and then fund studies which compare the optimum massage therapy for a given condition with other standard methods of care (medical, chiropractic, acupuncture, etc.). The MRAW suggested four primary prevention studies, two secondary prevention studies and replication studies.

3. **Fund studies of physiological (or other) mechanisms by which massage therapy achieves its effects.** The MRAW further suggested funding systematic documentation of physiological effects of massage and explorations of the dimensions and effects of "subtle energy."

4. **Fund studies stemming from a wellness paradigm.** Document what "wellness" means to stake holders. Establish the dimensions of the effects of massage therapy on "self-healing" and align these studies with the study of physiological mechanisms above. Explore the interaction of consciousness, wellness and the actual practice of massage therapists.

5. **Fund studies of the profession of therapeutic massage.** Fund studies which determine what makes a "good" or "great" massage therapist; document how massage therapists are perceived by themselves and others; evaluate the client assessment skills of massage therapists; and explore the dimensions of the therapeutic encounter.

Introduction

Rigorously controlled and replicated research is a key to the professionalization of any health care field. Reliable research findings are a prerequisite for access to many contexts in which massage therapists practice or would like to practice. For these reasons, the AMTA Foundation convened a three-day working conference of research scientists and massage therapists/bodyworkers in March 1999 to frame a research agenda for the field of therapeutic massage and bodywork. Without the active participation of members of the massage profession in deciding what research should be done, there is every possibility that knowledge generated from future research will not be relevant or of value to massage therapists or to their clients.

In preparation for the meeting, the Foundation recognized that various constituencies already held agendas, which would need to be articulated and addressed. Prior to the meeting, a web site survey and focus groups conducted by the Foundation revealed that massage therapists had three key goals that needed to inform the research agenda.

1. Massage therapists want more people to seek regular massage for health maintenance and well-being. What is the research agenda that might lead to this?

*This report was authored by Janet Kahn, Ph.D., who facilitated the Massage Research Agenda Workgroup in March 1999 during her tenure as AMTA Foundation President. This publication has been edited by the AMTA Foundation. © 2002 by the AMTA Foundation

Continued

BOX 10-1   MASSAGE THERAPY RESEARCH AGENDA — CONT'D

2. Massage therapists want to understand more clearly how and why their work is effective or ineffective. What is the research agenda that will lead to this understanding?

3. Some massage therapists want to be reimbursed by third party payers for their work. What is the research agenda most likely to lead to this? Other health care professionals also have concerns and questions that would drive their agenda for our field. For example, physicians and health care administrators want to know when to refer for massage and which kind of massage to recommend for which conditions. What is the research agenda that will help these health care professionals?

Thus the AMTA Foundation convened a Massage Research Agenda Workgroup (MRAW) which included physicians, clinical and experimental scientists, social scientists and massage therapists and bodyworkers all selected to represent a relatively broad spectrum of expertise in their fields. It included Americans, Canadians and Europeans.

All workgroups of the MRAW included at least one massage therapist, one clinical or survey research scientist, and one bench or biological scientist. Members of the MRAW were struck by how valuable these multi-disciplinary groups were. The MRAW cautioned against the all too frequent practice of research in CAM in general and therapeutic massage specifically, being designed and conducted without the benefit of any practitioners involved in conceptual roles. We highly recommend the creation of multi-disciplinary teams at least during the design phase.

In preparation for the meeting, the AMTA Foundation commissioned a background paper1 looking at issues of fit between the realities of massage treatment and the requirements of currently accepted research methodologies; examined claims made in major massage texts about the effects of massage and found many claims and little research cited; reviewed the existing massage research literature; and circulated to participants two recent reviews of the literature, noticing shortcomings and areas of promise. What follows is a review of the recommendations of the MRAW.

Arenas of Inquiry

The MRAW divided the general arena of **clinical research on safety and efficacy**, into two distinct categories:

- **studies that compare the relative effectiveness of specific massage modalities to one another**, seeking the strongest treatment for each condition/population/situation, and
- **studies that examine massage in comparison with other treatments** (e.g. massage therapy versus usual allopathic care or chiropractic treatment, etc.).

Studies of efficacy and outcome lead to **questions of mechanism**. There has been little done in this area for the field of massage. For example, premature infants gain more weight when they receive regular massage therapy than premature infants fed the same number of calories but not receiving regular massage therapy. Through what mechanism is massage therapy causing these results?

The final arena of inquiry that was identified is **socio-cultural knowledge**, which includes basic descriptive information about who seeks massage; how it is viewed by consumer, physicians, and others; and how massage therapists define the goals of treatment.

Specific Recommendations

The workgroup made a range of recommendations covering not only what kinds of studies ought to be done, but also how they might best be done, and what conditions must be met in order to move the agenda forward.

Build a Massage Research Infrastructure

The MRAW strongly emphasized that a field needs a research infrastructure in order to follow through on any research agenda. It is suggested that this infrastructure, crucial to the development of the profession, may be built through the following activities:

- Fund the education of researchers prepared to dedicate their careers to massage therapy research.
- Encourage the development of a research literate profession by teaching basic research literacy skills in massage schools and in continuing education contexts. This would include teacher training in this vital area. Continuing education could be supported through the creation of a self-study module, as well as workshops offered in research literacy, research methods and internships for participation on research teams.
- Work with the Commission on Massage Therapy Accreditation (COMTA), the AMTA Council of Schools (COS) and the National Certification Board for Therapeutic

Massage and Bodywork (NCBTMB) to establish research as a core competency in the professional education of massage therapists, as it is in many other professions.

- Create ways for people to be involved in research, including teaching massage therapists how to develop good case histories. A database of solid and informative cases would be a gold mine of ideas and evidence for later research. Encouraging more uniform training in systematic record keeping is also associated with this.

1Cassidy, C. (1999). Methodological issues in investigations of massage/bodywork therapy.

BOX 10-1   MASSAGE THERAPY RESEARCH AGENDA — CONT'D

- Foster collaboration and mutual education between medical schools and massage schools.
- Create pathways for the development of a massage research community including: ongoing workgroups; a virtual community or moderated chat room of massage research enthusiasts; research networks such as the hospital based massage research network; special interest groups on research within AMTA or across professional associations.
- Establish linkages between massage therapists and academics/researchers including those already interested and active in this field and those that we feel ought to be interested because of mutual concerns.
- Fund developmental grants to support the time it takes people to develop conceptually elegant experiments with sufficient statistical power to allow a definitive outcome.
- Disseminate this agenda as widely as possible to inform and stimulate interest among the health care research community.
- Fund, through the AMTA and/or AMTA Foundation, high priority studies that will both advance the knowledge in the field and establish the viability of massage as an area of inquiry.

Fund Research into Safety & Efficacy of Massage Therapy

Studies must be funded to identify those applications of massage therapy that are safe and have identifiable benefit and those that are not reliably effective and/or carry associated risk. The MRAW recommended as highest priority studies of the comparative efficacy of different kinds of massage therapy/bodywork in relation to a particular condition or goal, and then the utilization of the most effective massage protocol in clinical trials comparing massage with standard medical, chiropractic or other forms of care for the same conditions.

The following considerations went into identifying the specific safety and efficacy studies recommended below:

- Studies must preserve public health and safety.
- Studies must alleviate human suffering and associated costs.
- Studies should be undertaken when the expectation that massage therapy/bodywork will be beneficial in a particular situation rests on good anecdotal evidence, pilot data, and/or on a firm theoretical basis.
- Studies receive a higher priority when the current usual treatment is unacceptable in one or more ways including high cost, adverse side effects or pain and/or inconvenience of the treatment itself.
- The condition being studied should be sufficiently prevalent that the study will address a situation affecting many people's lives.
- Study subjects should be readily available.
- Study must have a clearly defined massage intervention and unambiguous outcomes/endpoints and also must be of import to stakeholders.
- The treatment, if successful, should be relatively easy to adopt.

It was acknowledged that high impact efficacy studies might focus on either primary or secondary prevention, within a clinically oriented pathology model, or draw more upon a "wellness agenda." Illustrative examples were generated during preliminary design sessions that utilized small teams including at least one massage therapist, one clinical researcher and one basic science researcher.

Suggested Primary Prevention Studies

WORKPLACE-BASED PRIMARY PREVENTION

Massage therapists often hear from clients that regular massage provides a host of benefits both in mood and physical health. Yet the effects of regular massage on a "healthy" population have never been studied. The MRAW endorsed as a priority a study that would examine (as key outcomes) the potential for regular massage to effect the frequency, duration and associated cost of injuries and illnesses common to a particular workplace, as well as exploring a range of promising outcomes including worker satisfaction with job, mental health outcomes, satisfaction with home life, etc.

MASSAGE TO PREVENT CONGESTIVE HEART FAILURE

This was offered as an example of a condition-specific primary care study. The goal of such a study would be to examine the potential for massage to prevent congestive heart failure among people who appear at high risk. Subjects might be patients 40+ years of age, diagnosed with moderate to severe hypertension and perhaps receiving medication for high blood pressure. They would be under the care of a physician and maintain regular visits to monitor their condition. Exclusion criteria would need to be developed and might include concurrent chronic diseases such as diabetes, kidney or liver failure, COPD, etc. Ideally the sample population would be ethnically diverse and include both males and females with sufficient sample size to allow for gender comparison. Subjects would be randomized to defined conditions such as a) normal care, b) normal care plus weekly massage, and c) a control group receiving normal care plus some other form of high contact care. Length of treatment would be determined by an examination of what is already known about the ability of massage to affect blood pressure. The principal outcomes would be BP, medication use, and of course, incidence of congestive heart failure.

Continued

BOX 10-1   MASSAGE THERAPY RESEARCH AGENDA — CONT'D

MASSAGE AND MUSCULOSKELETAL DISORDERS SUCH AS SCOLIOSIS

The lack of research on the use of massage in relation to musculoskeletal disorders is striking. In fact, musculoskeletal conditions may be the most promising arena for primary prevention investigations. Based on the experience of practitioners present at the MRAW, scoliosis was recommended as one study possibility.

The goal of such a study would be the prevention of a need for scoliosis surgery. It was stressed that this study should be done as a comparison of massage and usual care only after the within-massage/bodywork studies have been done to determine the most beneficial treatments for this condition. Subjects would be adolescents aged 12-18, recruited from a scoliosis clinic at the point when they are designated as candidates for future surgery. The length of treatment would be determined on the basis of existing data, but likely would be lengthy. The principal endpoint would be whether surgery was determined to be needed. The length of time to follow the subjects would be determined after consultation with experts in the field.

LOW BACK PAIN STUDIES

Studies on low back pain fit into two larger categories of investigation of the effects of massage on musculoskeletal disorders resulting in acute and/or chronic pain.

Initial work has begun in this field. Researchers at Group Health Center for Health Studies and Beth Israel Deaconess' Center for Alternative Medicine Research and Education are conducting high quality comparisons of massage and other treatments for lower back pain (both acute and persistent). Cherkin et al[2] indicate possible directions for additional work. For instance, given the relative success of massage compared to acupuncture and self-education shown in the Cherkin study, further investigations could attempt to determine whether there is a "best" massage treatment for persistent low back pain.

Suggested Secondary Prevention Studies

The MRAW recommended that attention be given to designing high quality studies examining the potential of massage in the area of secondary prevention. Two examples were given.

STUDY OF THE POTENTIAL FOR MASSAGE THERAPY TO PREVENT FALLING AMONG THE ELDERLY

Falling is a frequent occurrence among elderly persons, which results in both personal and social costs. With an aging population, such as exists in most industrialized countries, this issue will be of great interest.

It is often said by massage therapists that massage could be used to improve "groundedness" and balance. This could be tested in an elderly population. Subjects could be recruited through private physicians or medical centers after their first visit to a doctor for a fall. Age-related stratification of sample populations may be necessary. Subjects would be randomized to at least two conditions. One group would receive massage (the frequency and number of treatments to be set by the study team), and the other group would receive no massage treatment. Principle outcome measures could include both objective measures related to falling such as the time between falling episodes and the severity of injuries incurred, as well as measures related to quality of life.

SECONDARY PREVENTION OF DEPRESSION

Thousands of Americans experience depression and/or take antidepressant medications. This is a painful and costly condition, often accompanied by the unwanted side effects of antidepressants. Depression is affecting younger and younger populations. It is a worthy subject of investigation and preliminary data from studies done at the Touch Research Institute indicate massage may be an effective treatment. Subjects in such a study would be patients who already have experienced clinical depression and are deemed in remission. They would be randomly assigned to massage or no-massage treatment. The frequency and duration of treatment would be determined after examination of existing data. The principal outcome measure would be remission/relapse rate as indicated by future diagnoses of depression, use of antidepressants, and self-reports.

Suggested Replication Studies

One effect of the relative lack of funding for massage research, and the lack of acknowledged agenda for the work, is that few studies with promising results have been replicated. This is a serious, but easily remedied problem and the MRAW named replication of the best studies as one of the research priorities for the field of therapeutic massage and bodywork.

[2]Cherkin DC, Eisenberg D, Sherman KJ, et al (2001). Randomized trial comparing traditional Chinese medical acupuncture, therapeutic massage, and self-care education for chronic low back pain. Archives of Internal Medicine, 161, 1081–1088.

BOX 10-1 MASSAGE THERAPY RESEARCH AGENDA—CONT'D

Fund Studies of Physiological (or Other) Mechanisms by Which Massage Therapy Achieves its Effects

Inquiry into the avenues through which massage produces its effects is a pertinent and wide-open area for investigation. A myriad of studies could be conducted under this general heading.

Systematic Documentation of the Physiological Effects of Massage

It would be useful to conduct research designed to describe the physiological effects of massage separate from the matter of clinical impact. There are physiological effects that are regarded by many as established, but which have not been investigated since the advent of recent measurement tools. The claim that massage increases circulation of blood and lymph would be an example of this, as would investigation of the extent to which massage elicits sympathetic or parasympathetic response. Also, it would be useful to conduct research on the nature of fascia and its role in the effects of massage.

Seeking Explanations of Established Effects

Where certain effects of massage have been repeatedly demonstrated, it would be beneficial to establish how the body produces the effect. For instance, studies investigating the effects of massage on premature infants have consistently shown that those infants receiving massage have significantly greater weight gain than the unmassaged infants (a range of 28 47%), without any greater caloric intake. The mechanism of this weight gain has never been demonstrated.

Explorations of Subtle Energy

It was acknowledged by the MRAW that much is speculated or claimed, but little is actually known, about subtle energy and its role in healing in general and therapeutic massage in particular. Nonetheless, some massage schools and modalities teach "energy balancing" of one sort or another, and some massage education includes instruction in awareness of energy resonance and/or exchange between practitioner and client. While there are no agreed upon instruments of measurement for such subtle energy, the MRAW recognized the importance of the development of this field for a complete understanding of the effects of therapeutic massage and bodywork. We believe subtle energy should be studied both as a dimension of the therapeutic encounter and as a purposeful aspect of treatment.

Fund Studies Stemming from a Wellness Paradigm

Contemporary clinical research methodology and the questions it is designed to address have developed largely from within allopathic medicine, and thus, within a pathology-oriented framework. While therapeutic massage and bodywork is used to address such allopathically defined conditions, it is also, perhaps even more frequently, used for what clients and practitioners refer to as "wellness."

There are research questions that arise from a wellness paradigm that may not arise from a pathology paradigm and these, too, are important to pursue for an understanding of the effects of therapeutic massage. While wellness therapies may be the least "reimbursable" treatments at present, they may also be those most likely to ultimately change modern medicine and public health. The research needed includes qualitative studies aimed at eliciting operational definitions of heretofore vague terms (e.g. wellness, groundedness, centeredness, balance, etc.), descriptive studies, and "clinical" research. The following questions arose during MRAW discussions of these issues:

- What is wellness? According to client reports, more than 25% of visits to massage therapists are made for wellness. We need to know how clients define wellness when they seek it, and how they know when it has been achieved. We need to know how massage therapists define wellness when they say they offer treatments designed to enhance it.
- If we assume that the body is "self-healing" and that massage can somehow jump-start that healing process, how does this happen? Are the effects we see such as weight gain in premature infants, enhanced immune function among HIV+ men, etc. indications of this? What does jump-start mean?
- What is the interaction of consciousness and wellness? Do massage therapists practicing "wellness massage" tend to make suggestive comments during treatment? Are silent treatments more or less effective than treatments that include such suggestions?

Beyond "wellness," once it is defined, there lies the potential to investigate the role of massage in achieving peak performance. Such studies could include athletes, musicians and other performers already exploring the issues of human potential and peak performance. The issues can also be explored in relation to enhanced performance in other roles such as defense personnel, air traffic controllers, people in or just before high performance task situations (e.g. students taking exams), medical interns, 911 operators, children showing difficulty at school, care givers of all kinds, and those at the end of life.

Continued

BOX 10-1   MASSAGE THERAPY RESEARCH AGENDA — CONT'D

Fund Studies of the Profession of Therapeutic Massage

Despite its status as a healing modality that has existed for thousands of years across many cultures, there has been little systematic investigation of massage as a profession, including issues of training, public perception, and the like. The MRAW recommended strongly that this situation be remedied, and made a few specific suggestions.

The Search for Excellence

Little is known about what makes a "superior" massage therapist. This sentence has two separate meanings, both of which are important. First it reflects the fact that there is no agreed upon definition or description of a "good" massage therapist. The agreed upon training standards are stated in terms of hours of training (generally 500 hours in the United States, 2500 hours in Ontario, 3200 hours in British Columbia) rather than areas of competence, although this is about to change. Secondly it reflects the reality that there has been no systematic evaluation of educational practices in the profession. We do not know how one best trains a good massage therapist, or even the extent to which excellence in this field can be taught or is the result of a gift.

A range of studies could be designed to fill these gaps, from qualitative work to establish definitions of excellence in the field, to quantitative studies which ascertain whether such peer or client defined "excellence" corresponds to positive clinical results, to educational evaluation research geared to determining how both material and skills can be effectively transmitted. Furthermore, given the lack of uniformity in training in the United States today, it would be useful for the public to know how broad the range of skill or competence is among professional massage therapists who are trained at accredited institutions.

How Massage Therapists are Perceived by Themselves and Others

During the meetings of the MRAW, it became clear that the massage therapists regard client education as one of their critical roles and that the researchers did not initially share this view. This is a significant difference, and served to remind the MRAW that it would be of benefit to both the profession and the public to gather information about how massage therapists view their role and whether there is systematic variation in this by region, degree of training, years in practice, etc. It would also be of value to gather information on how the profession is perceived by the public, including clients, potential clients, referring health professionals, and health professionals in general. How do these groups view the work/role of massage therapists, and assess the effectiveness of massage therapists? How do all these groups view the role of clients? Are they thought of as passive recipients of a service or therapy? Do clients expect to learn from their massage therapists?

Evaluating Assessment Skills of Massage Therapists

Diagnosis falls outside the scope of practice of massage therapy. At the same time, massage therapists assess and reassess what is happening with clients in order to make decisions about treatment design. In part, because of the legal situation, our assessment has not been well studied, but it needs to be. In particular, it is important to study what is taught about assessment in comparison with what is practiced. Comparisons of this across regions with differing legal situations would be useful. In addition, it is vital to know whether there is inter-rater reliability in the area of assessment. That is, would different massage therapists, asked to assess the same clients, draw the same or different conclusions as to what is happening? Would they then design identical, similar, or widely varying treatment plans?

Dimensions of the Therapeutic Encounter

Finally, it was recognized that little investigation has been done on the therapeutic encounter itself within massage treatment. This is an important and potentially delicate area of inquiry, particularly within a climate in which much of what massage therapists may value as good practitioner/client interaction is seen, in another framework, as contamination or placebo effect. Nonetheless, or perhaps because of this, it is important to create ways of investigating the effects of everything from practitioner influence (both purposeful and accidental), to the influence of such environmental factors as music, lighting and so forth. What is the role of the practitioner/client relationship? How important is this attunement and how can one measure it? What therapist characteristics make a difference? How do you measure entrainment, e.g. EEG entrainment between client and therapist or pulse entrainment? Finally, assuming there is some "practitioner effect," it would be of value to determine ways of identifying characteristics that help match clients and therapists

Conclusion

The field of research in therapeutic massage and bodywork is just beginning to develop. This is an important step for a health care modality that is used widely but lacks extensive, rigorous data on its safety and efficacy. Many forms of research will be beneficial during this early, formative phase in the professionalization of massage in modern contexts. It is hoped that between federal and private funding sources, significant aspects of the work suggested here will be accomplished in the near future.

BOX 10-1   MASSAGE THERAPY RESEARCH AGENDA — CONT'D

Acknowledgments

The following individuals participated in the Massage Research Agenda Workgroup:

Researchers:

Alan Best, Ph.D., Senior Scientist, Centre for Clinical Epidemiology and Evaluation, Vancouver Hospital and Health Science Centre, Vancouver, British Columbia, Canada; Leon Chaitow, D.O., (In Absentia). Senior Lecturer, University of Westminster, London, England; Dan Cherkin, Ph.D., Senior Scientific Investigator, Group Health Center for Health Studies, Seattle, Washington; David Eisenberg, M.D., Director, Center for Alternative Medicine Research and Education, Beth Israel Deaconess Medical Center, Boston, Massachusetts; Robert L. Kahn, Ph.D. (In Absentia), Research Scientist, Institute for Social Research, Professor Emeritus of Psychology and Public Health, University of Michigan, Ann Arbor, Michigan; Brian Marcotte, Ph.D., (AMTA Foundation Trustee), CEO and Director, Strategic Analysis, Inc., Providence, Rhode Island; James Oschman, Ph.D., President, Nature's Own Research Association, Dover, New Hampshire; Candace Pert, Ph.D., Research Professor, Department of Physiology and Biophysics, Georgetown University Medical Center, Washington, D.C.

Massage Therapists:

Doug Alexander, Founding and Current Editor-in-Chief, Journal of Soft Tissue Manipulation, Ottawa, Ontario, Canada; Judith Aston, Founder and Director, Aston-Patterning, Incline Village, Nevada; Debra Curties, Executive Director, Sutherland-Chan School and Teaching Clinic, Toronto, Ontario, Canada; Deane Juhan, Instructor, Trager Institute, Mill Valley, California; George Kousaleos, (past AMTA Foundation Trustee,) Founder and Director, CORE Institute, Tallahassee, Florida; Carole Osborne-Sheets, Licensed Holistic Health Practitioner, Co-Founder and Instructor, International Professional School of Bodywork, San Diego, California; Lawrence E. Warnock, Ph.D., Executive Director and Owner, The Center for Health and Athletic Performance, Inc. and The Student-Athlete Educational Foundation, Reading, Massachusetts

Organization Representatives:

Janet Kahn, Ph.D., Foundation Past President, researcher, massage therapist; E. Houston LeBrun, Past President AMTA, massage therapist, Private Practice, Seattle, Washington; Martha Brown Menard, Ph.D., Foundation Past Vice President, researcher, massage therapist; Gini S. Ohlson, Foundation Director of Development and Foundation Manager; Deborah Worrad, CAE, Registrar, College of Massage Therapists of Ontario, Toronto, Ontario, Canada

From AMTA Foundation, & Kahn, J. (2002). *Massage therapy research agenda.* Evanston, IL: AMTA Foundation. Retrieved July 29, 2004, from www.massagetherapyfoundation.org/massageagenda.html.

ADVANCING MASSAGE THERAPY RESEARCH COMPETENCIES

The second document constituting this chapter proposes several dimensions or domains in which possibilities exist for advancing research competencies in the massage therapy profession (Hymel, 2003). These eight dimensions for thought and action represent somewhat of a sequel to the MRAW's recommendations. They also constitute an understandable follow-up to other contemporary developments in the profession regarding research publications, the evidence-based practice movement, expanded massage therapy education requirements, and accreditation issues.

Several of the major areas cited as being strategic to advancing research competencies cut across curricular, instructional, assessment, resource, and organizational domains. Others relate more directly to research problem areas, strategies, methods, and types of research documentation. There are several vantage points, then, from which the advancement of research competencies may be approached in the interest of the massage therapy profession and related health science professions.

Box 10-2 displays the published article that proposes a focus on eight related, yet diverse, dimensions or domains of thought and action with a view toward advancing research competencies (Hymel, 2003).

WHERE DO WE GO FROM HERE?

Our journey through this book's 10 chapters represents in many ways a modest starting point in terms of examining the many issues that bear on the

BOX 10-2   ADVANCING MASSAGE THERAPY RESEARCH COMPETENCIES: DIMENSIONS FOR THOUGHT AND ACTION

Glenn M. Hymel*

Abstract

Two major developments in the therapeutic massage and bodywork profession have recently brought to the forefront, in a most comprehensive fashion, the issue of research competencies. Specifically, the efforts of the American Massage Therapy Association (AMTA) Foundation's Massage Research Agenda Workgroup and the Commission on Massage Therapy Accreditation's **(COMTA)** expansion of competency-based standards to include a research component have both called the profession to a potentially heightened level of credibility. Accompanying such an opportunity for the massage/bodywork profession's development, though, are challenges still to be successfully deliberated and acted upon. One such challenge is that of coordinating the various curricular, instructional, organizational, and resource areas essential to advancing massage therapy research competencies. Accordingly, this paper suggests a multi-dimensional framework intended to initiate critical discussions of how the profession might now proceed. © 2003 Elsevier Science Ltd. All rights reserved.

Keywords

Massage therapy; Research competencies; Massage therapy research; Therapeutic massage and bodywork; Competency-based education

'I never faced a Problem which was more than the eternal problem of finding order'.
(Skinner, as cited in Gage, 1963, p. 88).

Introduction

Although the actual context of B. F. Skinner's quote was that of his dissenting from any overly formal view of the scientific method, its utterance comes to mind as one examines several recent documents leading to the massage/bodywork profession's current commitment to promoting massage therapy research competencies (MTRCs). Perhaps an explanation is in order.

The pioneering efforts of Tiffany Field (e.g. 1998, 2000a, b) in diverse areas of massage therapy research over the past decade have sounded a clarion call to all regarding the need for and ability to generate empirical evidence foundational to the profession's work.

Additionally, the strategic decision of the AMTA Foundation to convene the multidisciplinary Massage Research Agenda Workgroup (MRAW) in 1999 has provided an excellent basis from which to proceed in the effort to include *scientific inquiry* as still another feature of the profession's claim as a viable form of alternative medicine. Recent reports stemming from the MRAW's deliberations have appeared in various background papers, outcome summaries, and recommendations that have been characterized by AMTA Foundation President John Balletto (as cited in Kahn 2001a) as awe inspiring — a view with which many professionals might presumably agree.

Specifically, the MRAW-commissioned background paper by Cassidy (1998/1999, in press) indeed sets the stage by virtue of its exhaustive discussion of the complex and multidisciplinary journey on which the workgroup was embarking. Recently, Kahn's (2001a, b) two synthesizing articles and the AMTA Foundation's (2002) publication have served to report in a comprehensive way the outcomes and recommendations of the workgroup and, thereby, to acknowledge publicly the charge that now faces the profession. Another related work of recent vintage indeed germane to the above-cited reports is the comprehensive chapter on "Massage Therapy" by Freeman (2001) appearing in *Mosby's Complementary & Alternative Medicine: A Research-Based Approach*.

Dovetailing with the efforts of the MRAW has been the recent work of the Commission on Massage Therapy Accreditation (COMTA) as it reviewed various competency-based standards for massage therapy and bodywork education, and the implied professional skills that must be ensured as a precondition for licensing/certification. These developments have been reported in depth by Ostendorf and Schwartz (2001) in anticipation of their mandated implementation in 2003.

Among the newly established professional competencies is that of a research-based standard that is detailed as follows (C. Ostendorf, pers. comm. via e-mail, June 13, 2001; Ostendorf & Schwartz 2001, p 120):

Element 6.3: Demonstrate the ability to read and evaluate technical information found in articles in health-related journals and determine biases and limitations in the findings or premises the articles are based on.

I.   Explain the value of research to the profession.

II. Locate research literature on therapeutic massage.

*Glenn M. Hymel EdD, LMT

Dr. Hymel is Associate Professor and Former Chair, Department of Psychology, Loyola University New Orleans. His areas of specialization are educational psychology, research & statistics, and the psychology of personal adjustment. He is a graduate of the Blue Cliff School of Therapeutic Massage (Metairie, LA) and has a particular interest in the areas of stress management, chronic pain, chronic fatigue, and fibromyalgia. He is currently serving as Chair of the AMTA Foundation's Research Database Committee as well as the Research Proposal Review Committee.

Revised paper originally presented via poster session at the annual meeting of the American Massage Therapy Association, Quebec City, Quebec, Canada, October 2001.

BOX 10-2   ADVANCING MASSAGE THERAPY RESEARCH COMPETENCIES: DIMENSIONS FOR THOUGHT AND ACTION — CONT'D

III. Critically read and evaluate a published research article in the field of massage therapy/body-work.

IV. Access appropriate information resources as needed, and apply this information in practice.

It is to this particular standard that the remainder of this paper speaks. In so doing, it is critical to recognize that the intent here is to articulate those concepts, principles, and procedures that are foundational to understanding the nature of the scientific research process, regardless of whether one's goal is to function as (a) a *critical consumer* of the research literature already available or (b) a *competent investigator* engaged in the actual tasks of conducting original research. In both instances, the prerequisite knowledge base and research skills are identical and need to be present for either the informed evaluation of published research or the proficient implementation of an appropriately designed study.

Dimensions essential to advancing massage therapy research competencies

The research focus in this paper, admittedly, is on only a small segment of the newly established competencies; however, the implications for implementation are far-reaching and complex due to two basic realities:

1. Massage therapy and bodywork students appear to constitute an extremely heterogeneous group with respect to educational background, occupational experience, and professional goals. Accordingly, all aspects of educating pre-service therapists in the realm of research competencies must be informed by the reality of extensive student diversity.

2. In addition to pre-service therapists, another obvious population in need of research competency enhancement includes both massage therapy educators and in-service therapists already licensed/certified. The concern, then, must encompass not only curricular and instructional accommodations within massage therapy schools for pre-service therapists but also easily accessible opportunities for continuing educational experiences for colleagues already active in the field as practitioners and/or educators. In this latter regard, both in-service therapists and educators could benefit not only from research-focused continuing education seminars but even more from college/university-based courses on research methods, measurement techniques, and quantitative analyses.

Although these two concerns are indeed quite challenging, there are other realms that must be considered as one designs and implements strategies for advancing massage therapy research competencies (MTRCs). These additional considerations cut across not only other curricular and instructional issues but also matters pertinent to resource materials and personnel, varieties of research documents and strategies, areas of inquiry, and organizational contexts for supporting massage therapy research. With this in mind, then, Table 1 presents a framework from which one might begin the necessary work on those several dimensions suggested here as essential to advancing MTRCs. And even if Skinner is only partially correct in his view of "...the eternal problem of finding order," then certainly the massage/bodywork profession's task is well defined as it attempts to bring order and clarity to all that is implied within and across these eight dimensions.

Dimension 1 – curricular and instructional contexts for teaching MTRCs

This first dimension focuses on those curricular and instructional contexts in which MTRCs might be taught (see Table 2). Perhaps, the most basic context is that of a core research course being included in the massage therapy school's curricular offerings. Positioned among the initial courses

TABLE 1   OVERVIEW OF DIMENSIONS ESSENTIAL TO ADVANCING MASSAGE THERAPY RESEARCH COMPETENCIES (MTRCS)

Dimension 1 – Curricular and instructional contexts for teaching MTRCs

Dimension 2 – Application tasks for demonstrating MTRCs

Dimension 3 – Learning activities for enhancing MTRCs

Dimension 4 – Print, electronic and personnel resources for promoting MTRCs

Dimension 5 – Varieties of massage therapy research documents

Dimension 6 – Potential research strategies

Dimension 7 – Potential areas of inquiry in massage therapy research

Dimension 8 – Organizational contexts for supporting massage therapy research

TABLE 2   DIMENSION 1 – CURRICULAR AND INSTRUCTIONAL CONTEXTS FOR TEACHING MTRCS

1a. Research core course positioned in the massage therapy curriculum

1b. Research module embedded in specific massage therapy courses

1c. Continuing education workshops for massage therapy educators

1d. Continuing education workshops for in-service massage therapy practitioners

1e. Networking seminars for affiliated health care professionals

Continued

BOX 10-2   ADVANCING MASSAGE THERAPY RESEARCH COMPETENCIES: DIMENSIONS FOR THOUGHT AND ACTION — CONT'D

completed in a massage therapy program would allow for concurrent and subsequent coursework to build on those research skills developed at the outset of one's studies. A possible follow up to this core research course might be that of a research skills module as part of specific massage therapy courses.

Another possible context for teaching MTRCs is that of continuing education workshops. This would be an appropriate route not only for educators preparing to infuse their curriculum with research-focused modules, but also for in-service practitioners whose earlier education predated the current research emphasis. Finally, an additional context involves networking seminars for interested health care providers who might have overlapping interests in the research agendas of massage/bodywork professionals.

Whether the intended audience is that of pre-service therapists, educators, or in-service therapists, the reality still exists that the curricular and instructional tasks confronting the profession encompass a corpus of pre-requisite knowledge and skills essential to the critical evaluation of published research and the competent conduct of appropriately designed studies. Furthermore, each of the remaining seven dimensions likewise presumes this very same core of knowledge and skills necessary for both research consumers and active investigators.

Dimensions 2 — application tasks for demonstrating MTRCs
The second dimension involves those possible tasks by which one might demonstrate an application of research competencies appropriate to the profession (see Table 3). One fairly obvious tasks here is that of being able to "consume" — i.e., search, access, retrieve, critique, and use — the available massage/bodywork research literature. This, of course, would be a minimal type of activity in which all professionals would want to be proficient so as to position their own practice on a more informed-by-research basis. Perhaps an even more ambitious task in this dimension is that of individuals refining their research skills to the point of being able to contribute in an active fashion to the research literature as part of a multidisciplinary research team.

Dimension 3 — learning activities for enhancing MTRCs
This third dimension among eight centers on those learning activities most appropriate for enhancing MTRCs (see Table 4). The practice of actually conducting and evaluating professional literature searches is foundational to developing research competency in any profession or discipline. Essential to this activity — and actually building on it — is that of critiquing published massage therapy research documents in accordance with well-established criteria. These two foundational learning activities, in turn, make possible two additional activities at a more advanced level, viz., authoring a massage therapy proposal and participating in the implementation of a research study as a member of a professionally diversified team.

Dimension 4 — print, electronic, and personnel resources for promoting MTRCs
The fourth dimension essential to advancing MTRCs pertains to those print, electronic, and human resources appropriate to scientific inquiry within the profession. The elements listed here in Table 5 are fairly apparent; however, their acknowledgment certainly cannot hurt and does serve as a reminder of the vast array of resources — material and human — to which one can appeal.

TABLE 3   DIMENSION 2 — APPLICATION TASKS FOR DEMONSTRATING MTRCS

2a. Critical consumer of the massage therapy research literature
2b. Active contributor to the massage therapy research literature

TABLE 4   DIMENSION 3 — LEARNING ACTIVITIES FOR ENHANCING MTRCS

3a. Conducting and evaluating literature searches
3b. Critiquing published massage therapy research
3c. Authoring a massage therapy research proposal
3d. Participating as a multidisciplinary research team member

TABLE 5   DIMENSION 4 — PRINT, ELECTRONIC AND PERSONNEL RESOURCES FOR PROMOTING MTRCS

4a. Authored books
4b. Entries in edited books
4c. Journal articles
4d. Conference papers
4e. Theses and dissertations
4f. Technical reports
4g. Monographs, newsletters and bulletins
4h. Web- and electronic-based sources
4i. Professional colleagues and associations/organizations

Of special note in this dimension are several books that focus on the research process applied to the health sciences in general and/or manual therapies in particular. They span conventional as well as complementary and alternative interventions, and serve to accommodate a broad range of competency levels for readers and students. These resources might provide a starting point as one begins the complicated process of determining content coverage, instructional context, and learning activities most appropriate to both pre-service and in-service professionals. Although somewhat of a "sampler" at this point, these resources meriting particular attention are the following: Domholdt's (2000) *Physical Therapy Research;* Helewa and Walker's (2000); *Critical Evaluation of Research in Physical Rehabilitation;* Hicks' (1999); *Research Methods for Clinical Therapists;* Jenkins, Price, and Straker's (1998) *The Researching Therapist;* Kazdin's (1998) *Methodological Issues and Strategies in Clinical Research;* Menard's (2003) *Making Sense of Research: A Guide to Research Literacy for Complementary Practitioners;* Polzar and Thomas's (2000) *Introduction to Research in the Health Sciences;* and Rich's (2002) *Massage Therapy: The Evidence for Practice.*

Dimension 5 – types of massage therapy research documents

Dimension 5 specifies those varied types of massage therapy research documents that constitute the range of professional literature essential to promoting MTRCs (see Table 6). An obvious starting point is a genre of reference materials known as preliminary sources (e.g., Medline, PsycInfo, Sociological Abstracts, and the newly launched AMTA Foundation's Massage Therapy Research Database) that are accessible via on-line computer searches employing descriptor terms leading to bibliographic citations and accompanying abstracts. Empirical research reports, typically in the form of journal articles, provide both quantitative and qualitative analyses of research questions that have been operationalized and investigated via established scientific procedures ensuring both validity and reliability. Theoretical/conceptual works often represent a synthesis of earlier empirical studies in terms of explanatory themes and, in turn, provide a rationale for continued empirical research. Finally, state-of-the-art literature reviews provide an exhaustive coverage of both empirical and theoretical/conceptual studies in an attempt to synthesize past and current work in a given area of inquiry.

Dimension 6 – potential research strategies

The sixty dimension considered here is that of potential research strategies that may be used depending primarily on the nature of one's research question (see Table 7). A difference-oriented research strategy in its most basic form investigates the relationship between an independent variable (e.g. some form of treatment intervention) and a dependent variable (e.g., some outcome measure of interest), with its methodological options including true experimental, quasi-experimental, and ex post facto. The association-oriented research strategy employs methods typically labeled as correlational studies and predictive studies, each of which may function as a prelude to a difference-oriented study. The descriptive-oriented research strategy is frequently the initial focus in an evolving research problem area and span such methods as the following: case studies, observational studies, surveys, archival research, and content analyses. The complete array of research strategies, then, is available and should be reflective of the type of research question being investigated.

TABLE 7	DIMENSION 6 – POTENTIAL RESEARCH STRATEGIES
6a.	Difference-oriented research strategy
	6a.1 True experimental studies
	6a.2 Quasi-experimental studies
	6a.3 Ex post facto studies
6b.	Association-oriented research strategy
	6b.1 Correlational studies
	6b.2 Predictive studies
6c.	Descriptive-oriented research strategy
	6c.1 Case studies
	6c.2 Observational studies
	6c.3 Surveys
	6c.4 Archival studies
	6c.5 Content analyses

TABLE 6	DIMENSION 5 – TYPES OF MASSAGE THERAPY RESEARCH DOCUMENTS
5a.	Preliminary reference sources
5b.	Empirical research reports
5c.	Theoretical/conceptual treatises
5d.	State-of-the-art literature review documents

Continued

BOX 10-2 ADVANCING MASSAGE THERAPY RESEARCH COMPETENCIES: DIMENSIONS FOR THOUGHT AND ACTION—CONT'D

Dimension 7 — Potential Areas of Inquiry in Massage Therapy Research

The seventh dimension speaks to that vast array of potential areas of inquiry for massage therapy researchers. The recent works of Cassidy (1998/1999, in press), Freeman (2001), and Kahn (2001a, b) provide the backdrop for those varied areas listed in Table 8. Priority areas of safety and efficacy studies, along with primary and secondary prevention studies from both pathogenic and salutogenic (wellness) models, define to a large extent where we have been and where we need to expand. Inherent in each of these areas just cited is an underlying condition-treatment interface that ultimately must be addressed and understood in terms of explanatory mechanisms (see Field 2000b). And, of course, there is the realm of therapeutic massage profession studies so essential to our continued advancement and credibility, yet so lacking in past attention among researchers.

Dimension 8 — Organizational Contexts for Supporting Massage Therapy Research

The eighth and final dimension considered here is that of organizational contexts for supporting massage therapy research (see Table 9). From international, national, regional, and state massage/bodywork associations to highly focused special interest groups within a given association, the strength and support found in numbers of a collegial nature cannot be overestimated. Additionally, collaboration among massage therapy schools as well as accrediting associations can certainly further appropriate standards across diverse settings in the never-ending quest for professional excellence. And looking beyond the massage/bodywork profession per se, collaborative work can indeed be strengthened if and when alliances are forged with the schools, associations, and settings of other health care professionals.

Where Do We Go From Here?

The recent efforts of the MRAW and COMTA have provided a much-needed impetus for moving therapeutic massage and bodywork to a more research-oriented and evidence-based professional status. If the foundation thus laid by colleagues in these two groups is to bear fruit, then it is critical that appropriate follow-up work take place in a timely fashion. Such efforts would serve to provide therapists with the knowledge and skills that would allow them not only to evaluate critically the published research already available but also to function as active researchers if so inclined. Essentially, the prerequisites for understanding the nature of scientific inquiry and the investigative procedures involved are identical for both tasks.

The eight dimensions identified earlier as essential to addressing MTRCs represent a starting point for the work remaining to be done. Although the major areas covered relate to curricular, instructional, organizational, and resource themes, there is no one specific sequence that must be followed. Instead, it seems advisable to proceed "on all fronts" concurrently, yet with a keen awareness that each dimension informs — and is informed by — the others.

The diversity of individuals engaged in therapeutic massage and bodywork should serve everyone concerned quite well given the multi-faceted tasks that still need to be accomplished as the profession becomes more attuned to scientific inquiry. The agenda has been laid out with a collegial mandate to expand critical professional competencies. It is the responsibility of all professionals, then, to assess their individual gifts, bring them to bear on the issues at hand, and share the results of their efforts with others.

TABLE 8	DIMENSION 7 — POTENTIAL AREAS OF INQUIRY FOR MASSAGE THERAPY RESEARCHERS
7a.	Priority areas of safety and efficacy studies
7b.	Primary and secondary prevention studies from both pathogenic & salutogenic (wellness) models
7c.	Condition-treatment interface studies
7d.	Explanatory mechanism studies
7e.	Therapeutic massage profession studies

TABLE 9	DIMENSION 8 — ORGANIZATIONAL CONTEXTS FOR SUPPORTING MASSAGE THERAPY RESEARCHERS
8a.	International and national massage therapy associations
8b.	Regional and state massage therapy associations
8c.	Special interest groups (SIGs) within professional associations
8d.	Massage therapy schools and accrediting associations
8e.	Medical, nursing, chiropractic, physical therapy, and occupational therapy schools
8f.	Related health profession associations
8g.	Hospital and health clinic networks

BOX 10-2   ADVANCING MASSAGE THERAPY RESEARCH COMPETENCIES: DIMENSIONS FOR THOUGHT AND ACTION — CONT'D

References

AMTA Foundation (ed.) 2002 Massage Therapy Research Agenda. AMTA Foundation, Evanston, IL

Cassidy CM 1998/1999 Methodological issues in investigations of massage/bodywork therapy. Paper prepared for the AMTA Foundation's Massage Research Agenda Workshop. Paradigms Found Consulting, Bethesda, MD

Cassidy CM 2003 Methodological issues in investigations of massage/bodywork therapy (4-part series). Journal of Bodywork and Movement Therapies 7(1): 2–10

Domholdt E 2000 Physical Therapy Research: Principles and Applications 2nd edn. W. B. Saunders Co., Philadelphia

Freeman LW 2001 Massage therapy. In Freeman LW, Lawlis GF (eds). Mosby's Complementary & Alternative Medicine: A Research-based Approach Mosby, St. Louis 361–386

Field TM 1998 Massage therapy effects. American Psychologist 53: 1270–1280

Field TM 2000a Massage therapy research methods. In Lewith G, Wallack, Jonas (eds), Clinical Research Methodology for Complementary Therapies. Harcourt Brace, London

Field TM 2000b Touch therapy. Churchill Livingstone, New York

Gage NL 1963 Handbook of Research on Education. Rand McNally, Chicago

Helewa A & Walker JM 2000 Critical Evaluation of Research in Physical Rehabilitation: Towards Evidence-based Practice. W. B. Saunders Co. Philadelphia

Hicks CM 1999 Research Methods for Clinical Therapists: Applied Project Design and Analysis, 3rd edn. Churchill Livingstone, New York

Jenkins S, Price CJ & Straker L 1998 The Researching Therapist: A Practical Guide to Planning, Performing, and Communicating Research. Churchill Livingstone, New York

Kazdin AE (ed.) 1998 Methodological Issues & Strategies in Clinical Research, 2nd edn., American Psychological Association, Washington, DC

Kahn JR 2001a A new era for massage research. Massage Therapy Journal 40: 104–114

Kahn JR 2001b Research matters. Massage Magazine 93: 57–61

Menard MB 2003 Making Sense of Research: A Guide to Research Literacy for Complementary Practitioners. Curties-Overzet Publications, Inc., Moncton, New Brunswick

Ostendorf C & Schwartz J 2001 COMTA begins move toward competencies. Massage Therapy Journal 40: 116–120

Polzar S & Thomas SA (eds) 2000 Introduction to Research in the Health Science, 4th edn., Churchill Livingstone, New York.

Rich GJ (ed) 2002 Massage Therapy: The Evidence for Practice. Mosby, St. Louis

From Hymel, G.M. (2003). Advancing massage therapy research competencies: Dimensions for thought and action. *Journal of Bodywork and Movement Therapies*, *7*(3), 194–199.

research process. This initial exposure to the several research categories, strategies, methods, and so on has provided, we hope, at least the chance of allowing massage therapists and related health science professionals to become better prepared to function as consumers of, or active contributors to, research in one's chosen profession.

If indeed the topics covered in this book have given you a better understanding of the research process and the many options available for exploration, then only one of the book's two major objectives will have been met. Beyond your moving on from this experience with more knowledge and insight, it is equally important for something else to have occurred in what we might call the affective domain of learning. That "something else" falls in the realm of your having developed an appreciation of, an attraction to, a liking of the research process and all the excitement that scientific inquiry holds.

If that has been part of your experience with this book as well, then indeed the second of the two major objectives has likewise been accomplished. Beyond the *knowing* and the *appreciating*, it then becomes a matter of *acting* on what we understand and savor, and in that regard my sincere encouragement and best wishes are with you.

REFERENCES

AMTA Foundation, & Kahn, J. (2002). *Massage therapy research agenda.* Evanston, IL: AMTA Foundation. Retrieved July 29, 2004, from www.massagetherapy-foundation.org/massageagenda.html.

Hymel, G. M. (2003). Advancing massage therapy research competencies: Dimensions for thought and action. *Journal of Bodywork and Movement Therapies*, *7*(3), 194–199.

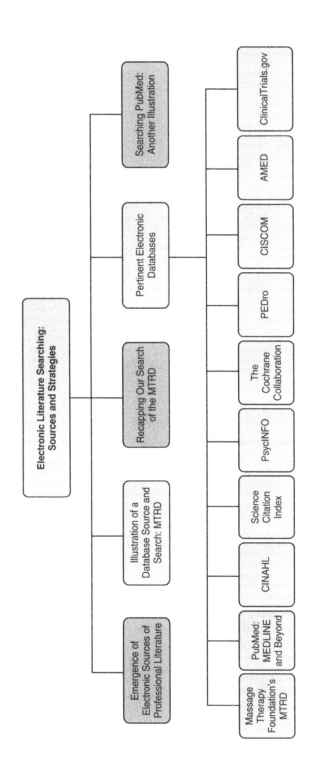

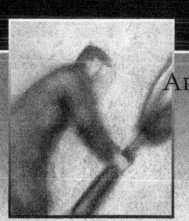

ELECTRONIC LITERATURE SEARCHING: SOURCES AND STRATEGIES

OUTLINE

OBJECTIVES

Upon completion of this appendix, the reader will have the information necessary to perform the following tasks:

1 Characterize the emergence of electronic sources of professional literature since the onset of the information technology revolution in the 1990s.

2 Perform an electronic search of the Massage Therapy Foundation's Massage Therapy Research Database (MTRD) using the Boolean operators AND, OR, and NOT.

3 Display by way of a Venn diagram the strategies used in a search of the MTRD as specified in Objective 2.

4 Characterize each of the following pertinent electronic databases as sources of professional literature: the Massage Therapy Foundation's MTRD; PubMed; CINAHL; the Science Citation Index; PsycINFO; the Cochrane Library and the Cochrane Complementary Medicine Field Registry, as components of the Cochrane Collaboration; PEDro; CISCOM; AMED; and ClinicalTrials.gov.

5 Perform an electronic search of PubMed using the Boolean operators AND, OR, and NOT.

AMED
Boolean operator AND
Boolean operator NOT
Boolean operator OR
Boolean operators
CAM on PubMed
CINAHL
CISCOM
ClinicalTrials.gov
Cochrane Collaboration

Cochrane Complementary Medicine Field
   Registry
Cochrane Library
Eliminator
Intersection
Massage Therapy Research Database (MTRD)
Medical subject headings (MeSH)
MEDLINE
Navigating the Web
PEDro

PsycINFO
PubMed
Science Citation Index (SCI)
Search engine
Search results
Search template
Union
Venn diagram
Web browser
World Wide Web

THE EMERGENCE OF ELECTRONIC SOURCES OF PROFESSIONAL LITERATURE

The information technology revolution of the 1990s resulted in an unprecedented proliferation of resources available in both personal and professional realms, and it appears that this quantum leap in the sheer volume of accessible information is going to continue unabated. No longer is the reliance solely on print resources; instead, the emergence of electronic sources of professional literature has come to the forefront and has contributed challenges of its own. These challenges exist not only in managing the volume of information now available, but also in assessing the quality of what is being generated. This type of management and assessment needs to occur regarding both electronic versions of journals and newsletters as well as the other vast resources available on the Internet.

The **World Wide Web** has evolved to a strategic point in terms of the role it plays as an interface to the seemingly innumerable resources of the Internet. Its goal of facilitating one's access to various Internet resources is advanced by the use of browsers (e.g., Microsoft Internet Explorer) and search engines (e.g., Google). These tools allow one to mine the Internet's diverse electronic sources of information, inclusive of specialized databases reflecting research in certain professional fields.

Of particular value in gaining insight regarding this mining of electronic resources in the health and behavioral sciences is MacBeckner and Berman's (2003) "Complementary Therapies on the Internet." Edwards's (2002) "The Internet for

Nurses and Allied Health Professionals" is likewise an informative source for learning about the various resources available and efficient strategies for accessing them. Another valuable resource is an article by Singer and Tan (2000) titled "Navigating the Internet Maze." Other highly recommended sources include the following: Guyatt and Rennie (2002); Nicoll (2001); Sackett, Straus, Richardson, Rosenberg, and Haynes (2000); Smith (2002); and Stave (2003).

The following is a discussion of a major database source of professional information electronically available to massage therapists and related complementary and alternative medicine (CAM) professionals.

AN ILLUSTRATION OF A DATABASE SOURCE AND A SEARCH STRATEGY: THE MASSAGE THERAPY FOUNDATION'S MASSAGE THERAPY RESEARCH DATABASE

The Massage Therapy Foundation (formerly known as the AMTA Foundation) maintains the **Massage Therapy Research Database (MTRD)**. This database is the only consolidated, comprehensive listing of citations to the scientific research literature on therapeutic massage and bodywork, and currently contains more than 4000 entries. It serves as a reference source to help one locate articles and other documents of relevance.

The MTRD originated in June 1998 via an initial grant from the AMTA to the AMTA Foundation.

This was in response to the absence at that time of a consolidated listing of research on massage and bodywork. Martha Menard Brown, PhD, and Janet Kahn, PhD, conceived the idea for the database as a supporting project in affiliation with the Massage Research Agenda Workgroup referenced earlier in this book. In early 2000, a team of massage therapists, physicians, and researchers serving as a peer-review committee started evaluating relevant citations for possible inclusion in the database. This effort is ongoing and results in quarterly upgrades to the database as new citations are peer-reviewed and judged to be appropriate for inclusion.

Details regarding the search terms used in compiling the quarterly set of citations subjected to peer review are available from the Massage Therapy Foundation. Likewise, information can be obtained from the Foundation identifying those various databases in the health and behavior sciences that are searched for the most relevant documents pertaining to massage and bodywork.

What follows over the next several pages is an introduction to (a) accessing the MTRD and (b) conducting an electronic search using standard procedures as well as certain activities specific to this particular database. We begin this introduction with an acknowledgment of certain terminology that has become almost a universal language since the onset of the information technology revolution.

A **Web browser** is computer software used to access various types of Internet resources (e.g., Web sites). Among some of the most prevalent Web browsers are Netscape and Microsoft Internet Explorer. Once a particular Web browser is opened, the Massage Therapy Foundation's Web site can be accessed by entering www.massagetherapyfoundation.org in the address box as illustrated in Figure A-1.

One may also use a **search engine** as another option for locating a Web site of interest. This course of action is usually taken if one does not know the actual URL for a particular Web site. Popular search engines include Alta Vista, Google,

Metacrawler, Northern Light, and YAHOO! Once on a particular search engine's Web site, the text of descriptive names, words, or expressions of interest is entered in the address box. This results in a listing of possible Web-based resources, inclusive of links to the Web sites of professional organizations and related sources.

Once on a chosen Web site accessed by using either a Web browser or a search engine, one typically has several options for **navigating the Web** through the different components or sections of the site. The section of interest is selected simply by clicking on the designated tab. For example, Figure A-2 shows the homepage for the Massage Therapy Foundation's Web site, along with the several options available for navigating within that Web site. One such option is the *Research Database* component.

As illustrated in Figure A-3, this *Research Database* component of the foundation's Web site provides the options of either accessing the *instructions* for using the database or going directly to the *search* page. More detailed information is provided within each of these two pages, as shown in Figures A-4 and A-5.

The various options available when using the **search template** are somewhat self-explanatory. The *default* regarding the first section covering author last name, article title, journal/book, year, and publication type is to leave everything blank with publication type designated as "any." This default allows for optimal inclusiveness when searching. In Figure A-6, only one key word, *massage,* is used in this search.

Figure A-7 displays the **search results** of the search using *massage* as the single key word. A total of 2596 citations was found matching the search directive of *massage.* The full bibliographic citation is given along with a listing of related key words for each of the 2596 sources found. In some cases, an abstract or summary may be provided as well. A researcher has the option also of clicking on the "Save Result" box for any given citation so

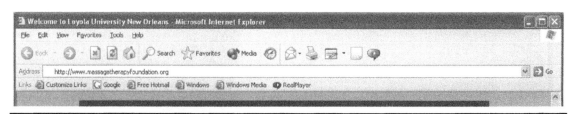

FIGURE A-1   ■   Example of a Web browser (Microsoft Internet Explorer) used to access the Massage Therapy Foundation's Web site at http://massagetherapyfoundation.org. (Courtesy Massage Therapy Foundation. Retrieved 2004.)

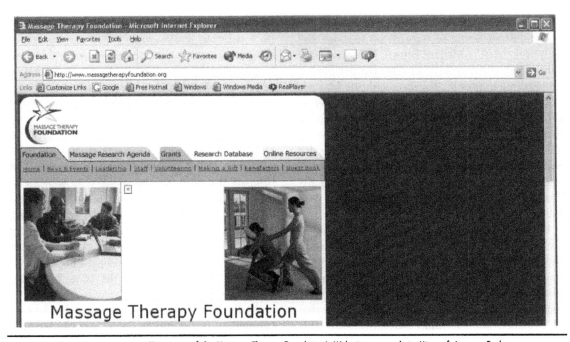

FIGURE A-2 ■ Homepage of the Massage Therapy Foundation's Web site accessed via Microsoft Internet Explorer. (Courtesy Massage Therapy Foundation. Retrieved 2004.)

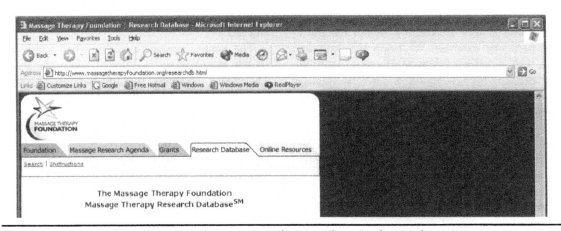

FIGURE A-3 ■ The research database component on the Massage Therapy Foundation's Web site. (Courtesy Massage Therapy Foundation. Retrieved 2004.)

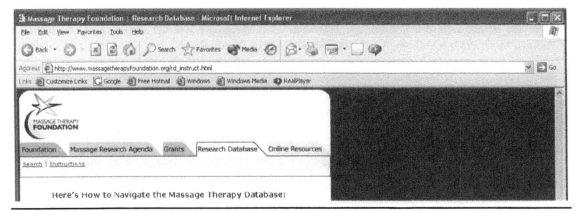

FIGURE A-4 ■ Instructions page in the research database section. (Courtesy Massage Therapy Foundation. Retrieved 2004.)

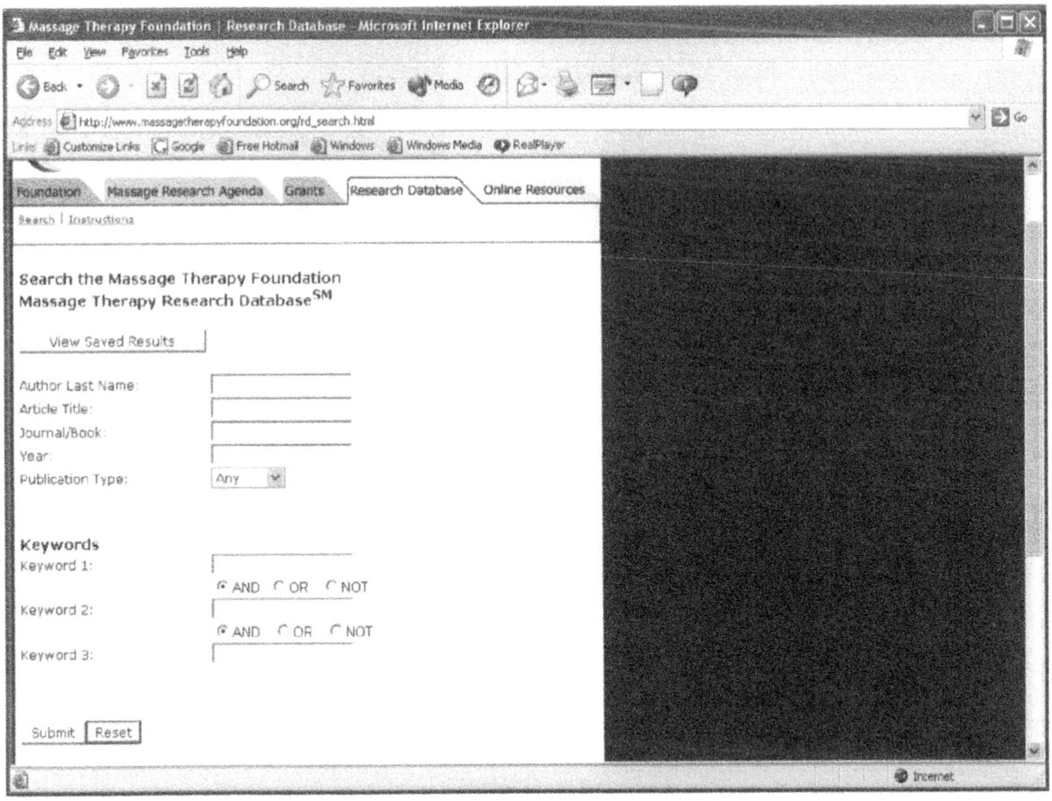

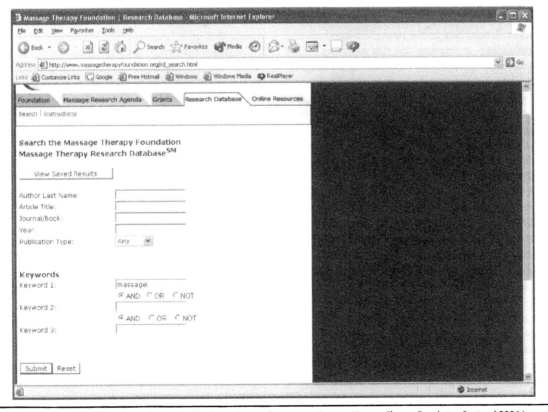

FIGURE A-5 ■ Search template page in the research database section. (Courtesy Massage Therapy Foundation. Retrieved 2004.)

FIGURE A-6 ■ Search template used with only one key word, *massage*. (Courtesy Massage Therapy Foundation. Retrieved 2004.)

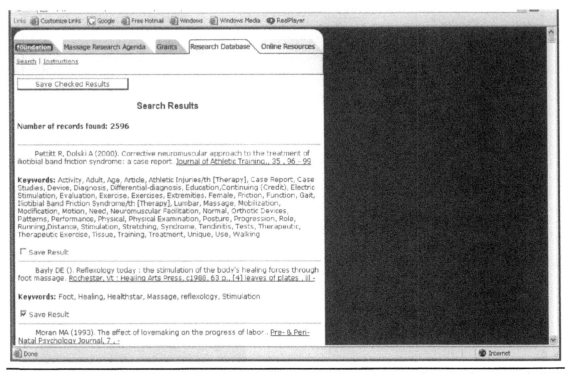

FIGURE A-7 ■ Display of 2596 hits or records found with *massage* as the key word. (Courtesy Massage Therapy Foundation. Retrieved 2004.)

as to identify the most promising subset of the 2596 hits. Once this subset of citations has been identified, the user would then click on the Save Checked Results box in the upper left-hand corner. Downloading or printing out this resulting subset then becomes possible, thereby making the original 2596 hits more manageable and useful.

Figures A-8 and A-9 display the search template and resulting 24 records found when the term *fibromyalgia* is used as the key word in the search. Likewise, Figures A-10 and A-11 indicate a total of 62 citations found in the massage research database when *hydrotherapy* is the basis for the search.

A fairly prevalent feature in the electronic searching of databases involves the use of what are known as **Boolean operators**. This simply refers to the use of words such as AND, OR, or NOT when employing two or more key words. Their function is to make a given search strategy either more exclusive or inclusive, depending on the Boolean operator used.

For example, using the **Boolean operator AND** to connect two key words has the effect of *restricting* the search to only those citations that include *both* of the two key words. This makes the search *more exclusive*–or *less inclusive*–than would be the case otherwise. Stated another way, *only those citations* that represent the **intersection** of the two key words

would be included in the listing of "hits," or records found. Accordingly, Figures A-12 and A-13 display the search template and only 15 hits when the Boolean search strategy is "massage AND fibromyalgia."

Another possibility is that of connecting two key words with the **Boolean operator OR**. This has the effect of *expanding* the search to all those citations that include one or the other of the two key words. This makes the search *more inclusive*–or *less exclusive*–than would be the case otherwise. Stated another way, *all those citations* that represent the **union** of the two key words would be included in the listing of hits or records found. Accordingly, Figures A-14 and A-15 display the search template and the total 2605 hits when the Boolean search strategy is "massage OR fibromyalgia."

The search template available here allows for the use of Boolean operators with as many as three key words. For example, another possible search strategy expression might be "massage OR fibromyalgia AND hydrotherapy." Some databases will use parentheses around two of three possible key words in a search. When this is the case, the key words within the parentheses are processed first, and that outcome is then followed by the processing of the third key word that was not captured by the parentheses. In the absence of parentheses being

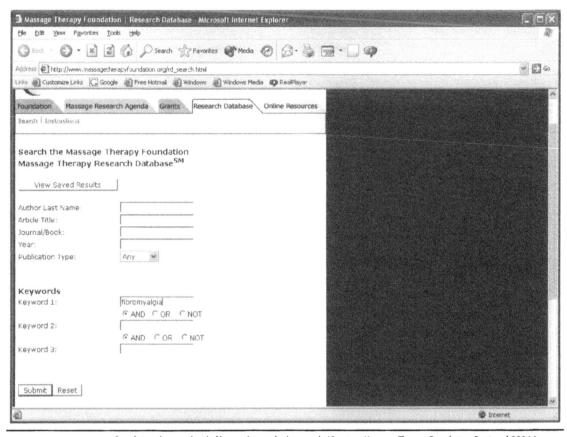

FIGURE A-8 ■ Search template used with *fibromyalgia* as the key word. (Courtesy Massage Therapy Foundation. Retrieved 2004.)

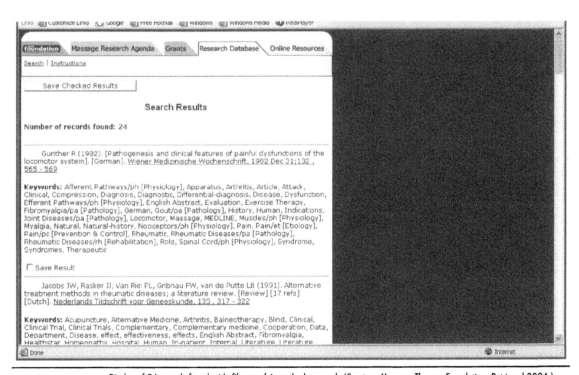

FIGURE A-9 ■ Display of 24 records found with *fibromyalgia* as the key word. (Courtesy Massage Therapy Foundation. Retrieved 2004.)

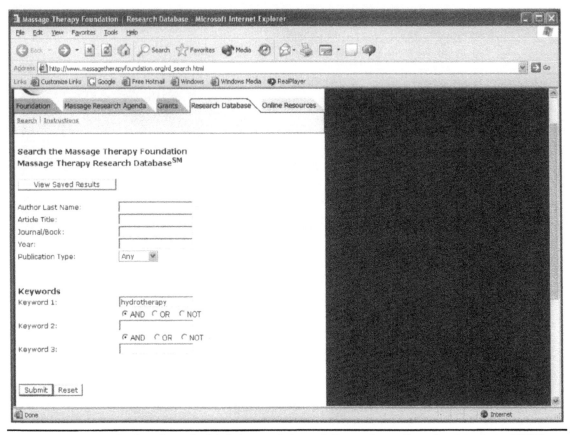

FIGURE A-10 ■ Search template used with *hydrotherapy* as the key word. (Courtesy Massage Therapy Foundation. Retrieved 2004.)

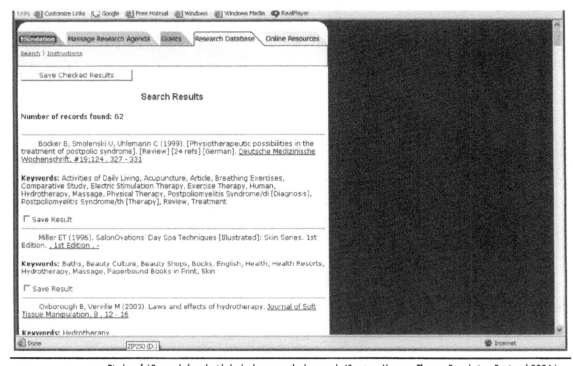

FIGURE A-11 ■ Display of 62 records found with *hydrotherapy* as the key word. (Courtesy Massage Therapy Foundation. Retrieved 2004.)

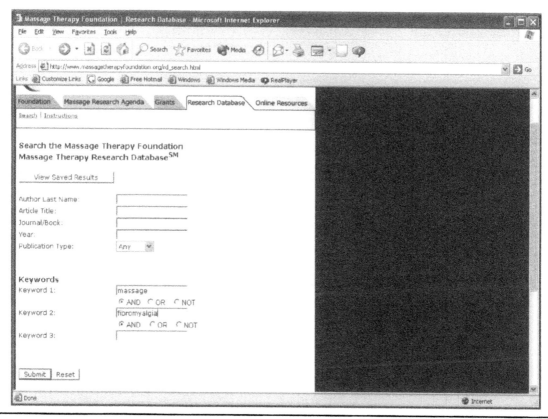

FIGURE A-12   ■   Search template used with "massage AND fibromyalgia" as the Boolean search strategy expression. (Courtesy Massage Therapy Foundation. Retrieved 2004.)

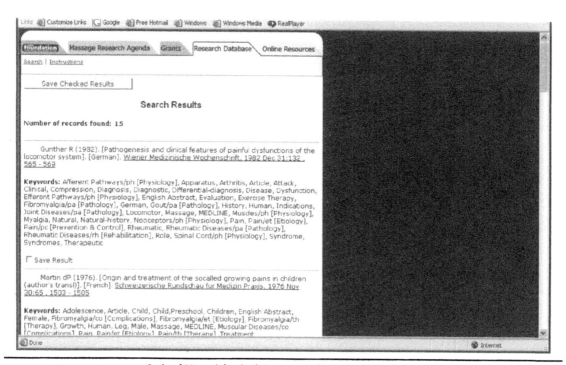

FIGURE A-13   ■   Display of 15 records found with "massage AND fibromyalgia" as the Boolean search strategy expression. (Courtesy Massage Therapy Foundation. Retrieved 2004.)

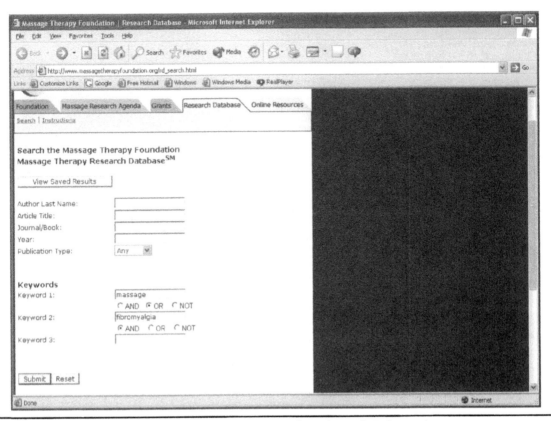

FIGURE A-14 ■ Search template used with "massage OR fibromyalgia" as the Boolean search strategy expression. (Courtesy Massage Therapy Foundation. Retrieved 2004.)

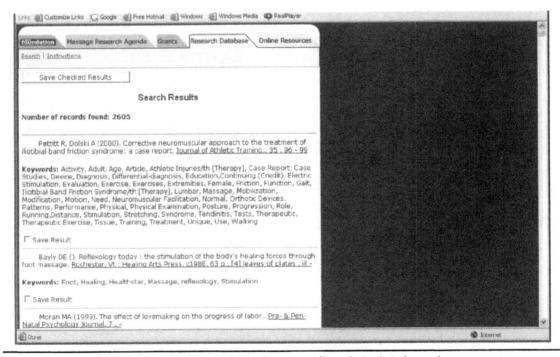

FIGURE A-15 ■ Display of 2605 records found with "massage OR fibromyalgia" as the Boolean search strategy expression. (Courtesy Massage Therapy Foundation. Retrieved 2004.)

used to structure a Boolean search strategy expression, it is standard procedure for the key words and their operators to be processed from left to right. Accordingly, Figures A-16 and A-17 show the search template and the total of 2596 hits when the Boolean search expression is "massage OR fibromyalgia AND hydrotherapy."

Using the operator OR to connect all three terms "massage OR fibromyalgia OR hydrotherapy" results in a search template and 2613 records found, as displayed in Figures A-18 and A-19.

A final consideration in this particular database where Boolean operators are concerned is the use of the **Boolean operator NOT**. Any key word preceded by NOT is a key word, which if mentioned in a citation, would result in that citation being excluded. The operator NOT is equivalent, then, to being an **eliminator**. Its function is to exclude certain citations based solely on the ground that the designated key word is present. Consequently, it has the effect of *restricting*, or limiting, a search in the manner just described. Figures A-20 and A-21 display the search template and the total of 2605

hits recorded when the Boolean search expression is "massage OR fibromyalgia NOT hydrotherapy."

RECAPPING OUR SEARCH OF THE MTRD: ESSENTIAL STEPS IN ANY ELECTRONIC DATABASE SEARCH

The basic procedures illustrated in using the Massage Therapy Foundation's MTRD are foundational to virtually any electronic search of a database. Different databases will vary somewhat in terms of the following essential features: navigating from a site's homepage, recognizing the options available within the database component of the site, using the instructions or tutorial provided at the outset prior to doing a search, recognizing the layout of the search template, using available pre-ordained search words or expressions specific to a particular database, employing Boolean operators with or without the parentheses option, specifying via a check-off option a subset of the original results generated, and engaging possible save or print features for retaining the results of one's search.

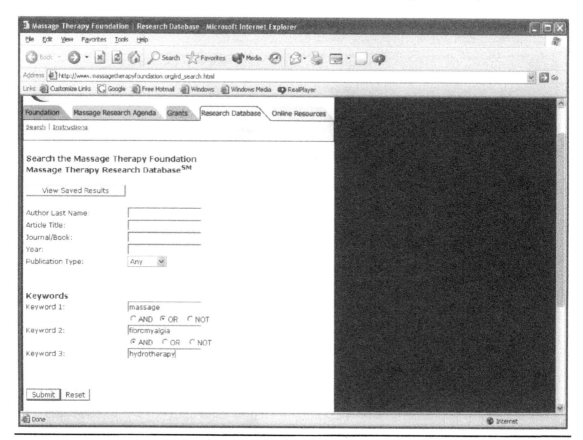

FIGURE A-16 ■ Search template used with "massage OR fibromyalgia AND hydrotherapy" as the Boolean search strategy expression. (Courtesy Massage Therapy Foundation. Retrieved 2004.)

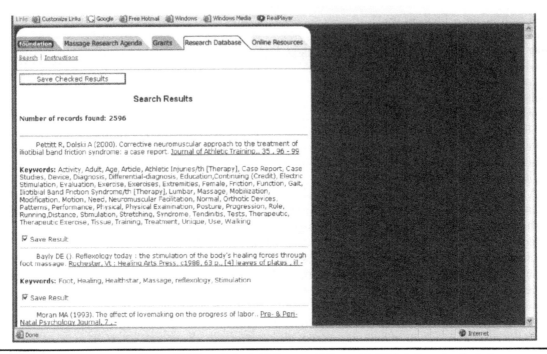

FIGURE A-17 ■ Display of 2596 records found with "massage OR fibromyalgia AND hydrotherapy" as the Boolean search strategy expression. (Courtesy Massage Therapy Foundation. Retrieved 2004.)

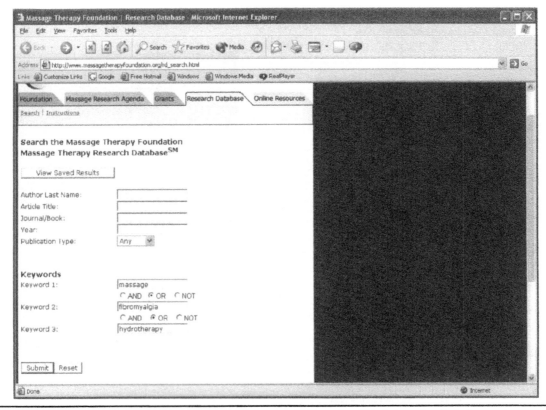

FIGURE A-18 ■ Search template used with "massage OR fibromyalgia OR hydrotherapy" as the Boolean search strategy expression. (Courtesy Massage Therapy Foundation. Retrieved 2004.)

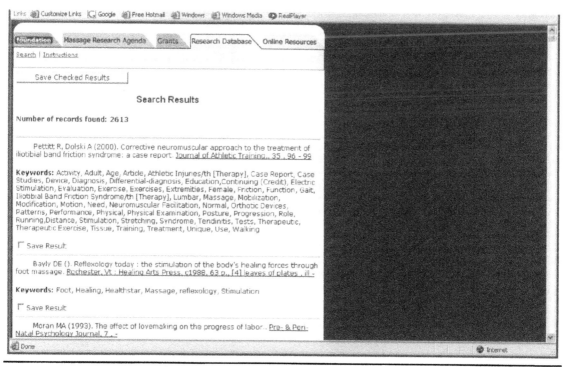

FIGURE A-19 ■ Display of 2613 records found with "massage OR fibromyalgia OR hydrotherapy" as the Boolean search strategy expression. (Courtesy Massage Therapy Foundation. Retrieved 2004.)

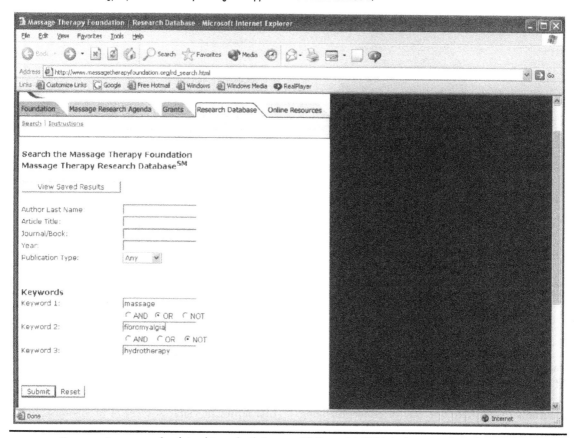

FIGURE A-20 ■ Search template used with "massage OR fibromyalgia NOT hydrotherapy" as the Boolean search strategy expression. (Courtesy Massage Therapy Foundation. Retrieved 2004.)

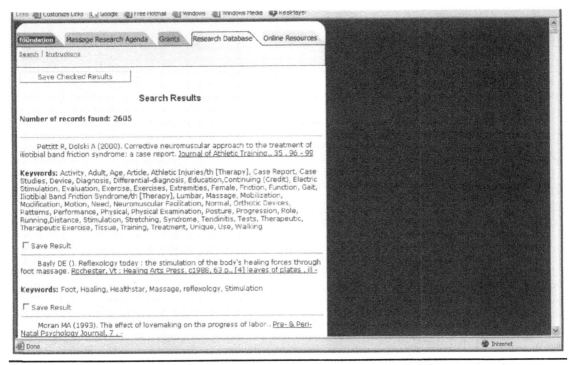

FIGURE A-21 ■ Display of 2605 records found with "massage OR fibromyalgia NOT hydrotherapy" as the Boolean search strategy expression. (Courtesy Massage Therapy Foundation. Retrieved 2004.)

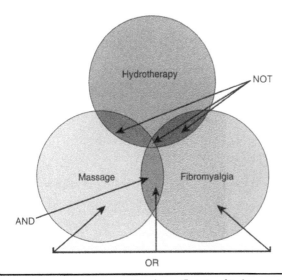

Note 1: "Massage AND Fibromyalgia" captures *only those citations* that contain *both* the keywords **massage** and **fibromyalgia** and is designated by the *intersection* of the massage circle and the fibromyalgia circle, thereby resulting in a *more exclusive*, or *less inclusive*, search.

Note 2: "Massage OR Fibromyalgia" includes *all those citations* that contain *one or the other* of the keywords **massage** and **fibromyalgia** and is designated by the *union* of the massage circle and the fibromyalgia circle, thereby resulting in a *more inclusive*, or *less exclusive*, search.

Note 3: Using "NOT Hydrotherapy" with either of the two search expressions above results in *excluding those citations* that have **hydrotherapy** as a keyword, thereby resulting in a *more restrictive* search than would be the case otherwise.

FIGURE A-22 ■ Venn diagram illustration of Boolean operators used with *massage, fibromyalgia,* and *hydrotherapy* terms.

Another consideration in recapping the procedure we followed earlier in searching the Foundation's MTRD is that of how one might visualize the use of Boolean operators. Figure A-22 uses **Venn diagrams** to illustrate one way of conceptualizing what is occurring as one uses the AND, OR, and NOT operators.

PERTINENT ELECTRONIC DATABASES AS SOURCES OF PROFESSIONAL LITERATURE

There are literally dozens of electronic databases that represent viable sources of professional literature for practitioners, educators, and researchers in various health and behavioral science areas. Each of the recommended resources cited at the beginning of this appendix provides detailed information that should enable you to identify and access those most germane to your interests and needs. The following is a listing of several of these databases that are most pertinent to the work of massage therapists and related health science professionals.

MTRD

We have reviewed in some detail the origin, nature, and search mechanism of the MTRD as well as the Web address for accessing it. This database represents the only consolidated electronic source that comprehensively includes bibliographic citations specific to therapeutic massage and bodywork. One of its principal values is the fact that several global databases (e.g., PubMed, HealthSTAR, and PsycINFO) in appropriate health and behavioral science areas are exhaustively searched on a quarterly basis for potential citations related to massage and bodywork. Each set of the resulting citations found is then subjected to a peer review to determine which titles are appropriate for inclusion in the MTRD. This process and the quarterly expanded database that results, therefore, accomplish for a prospective user what otherwise would require an individual's meticulous searching of the global databases using dozens of massage/bodywork-specific key words. The Foundation's Massage Therapy Research Database Committee performs this function as a professional service.

PUBMED: MEDLINE AND BEYOND

Stave (2003) provides an excellent resource titled "Field Guide to MEDLINE: Making Searching Simple." As indicated in the guide, **MEDLINE**, the electronic successor to the print-based *Index Medicus*, includes entries from 1966 to the present and is perhaps the most recognized and widely used of the biohealth databases. This resource currently contains 11 million records, is updated on a monthly basis, and associates with each citation approximately 10 to 12 **medical subject headings (MeSH)** for indexing and search retrieval purposes.

PubMed is an information system inaugurated by the National Library of Medicine (NLM) in 1997 to provide free Web access to MEDLINE via www.pubmed.gov. Although obviously inclusive of MEDLINE, PubMed contains additional entries that augment the MEDLINE records. Some examples of these additional entries include in-process records not yet assigned a MeSH as well as supplied-by-publisher records that likewise will eventually be given a MeSH. PubMed, then, is not technically synonymous with MEDLINE, in that these additional records augment the MEDLINE entries, which, admittedly, constitute by far the largest component of PubMed.

Another feature of PubMed specific to information on complementary and alternative medicine is **CAM on PubMed**, freely accessible via www.nlm. nih.gov/nccam/camonpubmed.html. This resource was developed by the NLM in tandem with the National Center on Complementary and Alternative Medicine (NCCAM). Its intent is to facilitate the search and retrieval of needed articles on CAM from the approximately 220,000 citations that constitute CAM on PubMed.

CUMULATIVE INDEX OF NURSING AND ALLIED HEALTH LITERATURE (CINAHL)

CINAHL is a database established in 1956 for the purpose of accommodating the professional literature needs of nonmedical health professionals (Helewa & Walker, 2000). It encompasses virtually all English-language nursing journals in addition to the primary journals from other health disciplines. Although a fee is required, CINAHL can be accessed via www.cinahl.com.

THE SCIENCE CITATION INDEX

Science Citation Index (SCI) approaches the search for literature sources in a unique way. The bibliographic information for a significant article of interest, say, is traced forward in time so as to identify those later or subsequent sources that cited the article in their reference lists. Consequently, someone using SCI can identify and retrieve those later or subsequent sources that are presumably germane to the area of interest because they cited the original significant article. Although a fee is required here as well, SCI can be accessed via www.isinet.com/ products/citation/sci or http://library.dialog.com/ bluesheets/html/b10034.html.

PsycINFO

PsycINFO is the computerized version of the print-based *Psychological Abstracts* maintained by the American Psychological Association (APA). PsycINFO is an excellent resource for the mind-body aspect of CAM in that it speaks directly to CAM interventions regarding mental disorders, stress management, and behavioral processes as well as neuroimmunology. Although a fee is required to use this database, it can be accessed via www.apa.org/ psycinfo.

THE COCHRANE COLLABORATION

The **Cochrane Collaboration** was initiated in 1993 by the National Health Service (NHS) in the United Kingdom and is organized around 15 Cochrane Centers established throughout the world. As indicated by Helewa and Walker (2000, p. 129), "the task of the Cochrane collaboration is to prepare, maintain, and disseminate systematic reviews of RCTs of health care or reviews of the most reliable evidence available."

The **Cochrane Library** is an electronic database produced by the Cochrane Collaboration to document and disseminate high-quality evidence for enhanced decision making by those providing and receiving health care as well as those engaged in health care research, education, and administration. Database components of the Cochrane Library include the following four: (a) the Cochrane Database of Systematic Reviews, (b) the Cochrane Controlled Trial Register in bibliographic form, (c) the Database of Abstracts of Reviews of Effectiveness, and (d) the Cochrane Review Methodology Database in bibliographic form regarding the science of research synthesis. This electronic database comprising the Cochrane Library is made available by subscription on a quarterly basis, and is distributed via CD-ROM as well as the Internet at www.cochrane.org/reviews/clibintro.htm.

The **Cochrane Complementary Medicine Field Registry** is another aspect of the Cochrane Collaboration that "promotes and facilitates the production and collection of systematic reviews in complementary medicine and continually maintains and updates a registry of randomized controlled trials" (MacBecker & Berman, 2003, p. 31). This registry is located at the University of Maryland Complementary Medicine Program and can be accessed free at www.compmed.umm.edu/cochrane/index.html.

PEDro

PEDro is an electronic database that provides a broad range of reviews and rated trials in rehabilitation and physiotherapy. This database is free and can be accessed via www.cchs.usyd.edu.au/pedro.

CENTRALIZED INFORMATION SERVICE FOR COMPLEMENTARY MEDICINE (CISCOM)

CISCOM is an electronic database maintained by the Research Council for Complementary Medicine, UK. It contains randomized trials and bibliographic citations and abstracts pertaining to major complementary therapies. A fee is required for using this database, which can be accessed at www.rccm.org.uk/cisc.html.

ALLIED AND COMPLEMENTARY MEDICINE (AMED)

AMED is a database that appears in various print and electronic formats. It addresses resources available in complementary medicine, palliative care, and numerous professions allied with medicine. Maintained by the Health Care Information Service of the British Library, AMED requires a fee for use and can be accessed at www.bl.uk.

CLINICALTRIALS.GOV

ClinicalTrials.gov is a source that provides disease treatment information, inclusive of CAM-oriented therapies, modalities, and substances. It can be accessed free of charge at http://clinicaltrials.gov.

SEARCHING PUBMED: ANOTHER ILLUSTRATION OF AN ELECTRONIC DATABASE SEARCH OPTION

Our earlier discussion of PubMed as one of several pertinent electronic databases sets the stage for this brief demonstration of a PubMed search. As a reminder of an excellent resource cited earlier, the *Field Guide to MEDLINE* by Stave (2003) provides a focused discussion of the intricacies of using PubMed and should augment our current brief tour quite well.

Using the Microsoft Internet Explorer browser, we access the PubMed homepage by entering the Web address www.pubmed.gov. Figure A-23 displays the resulting homepage that represents our starting point in implementing a search in this database.

Figure A-24 displays the PubMed page that results from having selected the Preview/Index option. As you can see, this page indicates that 7048 citations have been located using the search term *massage*.

Figure A-25 shows the resulting PubMed page that is displayed as a consequence of our having initiated a second search (i.e., search #2), which was driven by the search expression "massage AND fibromyalgia." Having clicked Preview earlier, we get an update on the number of citations (i.e., 23) found in this second search before actually viewing the listing of the citations.

Figure A-26 displays the first of two PubMed pages that list the 23 citations actually uncovered in our search using the expression "massage AND fibromyalgia."

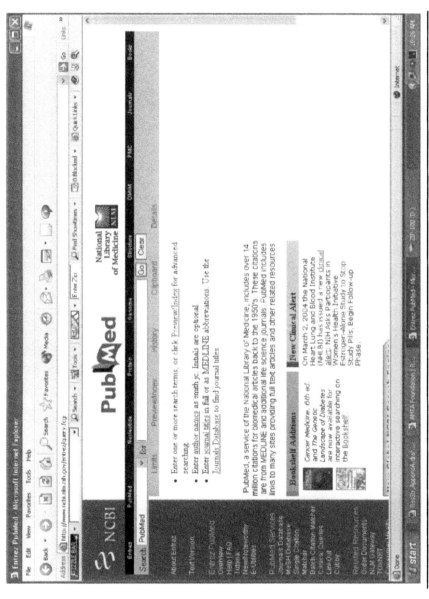

FIGURE A-23 ■ Homepage of PubMed accessed via Microsoft Internet Explorer using www.pubmed.gov. *Note:* Immediately to the right of the Search PubMed box, we next enter the search term *massage* in the blank query box. Before clicking the Go button, we have the choice of clicking the Preview/Index option in the Features bar immediately below the query box. By doing so we can find out the number of retrieved citations before actually having them listed. (Courtesy PubMed, a product of the National Center for Biotechnology Information and the U.S. National Library of Medicine.)

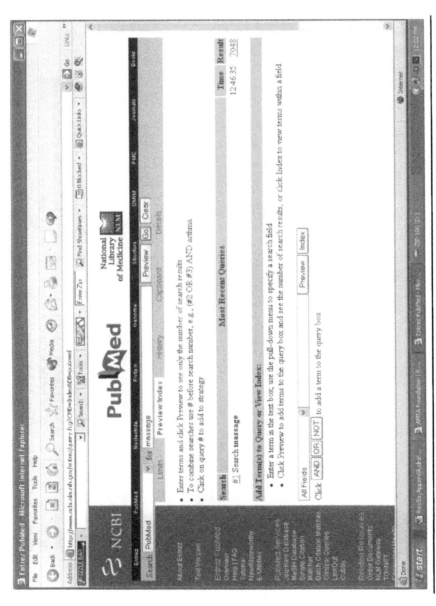

FIGURE A-24 ■ Display of Preview/Index option after using *massage* as a search term. *Note:* As indicated, a total of 7048 citations was found using the search term *massage* in what is recorded as "Search 1." To make the search more specific to our interest, we can now click the AND option and also enter "fibromyalgia" in the blank query box, both of which are located in the Add Term(s) to Query or View Index section at the bottom of the current PubMed page displayed here. We then click Preview to the right of the query box wherein we just entered "fibromyalgia." (Courtesy PubMed, a product of the National Center for Biotechnology Information and the U.S. National Library of Medicine.)

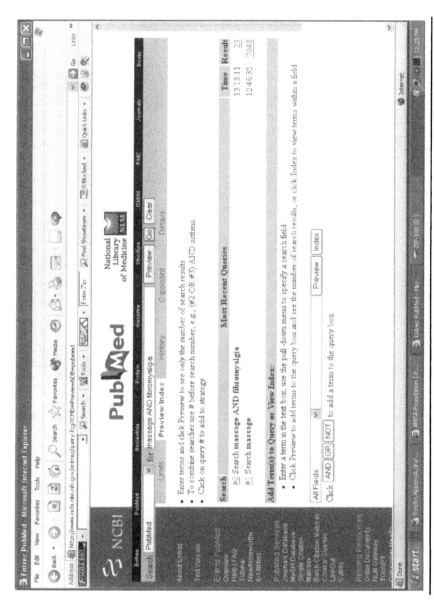

FIGURE A-25 ■ Display of Preview option after using "massage AND fibromyalgia" as a search expression. *Note:* The use of "massage AND fibromyalgia" as a search expression restricted our search to only those citations that include *both* the terms *massage* and *fibromyalgia*. As indicated, this resulted in a substantially more limited collection of pertinent citations numbering only 23. We now have a more manageable number of citations that lends itself to displaying the listing of the actual citations found. This listing is generated by clicking the Go box to the right of the query box that shows the expression "massage AND fibromyalgia." (Courtesy PubMed, a product of the National Center for Biotechnology Information and the U.S. National Library of Medicine.)

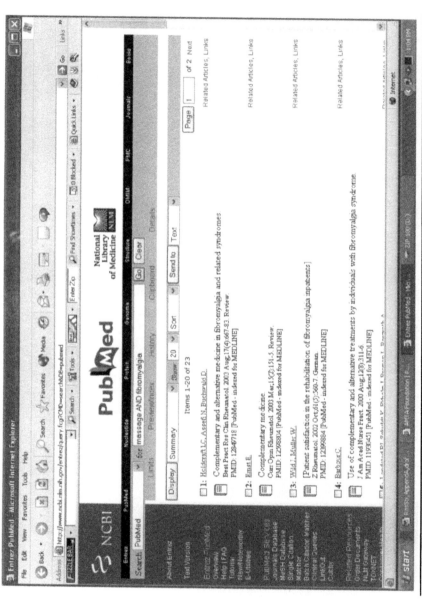

FIGURE A–26 ■ Display of listing of 23 citations found using "massage AND fibromyalgia" as a search expression. *Note:* This PubMed page is the first of two pages listing the citations for the 23 documents found by using the "massage AND fibromyalgia" search expression. We can attempt to further restrict the search by introducing the Boolean operator NOT with the term *hydrotherapy* into the search strategy. By using the expression "massage AND fibromyalgia NOT hydrotherapy," we can eliminate from our current listing of 23 citations any that contain the key word *hydrotherapy*. One way to accomplish this is by adding to the query box the expression "NOT hydrotherapy." As the next figure indicates, when this is done there is no reduction in the number of citations listed. (Courtesy PubMed, a product of the National Center for Biotechnology Information and the U.S. National Library of Medicine.)

Figure A-27 shows that by introducing the expression "NOT hydrotherapy" there was no elimination of citations from our previous subset of 23. We may surmise, then, that none of the 23 citations found in the "massage AND fibromyalgia" search has the key word *hydrotherapy* in the fields searched.

Figure A-28 displays the search history generated when the "History" option is selected, along with the possibility of building on our search history to continue refining the search strategy.

As promised, Figure A-29 displays the combination of search #2 and the Boolean addition of "NOT medication."

Figure A-30 shows the resulting listing of 20 rather than 23 citations brought about by augmenting our previous search #2 (i.e., "massage AND fibromyalgia") with "NOT medication."

Figures A-23 through A-30 provide a basic introduction to only a few of the many features inherent in PubMed. In terms of mastering the intricacies of this massive database, there is really no substitute for actually accessing the PubMed site, completing the tutorial listed in the left-hand sidebar on each page, and then actually practicing search strategies.

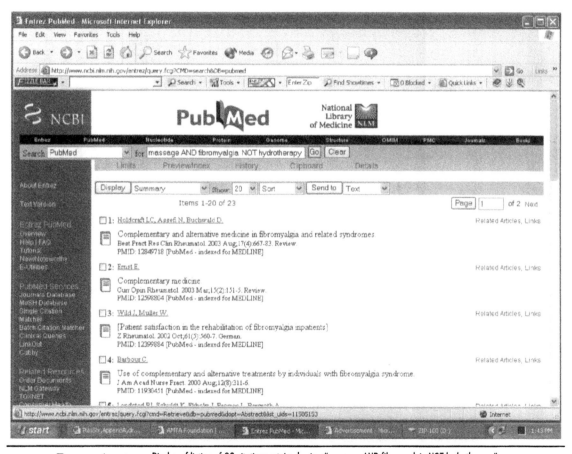

FIGURE A-27 ■ Display of listing of 23 citations retained using "massage AND fibromyalgia NOT hydrotherapy" as a search expression. *Note:* If the term *hydrotherapy* had been present in the searched fields of any of the 23 citations originally found using "massage AND fibromyalgia," then they would have been eliminated in this current search. That, however, was not the case. In the interest of illustrating such a possible outcome, we might explore the Boolean operator NOT in combination with the term *medication*. To demonstrate yet another way to combine terms in a search, we will now appeal to the History option appearing directly under the query box. This option may be used to combine a previously numbered search with a new search term. That is precisely what we will do by combining our earlier search #2 with the expression "NOT medication." The next three figures in this sequence display that option and the resulting outcome of 20 instead of 23 citations found. (Courtesy PubMed, a product of the National Center for Biotechnology Information and the U.S. National Library of Medicine.)

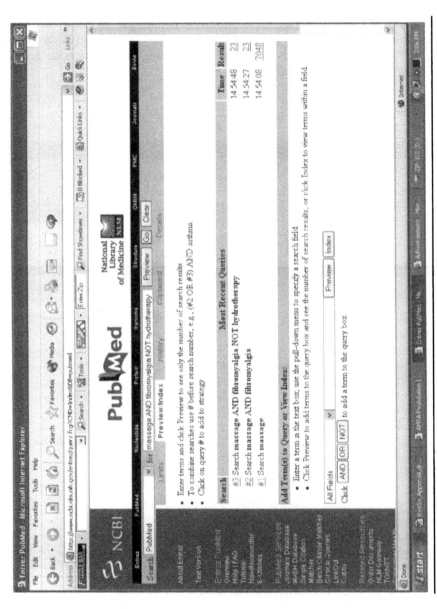

FIGURE A-28 ■ Display of search history after three previous searches and possibility of building on a previous search. *Note:* Search #2 identified in the middle of this page allows us to build on a previous search to include "NOT medication." By clicking the Clear box at the top and then entering "#2 NOT medication" in the resulting blank query box, we thereby engage yet another search using essentially the expression "massage AND fibromyalgia NOT medication." Figures A-29 and A-30 show this use of the search history and the resulting list of 20 rather than 23 citations. (Courtesy PubMed, a product of the National Center for Biotechnology Information and the U.S. National Library of Medicine.)

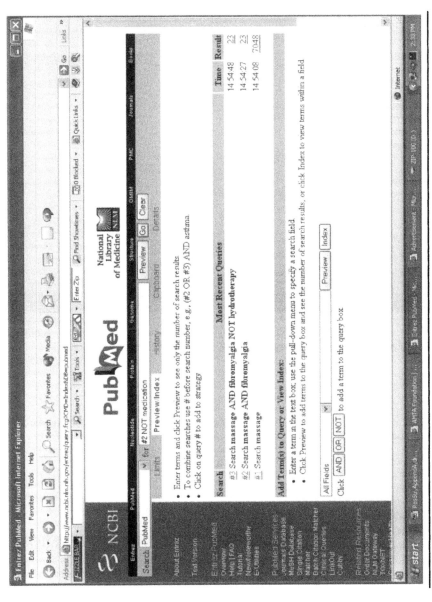

FIGURE A-29 ■ Display of search history used in combination with added Boolean operator to continue the search. *Note:* As indicated earlier, this PubMed page allows us to add to our previous search #2 the expression "NOT medication." (Courtesy PubMed, a product of the National Center for Biotechnology Information and the U.S. National Library of Medicine.)

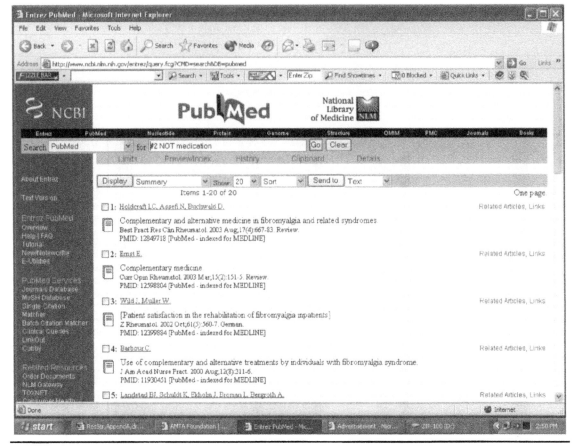

FIGURE A-30 ■ Display of results from search #2 combined with Boolean operator "NOT medication." (Courtesy PubMed, a product of the National Center for Biotechnology Information and the U.S. National Library of Medicine.)

REFERENCES

Edwards, M. J. A. (2002). *The Internet for nurses and allied health professionals* (3rd ed.). New York: Springer.

Guyatt, G., & Rennie, D. (Eds.). (2002). *Users' guide to the medical literature: Essentials of evidence-based clinical practice.* Chicago, IL: AMA Press.

Helewa, A., & Walker, J. M. (2000). *Critical evaluation of research in physical rehabilitation: Towards evidence-based practice.* Philadelphia: W. B. Saunders.

MacBeckner, W., & Berman, B. M. (2003). *Complementary therapies on the Internet.* St. Louis, MO: Churchill Livingstone.

Nicoll, L. H. (2001). *Nurses' guide to the Internet* (3rd ed.). Philadelphia: Lippincott Williams & Wilkins.

Sackett, D. L., Straus, S. E., Richardson, W. S., Rosenberg, W., & Haynes, R. B. (2000). *Evidence-based medicine: How to practice and teach EBM* (2nd ed.). New York: Churchill Livingstone.

Singer, K. P., & Tan, B. K. (2000). Navigating the Internet maze. *Manual Therapy, 5*(3), 165–172.

Smith, R. P. (2002). *The Internet for physicians* (3rd ed.). New York: Springer.

Stave, C. D. (2003). *Field guide to MEDLINE: Making searching simple.* Philadelphia: Lippincott Williams & Wilkins.

ADDITIONAL RECOMMENDED RESOURCES

Anderson, T., & Kanuka, H. (2003). *E-research: Methods, strategies, and issues.* Boston: Allyn & Bacon.

Bero, L., & Rennie, D. (1995). The Cochrane collaboration. *Journal of the American Medical Association, 274*(24), 1935–1938.

Clegg, B. (2001). *The professional's guide to mining the Internet: Information gathering and research on the net* (2nd ed.). Sterling, VA: Stylus.

Dumholdt, E. (2000). *Physical therapy research: Principles and applications* (2nd ed.). Philadelphia: W. B. Saunders.

Greenhalgh, T. (2001). *How to read a paper: The basics of evidence based medicine* (2nd ed.). London: BMJ Books.

Mascara, C., Czar, P., & Hebda, T. (2001). *Internet resource guide for nurses and health care professionals* (2nd ed.). Upper Saddle River, NJ: Prentice-Hall.

Sherrington, C., Herbert, R. D., Maher, C. G., & Moseley, A. M. (2000). PEDro: A database of randomized trials and systematic reviews in physiotherapy. *Manual Therapy, 5*(4), 223–226.

Smith, P., James, T., Lorentzon, M., & Pope, R. (2004). *Shaping the facts: Evidence-based nursing and health care.* New York: Churchill Livingstone.

Young, K. M. (2000). *Informatics for healthcare professionals.* Philadelphia: F. A. Davis.

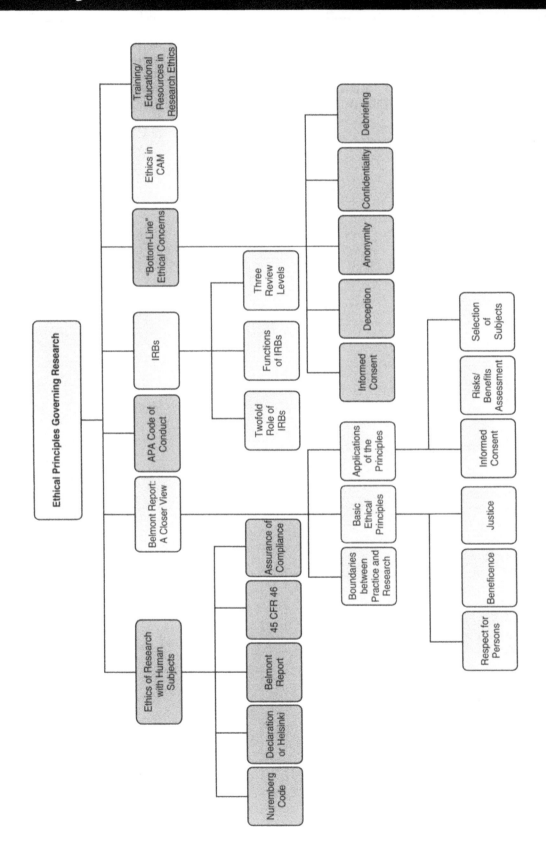

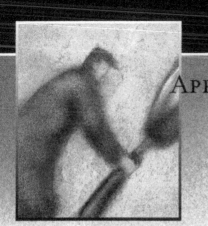

APPENDIX

B

ETHICAL PRINCIPLES GOVERNING RESEARCH IN THE BIOMEDICAL AND BEHAVIORAL SCIENCES

OUTLINE

OBJECTIVES

Upon completion of this appendix, the reader will have the information necessary to perform the following tasks:

1 Discuss the historical background and current contexts regarding the ethics of human subjects research with particular attention to the following:
  a. the Nuremberg Code
  b. the World Medical Association's Declaration of Helsinki
  c. the Belmont Report
  d. Title 45, Code of Federal Regulations, Part 46, Protection of Human Subjects (45 CFR 46)
  e. Assurance of Compliance with 45 CFR 46

2 Regarding the Belmont Report, discuss the distinctions that exist among the following:
  a. boundaries between practice and research
  b. basic ethical principles of respect for persons, beneficence, and justice
  c. applications of the ethical principles with respect to informed consent, assessment of risks and benefits, and selection of subjects

3 Characterize the positions taken in the American Psychological Association's Ethical Principles of Psychologists and Code of Conduct regarding the following issues: institutional approval; informed consent to research; informed consent for recording voices and images in research; client/patient, student, and subordinate research participants; dispensing with informed consent for research; offering inducements for research participation; deception in research; and debriefing.

KEY TERMS

45 CFR 46
Active deception
Anonymity
APA Code of Conduct
Assessment of risks and benefits
Assurance of compliance
Belmont Report (1979)
Beneficence
Common Rule
Confidentiality
Debriefing
Deception

Declaration of Helsinki
  (1964/2000)
Department of Health and Human Services
Ethical principles
Exempt from review
Expedited review
Full board review
Independent ethics committee
Informed consent
Institutional review board
Justice
National Cancer Institute

National Institutes of Health
Nuremberg Code (1947)
Office for Human Research Protections
Office of Human Subjects Research
Passive deception
Practice
Research
Respect for persons
Selection of subjects
World Medical Association

4 Regarding an institutional review board (IRB), discuss the
   following issues:
   a. expectations of the Department of Health and Human
       Services' Office of Human Research Protections;
   b. twofold role of an IRB;
   c. functions of an IRB; and
   d. three levels of IRB research proposal review.
5 Characterize the meaning and intent associated with each of the
   following bottom-line ethical concerns regarding research with
   human subjects: informed consent; deception, both passive and
   active; anonymity; confidentiality; and debriefing.
6 Identify and discuss at least five characteristics of and/or
   controversies surrounding complementary and alternative
   medicine (CAM) that relate to ethical concerns in CAM research.
7 Identify and discuss at least three nonprint resources available
   for training/educational purposes in research ethics.

ETHICS OF RESEARCH WITH HUMAN SUBJECTS: HISTORICAL BACKGROUND AND CURRENT CONTEXTS

An understanding and appreciation of the **ethical principles** of research with human subjects depends largely on one's familiarity with the historical precedents leading us to where we are today. In that regard, the following sections speak to certain historical and contemporary developments.

THE NUREMBERG CODE (1947)

In 1946, 23 Nazi physicians were tried before the Nuremberg Military Tribunal for crimes committed against prisoners of war. One outcome of the trial was the codification of basic ethical standards for conducting research with human subjects. This codification, known as the **Nuremberg Code**, identifies 10 conditions that must be met in order to justify research with human subjects. Of the 10 conditions cited, the two most critical are (a) the need for voluntary informed consent of the subjects and (b) a scientifically justifiable research design capable of potentially beneficial outcomes for the good of society. The **National Institutes of Health's** (NIH's) **Office of Human Subjects Research** Web site lists these 10 *Directives for Human Experimentation* (NIH, 2004c, http://ohsr.od.nih.gov/guidelines/nuremberg.html).

THE WORLD MEDICAL ASSOCIATION'S DECLARATION OF HELSINKI (1964/2000)

Because of the need for guidelines more comprehensive than the Nuremberg Code, the **World Medical Association** (WMA) adopted in 1964 the **Declaration of Helsinki**, which articulates certain ethical principles and guidelines for biomedical research involving human subjects. This declaration identifies 12 basic ethical principles as well as specific guidelines pertaining to (a) medical research combined with clinical care (clinical research) and (b) nontherapeutic biomedical research involving human subjects (nonclinical biomedical research). The WMA has amended this declaration several times since 1964, with the most recent occurring in 2000. The full text is likewise accessible through the NIH's Office of Human Subjects Research Web site (NIH, 2004e, http://ohsr.od.nih.gov/guidelines/helsinki.html).

THE BELMONT REPORT (1979)

One outcome of the signing of the National Research Act (Pub. L. 93-348) in 1974 was the formation of the National Commission for the Protection of Human Subjects of Biomedical and Behavioral Research. Part of this commission's work started in 1976 at the Smithsonian Institution's Belmont Conference Center, continued on a monthly basis through 1979, and finally resulted in the publication of the **Belmont Report**. This document speaks to several ethical principles and guidelines for the protection of human subjects of research. More specifically, it covers three major areas: (a) the boundaries between practice and research; (b) basic ethical principles pertaining to respect for persons, beneficence, and justice; and (c) applications of these principles in terms of informed consent, the assessment of risk and benefits, and the selection of subjects. This report is available through the NIH (2004a, http://ohsr.od.nih.gov/guidelines/belmont.html).

TITLE 45, CODE OF FEDERAL REGULATIONS, PART 46, PROTECTION OF HUMAN SUBJECTS (45 CFR 46, 1981/1991)

The federal government's role regarding the protection of human research subjects continued into the 1980s in the form of approval given to *Title 45, Code of Federal Regulations, Part 46*. Also known as the **Common Rule, 45 CFR 46** originally applied only to research conducted or supported by the **Department of Health and Human Services** (DHHS);

however, in 1991 the regulations were revised and made applicable to all federally supported research.

Subpart A of 45 CFR 46 delineates the basic DHHS policy for the protection of human research subjects. Principal areas addressed in this subpart include—but are not limited to—the following: mechanisms for assuring compliance; IRB membership, functions, operations, criteria for approval of research, and records; expedited review procedures; requirements for and documentation of informed consent; and use of federal funds. Subpart B of the Common Rule builds on the basics of Subpart A and delineates additional protections for pregnant women, human fetuses, and neonates involved in research. Subpart C provides additional DHHS protections for biomedical and behavioral research involving prisoners as subjects, whereas Subpart D does likewise for children involved as subjects in research.

This legislation represents a framework, rather than a set of rigidly applied rules, for ensuring the rights and welfare of human research subjects. The most recent revision occurred in 2001. These regulations are accessible via the NIH (2004d, http://ohsr.od.nih.gov/guidelines/45cfr46.html).

ASSURANCE OF COMPLIANCE WITH 45 CFR 46 (1998)

Given that 45 CFR 46 is an overarching framework, its actual implementation is overseen by the DHHS's **Office for Human Research Protections** (OHRP). Any institution engaged in human subjects research that is conducted or supported by any agency of the DHHS must have an OHRP-approved **assurance of compliance** (or simply *assurance*). This is a statement of the institution's policy and procedures for protecting human subjects that assures compliance with 45 CFR 46. The OHRP currently offers institutions four assurance options: Federalwide Assurance (FWA), Multiple Project Assurance (MPA), Cooperative Project Assurance (CPA), and Single Project Assurance (SPA). Of these four possibilities, the OHRP encourages institutions that need OHRP-approved assurance to submit an FWA. This is due primarily to the following two reasons: (a) it is the simplest type of assurance to complete, and (b) it applies broadly not only to all human subjects research conducted or supported by the DHHS, but also to human subjects research conducted or supported by most other U.S. federal departments and agencies. Further information is available via the OHRP (2004a, www.hhs.gov/ohrp/assurances/assurances_index.html).

NIH GUIDELINES FOR THE CONDUCT OF RESEARCH INVOLVING HUMAN SUBJECTS: SUMMARY RESOURCE

The historical/contemporary review provided in the preceding sections is summarized in a document published by the NIH (2004b). It is titled "Guidelines for the Conduct of Research Involving Human Subjects at the National Institutes of Health" and is accessible via http://ohsr.od.nih.gov/guidelines/graybook.html.

THE BELMONT REPORT: A CLOSER VIEW

As mentioned earlier, the Belmont Report addresses three major themes: (a) boundaries between practice and research, (b) ethical principles, and (c) applications of the principles. In the context of protecting human subjects of research, these three themes are discussed as follows.

BOUNDARIES BETWEEN PRACTICE AND RESEARCH

Practice here refers to biomedical or behavioral interventions providing diagnosis, preventive treatment, or therapy to a patient or client with a reasonable expectation of enhancing the individual's well-being. In contrast, **research** is an activity implemented to investigate a hypothesis, allow conclusions to be drawn, and consequently advance generalizable knowledge typically conveyed in theories, principles, and statements of relationships uncovered. Admittedly, research and practice may conceivably be addressed in tandem as is the case when research aims to evaluate a given therapy's safety and efficacy. As a general guideline, if an activity entails any aspect of the research process, then it must be reviewed to ensure the protection of the human subjects involved.

BASIC ETHICAL PRINCIPLES

These are general judgments reflective of our cultural tradition that represent the underlying rationale for specific ethical prescriptions and evaluations of human behavior. Particularly relevant to the ethical aspects of human subjects research are the principles of respect for persons, beneficence, and justice.

Respect for persons requires, at the very least, a twofold obligation. One is to accommodate the autonomy of individuals by acknowledging their opinions and choices and refraining from impeding their behavior unless their actions are harmful to others. The other is to safeguard those individuals who suffer diminished autonomy due to their being immature or incapacitated to an extent that seriously compromises their capacity for self-determination.

Beneficence as an ethical principle here refers to an obligation to ensure the well-being of individuals. In this document, beneficent actions are expressed as two complementary forms of behavior, namely, the obligations to do no harm and to maximize potential benefits while minimizing possible harm.

Justice is understood here in the context of "fairness in distribution" or "what is deserved" regarding the possible benefits of research as well as the assumption of its burdens. Inherent in this principle is the notion that equals ought to be treated equally with respect to certain properties on which the distribution of benefits and burdens should be based. In this regard, these properties or bases for the distribution of benefits and burdens to each person must be considered in terms of equal share and according to individual need, individual effort, societal contribution, and merit.

APPLICATIONS OF THE PRINCIPLES

Applying these three principles in the actual conduct of research requires that consideration be given to the following: informed consent, assessment of risks and benefits, and the selection of subjects.

The moral requirement of **informed consent** by research subjects derives primarily from the ethical principle of respect for persons discussed earlier. A certain amount of controversy and debate exists regarding not only the nature of informed consent but also whether it is actually possible on the part of a research subject. There is consensus, though, that three critical elements must be present as we attempt to give research subjects the opportunity to decide what shall or shall not happen to them. The first element concerns the extent and nature of *information* that should be provided such that individuals, knowing that the procedure is neither essential for their care nor perhaps fully understood by them, can still decide whether they wish to participate in a study aimed at advancing knowledge. The second element of *comprehension* mandates that the study-related information be provided to the research subjects in a manner and context that accommodate their ability to understand. The third critical element is that the informed consent must be *voluntary*. Implicit in this element is the absence of both (a) coercion in the form of any overt threat to obtain compliance and (b) undue influence in the form of any type of inappropriate reward or overture designed to encourage compliance.

The moral requirement of an **assessment of risks and benefits** emanates primarily from the ethical principle of *beneficence*. This application of beneficence should be viewed not only as a responsibility but also as an opportunity for the investigator, a review committee, and a prospective subject. For all three parties involved it allows for the systematic gathering of comprehensive information about the research being proposed. In so doing, it provides the investigator with a means to examine critically if indeed the planned research is optimally designed. For a review committee, it allows a means for ascertaining if the research subjects will encounter justifiable risks. And for the prospective research subjects themselves, the assessment provides essential information to help them decide whether or not to actually participate in the study.

The moral requirement of the **selection of subjects** in a fair manner stems primarily from the ethical principle of justice, which here is considered at two levels. Individual justice mandates the selection of subjects in an equitable manner such that preferential or biased factors do not come into play. Social justice speaks to the issue of classes or groups of subjects, and the distinction that must be made regarding which classes ought or ought not participate in certain kinds of research based on ability to bear the burdens of research. The moral requirement here also mandates that researchers be vigilant against socially institutionalized injustices that may reflect social, economic, racial, sexual, and cultural biases.

AMERICAN PSYCHOLOGICAL ASSOCIATION: ETHICAL CONSIDERATIONS FOR RESEARCH WITH HUMAN PARTICIPANTS

The research methodology and ethical concerns of this book focus on investigative inquiry in both the biomedical and behavioral science arenas. In the behavioral science realm, the American Psychological Association (APA, 2002) updated its Ethical Principles of Psychologists and Code of Conduct to include ethical standards in 10 areas.

This most recent document is available at www.apa.org/ethics. Standard 8 in the APA ethical guidelines relates to the conduct of research with human participants and is excerpted in Box B-1.

The inclusion of this excerpt from the **APA Code of Conduct** reflects to a large extent the similarity of concerns that exists among researchers, practitioners, and educators across the several biomedical and behavioral science disciplines. The specialty of health psychology, for example, is directly related to several aspects of the complementary and alternative medicine (CAM) professions, not the least of which is the emphasis on the mind-body connection (cf. Nezu, Tsang, Lombardo, & Baron, 2003). Also, many of the challenges that psychologists encounter in researching different psychotherapeutic interventions are indeed shared by manual therapists (cf. Wampold, 2001). Examples involve such issues as identifying viable comparison groups/treatments and exploring the underlying mechanisms of a particular intervention. Accordingly, it is not surprising that basic ethical concerns and mandates of a multidisciplinary nature will surface and assume a major role whether one's orientation is from a biomedical or behavioral science perspective.

INSTITUTIONAL REVIEW BOARD

As mentioned earlier in our discussion of federal requirements regarding human research subjects, the role of an **institutional review board** (IRB) is critical to protecting both the scientific and ethical integrity of the investigative effort. The DHHS requires such a review by any agency or institution receiving government funding for human-participant research. This essentially includes all colleges, universities, hospitals, and clinics wherein the research endeavor involves human subjects. Directions for registering an institution's IRB (or **independent ethics committee** [IEC]) with the DHHS's Office of Human Research Protections (2004b) are available at www.hhs.gov/ohrp/assurances. Affiliated with an IRB is a twofold role that is assumed as well as corresponding functions and levels at which the review process is completed.

TWOFOLD ROLE OF THE IRB

The IRB is external to the research team whose proposal is being examined. This is critical given the following twofold role assumed by any IRB: (a) It is *ethically guided* by the requirements of the Common

BOX B-1   AMERICAN PSYCHOLOGICAL ASSOCIATION'S ETHICAL STANDARD 8 FOR THE CONDUCT OF RESEARCH WITH HUMAN PARTICIPANTS

8.01 Institutional Approval

When institutional approval is required, psychologists provide accurate information about their research proposals and obtain approval prior to conducting the research. They conduct the research in accordance with the approved research protocol.

8.02 Informed Consent to Research

(a) When obtaining informed consent as required in Standard 3.10, Informed Consent, psychologists inform participants about (1) the purpose of the research, expected duration, and procedures; (2) their right to decline to participate and to withdraw from the research once participation has begun; (3) the foreseeable consequences of declining or withdrawing; (4) reasonably foreseeable factors that may be expected to influence their willingness to participate such as potential risks, discomfort, or adverse effects; (5) any prospective research benefits; (6) limits of confidentiality; (7) incentives for participation; and (8) whom to contact for questions about the research and research participants' rights. They provide opportunity for the prospective participants to ask questions and receive answers. (See also Standards 8.03, Informed Consent for Recording Voices and Images in Research; 8.05, Dispensing With Informed Consent for Research; and 8.07, Deception in Research.)

(b) Psychologists conducting intervention research involving the use of experimental treatments clarify to participants at the outset of the research (1) the experimental nature of the treatment; (2) the services that will or will not be available to the control group(s) if appropriate; (3) the means by which assignment to treatment and control groups will be made; (4) available treatment alternatives if an individual does not wish to participate in the research or wishes to withdraw once a study has begun; and (5) compensation for or monetary costs of participating including, if appropriate, whether reimbursement from the participant or a third-party payor will be sought. (See also Standard 8.02a, Informed Consent to Research.)

8.03 Informed Consent for Recording Voices and Images in Research

Psychologists obtain informed consent from research participants prior to recording their voices or images for data collection unless (1) the research consists solely of naturalistic observations in public places, and it is not anticipated that the recording will be used in a manner that could cause personal identification or harm, or (2) the research design includes deception, and consent for the use of the recording is obtained during debriefing. (See also Standard 8.07, Deception in Research.)

8.04 Client/Patient, Student, and Subordinate Research Participants

(a) When psychologists conduct research with clients/patients, students, or subordinates as participants, psychologists take steps to protect the prospective participants from adverse consequences of declining or withdrawing from participation.

(b) When research participation is a course requirement or an opportunity for extra credit, the prospective participant is given the choice of equitable alternative activities.

| BOX B-1 | AMERICAN PSYCHOLOGICAL ASSOCIATION'S ETHICAL STANDARD 8 FOR THE CONDUCT OF RESEARCH WITH HUMAN PARTICIPANTS — CONT'D |

8.05 Dispensing With Informed Consent for Research

Psychologists may dispense with informed consent only (1) where research would not reasonably be assumed to create distress or harm and involves (a) the study of normal educational practices, curricula, or classroom management methods conducted in educational settings; (b) only anonymous questionnaires, naturalistic observations, or archival research for which disclosure of responses would not place participants at risk of criminal or civil liability or damage their financial standing, employability, or reputation, and confidentiality is protected; or (c) the study of factors related to job or organization effectiveness conducted in organizational settings for which there is no risk to participants' employability, and confidentiality is protected or (2) where otherwise permitted by law or federal or institutional regulations.

8.06 Offering Inducements for Research Participation

(a) Psychologists make reasonable efforts to avoid offering excessive or inappropriate financial or other inducements for research participation when such inducements are likely to coerce participation.

(b) When offering professional services as an inducement for research participation, psychologists clarify the nature of the services, as well as the risks, obligations, and limitations. (See also Standard 6.05, Barter With Clients/Patients.)

8.07 Deception in Research

(a) Psychologists do not conduct a study involving deception unless they have determined that the use of deceptive techniques is justified by the study's significant prospective scientific, educational, or applied value and that effective nondeceptive alternative procedures are not feasible.

(b) Psychologists do not deceive prospective participants about research that is reasonably expected to cause physical pain or severe emotional distress.

(c) Psychologists explain any deception that is an integral feature of the design and conduct of an experiment to participants as early as is feasible, preferably at the conclusion of their participation, but no later than at the conclusion of the data collection, and permit participants to withdraw their data. (See also Standard 8.08, Debriefing.)

8.08 Debriefing

(a) Psychologists provide a prompt opportunity for participants to obtain appropriate information about the nature, results, and conclusions of the research, and they take reasonable steps to correct any misconceptions that participants may have of which the psychologists are aware.

(b) If scientific or humane values justify delaying or withholding this information, psychologists take reasonable measures to reduce the risk of harm.

(c) When psychologists become aware that research procedures have harmed a participant, they take reasonable steps to minimize the harm.

From American Psychological Association. (2002). Ethical principles of psychologists and code of conduct. *American Psychologist, 57*, 1060–1073.

Rule in evaluating and making recommendations regarding a proposed study. (b) It is *legally required* to uphold those same requirements by virtue of the *assurance of compliance* statement furnished by the research team's institution. Critical guidelines, then, must be followed in an objective, unbiased, and comprehensive manner to ensure not only the scientific sophistication of the proposed study, but also the ethical integrity of its implementation.

FUNCTIONS OF THE IRB

In discharging its twofold role that entails both ethical and legal responsibilities, the IRB addresses several functions. These functions relate to both reviewing and monitoring the research effort. As discussed by Lo (2001), the IRB's principal functions address the following concerns: (a) Risks to participants are minimized and are considered reasonable relative to the anticipated benefits and importance of the knowledge that is expected to accrue. (b) Selection of participants is fair and equitable. (c) Informed consent is received from the participants or their legal representatives. (d) Confidentiality is appropriately maintained.

THREE LEVELS OF IRB RESEARCH PROPOSAL REVIEW

The IRB's role and functions may be addressed at three levels. Stommel and Wills (2004, p.385) have summarized these three possibilities as follows:

> *'Exempt from review'* The proposed research involves no more than minimal risk. "Exempt from review" refers specifically to exemption from full board review. Researchers should never decide independently that their research is exempt from IRB review. All research must be submitted for IRB review. If the IRB concurs that the research meets the criteria for exemption, the IRB issues an exemption approval letter to the researcher.
>
> *'Expedited review'* The proposed research involves no more than minor risk. If there is any question about the level of risk involved in a proposed research project, the proposed project should undergo full board review.
>
> *'Full board review'* All research that cannot be categorized as exempt or expedited must undergo full review.

ETHICAL CONCERNS REGARDING RESEARCH WITH HUMAN SUBJECTS: THE BOTTOM LINE

We have been surveying several ethical principles and their practical applications regarding research with human subjects. The following is a listing of those bottom-line concerns that must be addressed in any research setting involving the participation of human subjects.

As discussed earlier in our coverage of the Belmont Report, the ethical mandate of *informed consent* speaks to the need for an investigator to ensure that prospective subjects have all of the required information necessary to make a rational decision regarding their participation in a study. The information, comprehension, and voluntary elements required here always necessitate documentation via an informed consent form.

Deception involves the researcher either intentionally withholding information about the study from participants (an act of *omission*, or **passive deception**) or intentionally misleading the participants regarding the true nature of a study (an act of *commission*, or **active deception**). Naturally, a risks/benefits assessment is critical in this regard and certainly relates to the principle of beneficence as covered earlier in the Belmont Report.

Related, but distinctly different, are the concepts of anonymity and confidentiality. **Anonymity** ensures that the researcher has no way of associating a research subject's identity with any information received from that individual. **Confidentiality** means that although the researcher potentially or actually can associate a research subject's identity with information received from that individual, assurances are given that such associations of one's identity and information will be kept secret, private, and undisclosed. Any potential limits to confidentiality in a study, however, must be acknowledged in the informed consent form.

Debriefing refers to the planned post-investigation explanation of a study's purpose given to the research participants. This is particularly important in studies that involve any form of deception. One possible—though unlikely—outcome of a debriefing session may be that some subjects may decide to withdraw their earlier consent to use the data generated by their participation.

ETHICS IN CAM RESEARCH AND TRAINING/ EDUCATIONAL OPTIONS IN RESEARCH ETHICS: ADDITIONAL RESOURCES

ETHICS IN CAM RESEARCH

One of two helpful resources on the ethics of CAM-related research is an article by Miller, Emanuel,

Rosenstein, and Straus (2004) titled "Ethical Issues Concerning Research in Complementary and Alternative Medicine." The authors address the paucity of attention to the ethics of research studies investigating CAM treatments and several controversial issues bearing on such ethical considerations. These issues include the value of rigorous CAM research; the validity of randomized, placebo-controlled clinical trials of CAM interventions; the justification for such clinical trials of CAM treatments for medical conditions in the face of demonstrated effective conventional treatment; and the practice and policy implications of CAM and conventional treatments found to be no better than placebo. Miller at al. (2004) concluded their review of these controversies as follows:

> Growing use of CAM treatments in the United States and increased appreciation of the role of traditional, indigenous healing practices in developing nations necessitate rigorous, ethically sound clinical research to assess their therapeutic value. The standards of evidence-based medicine, developed over the years to understand and evaluate conventional medical therapies, apply equally to CAM. The arguments that placebo-controlled RCTs are not appropriate for evaluating most CAM treatments lack merit. Although the use of placebo-controlled trials raises ethical concerns when proven effective treatment exists for the condition under investigation, they are ethically justified, provided that stringent criteria for protecting research subjects are satisfied. Conceptual and empirical research should focus on whether CAM and conventional treatments that are demonstrated to be no better than placebo may still have therapeutic value, provided that their risks are minor and their benefit can be reliably attributed to the placebo effect. (p. 604)

Another informative piece appearing in the *Journal of Medical Ethics* is by Ernst, Cohen, and Stone (2004). These authors explore some of the characteristics of CAM that seem to give rise to many of the ethical problems associated with evidence-based CAM. One such characteristic involves the conceptual and pragmatic distinctions between CAM and conventional medicine. Others include the view of CAM as private medicine as well as the observation that providers of CAM are often not medically trained. Remaining features of CAM that tend to prompt ethical debate include the following: CAM (at least in the United Kingdom) is not regulated as rigorously as conventional medicine; CAM effectiveness and safety are often considered unproven; CAM research funds are relatively scarce; CAM has an underdeveloped research culture; and CAM is holistic and, hence, may have some

therapeutic benefits not readily amenable to quantitative measurement. Against the backdrop of these CAM characteristics, though, the authors maintain that (a) such features and challenges are not a viable deterrent to good CAM research, and (b) there are no reasons in principle why rigorous CAM research cannot be pursued.

TRAINING/EDUCATIONAL RESOURCES FOR RESEARCH ETHICS

The various print and electronic sources already cited in this appendix represent a starting point for practitioners, educators, and researchers interested in delving more deeply into the principles and procedures governing the ethics of research with human subjects.

Another highly recommended source is an online tutorial by the NIH's **National Cancer Institute** (2004) titled *Human Participation Protections: Education for Research Teams.* Beginning in October 2000, the NIH has required education in the protection of human research subjects for all investigators and related personnel submitting NIH applications for grants or proposals for contracts or receiving new or noncompeting awards. This online course represents one available option for fulfilling this obligation for education in the realm of human participant protection. The online tutorial is accessible via http://cme.nci.nih.gov and provides the option of selecting a "completion certificate only, no continuing education credit" route. Other training resources are available at the following locations:

University of Washington School of Medicine (http://eduserv.hscer.washington.edu/bioethics/topics)

The University of Minnesota (www.research.umn.edu/consent)

The University of California at Irvine (http://tutorials.rgs.uci.edu)

DHHS, Office for Human Research Protection (www.hhs.gov/ohrp)

National Human Genome Research Institute (www.nhgri.nih.gov/PolicyEthics)

University of Michigan (www.responsibility.research.umich.edu/casematerialsdir.html)

In addition to these print and online resources, still another option available is a three-part videotape reissued by the NIH's Office of Human Research Protections in 2001. The appropriate bibliographic information indicating the topics covered in the three instructional segments follows: Office of Human Research Protections. (Producer). (2001). *Protecting human subjects: Part I, Evolving concerns–Protection for human subjects* (22 mins.); *Part II, Balancing society's mandates–IRB review criteria* (36 mins.); *Part III, The Belmont Report–Basic ethical principles and their applications* (28 mins.), Washington, DC: National Institutes of Health.

A final resource that should prove helpful is the Web link to the document titled *Human Subjects Institutional Review Board Policy and Procedures*. It is available via the Office of Grants and Research (2004) at Loyola University New Orleans (www.loyno.edu/org/human.subjects.html). This document speaks to such issues as the discharge of responsibilities for the protection of the rights and welfare of human subjects; committee structure and committee procedures; applicant's procedures; subject's procedures; and instructions to principal investigators/project directors regarding subjects at risk, protocol, and informed consent.

REFERENCES

American Psychological Association. (2002). Ethical principles of psychologists and code of conduct. *American Psychologist, 57,* 1060–1073. (Also available at ww.apa.org/ethics.)

Ernst, E., Cohen, M. H., & Stone. J. (2004). Ethical problems arising in evidence based complementary and alternative medicine. *Journal of Medical Ethics, 30,* 156–159.

Lo, B. (2001). Addressing ethical issues. In S. B. Hulley, S. R. Cummings, W. S. Browner, D. Grady, N. Hearst, & T. B. Newman (Eds.), *Designing clinical research* (2nd ed.). (pp. 215–230). Philadelphia: Lippincott Williams & Wilkins.

Miller, F. G., Emanuel, E. J., Rosenstein, D. L., & Straus, S. E. (2004). Ethical issues concerning research in complementary and alternative medicine. *Journal of the American Medical Association, 291,* 599–604.

National Cancer Institute. (2004). *Human participation protections: Education for research teams* (Online tutorial). Washington, DC: NIH, NCI. (Accessible at http://cme.nci.nih.gov.)

National Institutes of Health. (2004a). *The Belmont report: Ethical principles and guidelines for the protection of human subjects of research.* Washington, DC: NIH. Retrieved August 5, 2004, from http://ohsr.od.nih.gov/guidelines/belmont.html.

National Institutes of Health. (2004b). *Guidelines for the conduct of research involving human subjects at the National Institutes of Health.* Washington, DC: NIH. Retrieved August 5, 2004, from http://ohsr.od.nih.gov/guidelines/graybook.html.

National Institutes of Health. (2004c). *Nuremberg code: Directives for human experimentation.* Washington, DC: NIH. Retrieved August 5, 2004, from http://ohsr.od.nih.gov/guidelines/nuremberg.html.

National Institutes of Health. (2004d). *Title 45, code of federal regulations, part 46, protection of human subjects.* Washington, DC: NIH. Retrieved August 5, 2004, from http://ohsr.od.nih.gov/guidelines/45cfr46.html.

National Institutes of Health. (2004e). *World Medical Association Declaration of Helsinki: Ethical principles for medical research involving human subjects.* Washington, DC: NIH. Retrieved August 5, 2004, from http://ohsr.od.nih.gov/guidelines/helsinki.html.

Nezu, C. M., Tsang, S., Lombardo, E. R., & Baron, K. P. (2003). Complementary and alternative therapies. In A. M. Nezu, C. M. Nezu, & P. A. Geller (Eds.), *Handbook of psychology: Vol. 9. Health psychology* (pp. 591–614). Hoboken, NJ: John Wiley & Sons.

Office for Human Research Protections. (Producer). (2001). *Protecting human subjects: Part I, Evolving concerns–Protection for human subjects* (22 mins.); *Part II, Balancing society's mandates–IRB review criteria* (36 mins.); *Part III, The Belmont Report–Basic ethical principles and their applications* (28 mins.). Washington, DC: National Institutes of Health.

Office for Human Research Protections. (2004a). *Assurances.* Washington, DC: DHHS, OHRP. Retrieved August 11, 2004, from www.hhs.gov/ohrp/assurances/assurances_index.html.

Office for Human Research Protections. (2004b). *Registration of an institutional review board (IRB) or independent ethics committee (IEC).* Washington, DC: DHHS, OHRP. Retrieved August 11, 2004, from www.hhs.gov/ohrp/assurances.

Office of Grants and Research, Loyola University New Orleans. (2004). *Human subjects institutional review board policy and procedures.* New Orleans: Loyola University, Office of Grants and Research. Retrieved August 5, 2004, from www.loyno.edu/org/human.subjects.html.

Stommel, M., & Wills, C. E. (2004). *Clinical research: Concepts and principles for advanced practice nurses.* Philadelphia: Lippincott Williams & Wilkins.

Wampold, B. E. (2001). *The great psychotherapy debate: Models, methods, and findings.* Mahwah, NJ: Lawrence Erlbaum Associates.

ADDITIONAL RECOMMENDED RESOURCES

Domholdt, E. (2000). *Physical therapy research: Principles and applications* (2nd ed.). Philadelphia: W. B. Saunders.

Elmes, D. G., Kantowitz, B. H., & Roediger, H. L. (2003). *Research methods in psychology* (7th ed.). Belmont, CA: Thomson Wadsworth.

Gillis, A., & Jackson, W. (2002). *Research for nurses: Methods and interpretation.* Philadelphia: F. A. Davis.

Goodwin, C. J. (2005). *Research in psychology: Methods and design* (4th ed.). Danvers, MA: John Wiley & Sons.

Gravetter, F. J., & Forzano, L. B. (2003). *Research methods for the behavioral sciences.* Belmont, CA: Thomson Wadsworth.

Kazdin, A. E. (2003). *Research design in clinical psychology* (4th ed.). Boston: Allyn & Bacon.

La Vaque, T. J., & Rossiter, T. (2001). The ethical use of placebo controls in clinical research: The Declaration of Helsinki. *Applied Psychophysiology and Biofeedback, 26*(1), 23–37.

Polit, D. F., & Beck, C. T. (2004). *Nursing research: Principles and methods* (7th ed.). Philadelphia: Lippincott Williams & Wilkins.

Portney, L. G., & Watkins, M. P. (2000). *Foundations of clinical research: Applications to practice* (2nd ed.). Upper Saddle River, NJ: Prentice-Hall Health.

Smith, R. A., & Davis, S. F. (2003). *The psychologist as detective: An introduction to conducting research in psychology* (3rd ed.). Upper Saddle River, NJ: Prentice-Hall/Pearson Education.

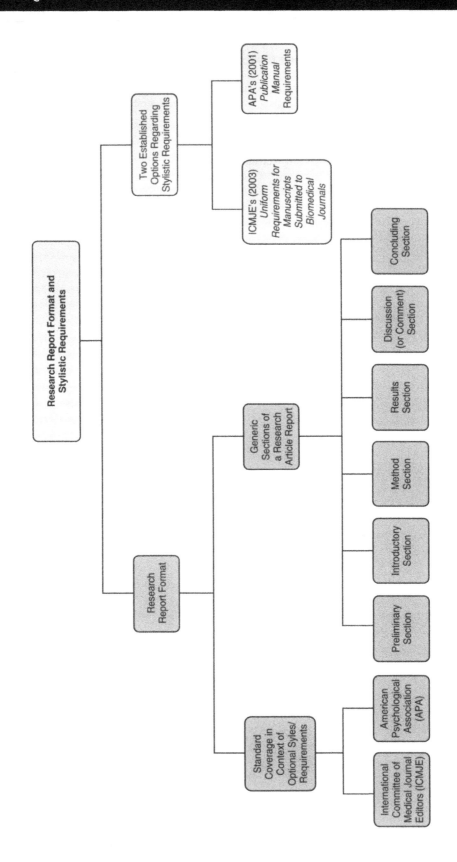

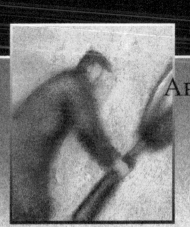

APPENDIX

C

RESEARCH REPORT FORMAT AND STYLISTIC REQUIREMENTS

OUTLINE

OBJECTIVES

Upon completion of this appendix, the reader will have the information necessary to perform the following tasks:

1 Identify the two major stylistic guides for health science and behavioral science researchers that provide the basis for (a) the standard topical coverage format in a research report and (b) requirements for manuscript preparation.

2 Identify the six generic sections of a research article report.

3 For each of the six generic sections of a research article report, characterize the features or contents covered.

4 Regarding the International Committee of Medical Journal Editors' most recent (2003) update of the *Uniform Requirements for Manuscripts Submitted to Biomedical Journals,* (a) state the purpose of the document and (b) recognize appropriate applications of the guidelines for manuscript preparation and submission.

5 Regarding the American Psychological Association's most recent edition (5th ed., 2001) of the *APA Publication Manual,* (a) state the purpose of the manual and (b) recognize appropriate applications of the guidelines for organizing and preparing a manuscript for submission.

American Psychological Association
Concluding section
Discussion/Comments section
International Committee of Medical Journal
    Editors

Introductory section
Method section
Preliminary section
Publication Manual of the American
    Psychological Association

Results section
Stylistic requirements
Uniform Requirements for Manuscripts
    Submitted to Biomedical Journals

RESEARCH REPORT FORMAT

The type of research report we are mainly concerned with in this appendix is that of a manuscript that will eventually take the form of a printed journal article appearing in a health science or behavioral science publication. More specifically, we are speaking of an empirical study wherein data pertinent to the research question at hand have been collected and analyzed, and are now being disseminated to the professional community. With this context in mind, the research report format must (a) adhere to certain **stylistic requirements** and (b) typically encompass certain generic sections that conventionally define the structure of an empirical research article. In addition to the two stylistic resources we will be emphasizing in this appendix, other helpful aids regarding scientific communication are works by Browner (1999) and Byrne (1998).

STANDARD COVERAGE IN CONTEXT OF OPTIONAL STYLES/REQUIREMENTS

As just mentioned, the standard structure or coverage of a research article is rather generic and conventional across the various health science and behavioral science professions, and this standard coverage is our focus in the next section. Before considering that structure, though, it is important to acknowledge two available options regarding stylistic requirements that give direction to standardizing scientific communication.

One such option is the *Uniform Requirements for Manuscripts Submitted to Biomedical Journals* produced by the International Committee of Medical Journal Editors (ICMJE, 2003). The other alternative is the *Publication Manual of the American Psychological Association* (APA, 2001, 2004). The following section reflects both of these sources and details the standard coverage found in the vast majority of research articles appearing in health science and behavioral science journals. Furthermore, later in this appendix we will

address some of the specific requirements of these two styles by way of excerpts from their actual guidelines.

GENERIC SECTIONS OF A RESEARCH ARTICLE REPORT

Although slight variations exist, both the ICMJE and the APA guidelines identify a generic structure for research articles. This conventional structure, in turn, allows for certain functions to be addressed in our attempts at scientific communication. The typical sections constituting this structure are discussed next.

Preliminary Section

The **preliminary section** encompasses such features as the title page, abstract, and key words. The principal types of information provided on the title page include the title of the article, authors' names and institutional affiliations, disclaimers, corresponding authors, sources of support, running head, word count, and designation of number of figures and tables. The length and structured format of the abstract synthesizing the content of the article vary depending on the editorial policy of a given journal. Many journals require a specification of 3 to 10 key words or short phrases that identify the main topics of the report.

Introductory Section

The major intent of the **introductory section** is to provide a literature-based context for the study being reported. This serves partly to establish the nature and significance of the problem investigated, inclusive of the study's subjects, setting, and variables. It also operationalizes the research question studied as well as the rationale for the hypotheses tested.

Method Section

The **method section** does precisely what the name implies—it communicates the research procedures employed in the conduct of the study. This typically spans such concerns as the description and selection of participants, the nature of the research design, the manipulation and/or measurement of the study's variables, and the instrumentation used for manipulation and/or measurement purposes. In certain biomedical journals, this section also includes an identification of the data analysis techniques used. One of the most important considerations in the method section is that accurate and precise information must be provided so as to allow for the possible replication of the study by future researchers.

Results Section

The **results section** communicates the outcomes of the study by way of logically sequenced text, tables, and figures (illustrations). The outcomes emanate from the nature of the data analyses conducted in the attempt to test the study's hypotheses. Descriptive and inferential statistics usually provide the context within which the results are framed, although in the instance of qualitative studies the reliance on verbal data may dictate otherwise. To avoid interrupting the flow of the results section, any extra or detailed supplementary information may be provided in the report's appendix or in an electronic version of the article if such a journal format is available.

Discussion (or Comment) Section

The **discussion/comments section** provides the opportunity not only to synthesize the main findings but to address viable explanations for the findings. Part of this effort should involve comparing and contrasting the study's results with relevant studies acknowledged earlier in the introductory section. The discussion section also provides the opportunity for study limitations to be cited as well as for implications to be explored regarding future research and/or clinical practice.

Concluding Section

The report's **concluding section** includes such items as references, appendixes, notes/acknowledgments, tables, and figures. The bibliographic format for citations included in the references will vary somewhat across different journals. Likewise, journal distinctions might also be made regarding the other features of the concluding section.

TWO ESTABLISHED OPTIONS REGARDING STYLISTIC REQUIREMENTS

As introduced earlier, the two most recognized and established stylistic formats for scientific

communication in the health science and behavioral science arenas are (a) the ICMJE's (2003) *Uniform Requirements for Manuscripts Submitted to Biomedical Journals* and (b) the APA's (2001, 2004) *Publication Manual*. The two sections that follow provide excerpts related to these two sources and are intended simply as an introduction. Professional reliance on these two sets of stylistic requirements necessitates, of course, access to and study of the documents in their entirety.

ICMJE'S (2003) UNIFORM REQUIREMENTS FOR MANUSCRIPTS SUBMITTED TO BIOMEDICAL JOURNALS

The **International Committee of Medical Journal Editors** (ICMJE) most recently updated this set of stylistic guidelines in November 2003. The **Uniform Requirements for Manuscripts Submitted to Biomedical Journals** document covers the following nine sections: I. Statement of Purpose; II. Ethical Considerations in the Conduct and Reporting of Research; III. Publishing and Editorial Issues Related to Publication in Biomedical Journals; IV. Manuscript Preparation and Submission; V. References; VI. About the International Committee of Medical Journal Editors; VII. Authors of the Uniform Requirements; VIII. Use, Distribution, and Translation of the Uniform Requirements; and IX. Inquiries.

Sections I and IV of the document are the most pertinent to our present concerns. Accordingly, these two sections appear as excerpts in Box C-1 that follows. Access to the complete document is available electronically at www.icmje.org/index.html.

APA'S (2001, 2004) PUBLICATION MANUAL

The *Publication Manual of the American Psychological Association* (2001) is a definitive stylistic resource in the behavioral and social sciences that is used extensively beyond the discipline and profession of psychology per se. The current fifth edition of the **American Psychological Association's** (APA's) *Publication Manual* addresses the following nine sections: 1. Content and Organization of a Manuscript; 2. Expressing Ideas and Reducing Bias in Language; 3. APA Editorial Style; 4. Reference List; 5. Manuscript Preparation and Sample Paper to Be Submitted for Publication; 6. Material Other Than Journal Articles; 7. Manuscript Acceptance and Production; 8. Journals Program of the APA; and 9. Bibliography. This document also spans the following five appendixes: A. Checklist for Manuscript Submissions; B. Checklist for Transmitting Accepted Manuscripts for Electronic Production; C. Ethical

Text continued on p. 280

BOX C-I   EXCERPT FROM UNIFORM REQUIREMENTS FOR MANUSCRIPTS SUBMITTED TO BIOMEDICAL JOURNALS: WRITING AND EDITING FOR BIOMEDICAL PUBLICATION

Updated October 2004
International Committee of Medical Journal Editors

I. Statement of Purpose
I.A. About the Uniform Requirements
A small group of editors of general medical journals met informally in Vancouver, British Columbia, in 1978 to establish guidelines for the format of manuscripts submitted to their journals. The group became known as the Vancouver Group. Its requirements for manuscripts, including formats for bibliographic references developed by the National Library of Medicine, were first published in 1979. The Vancouver Group expanded and evolved into the International Committee of Medical Journal Editors (ICMJE), which meets annually. The ICMJE gradually has broadened its concerns to include ethical principles related to publication in biomedical journals.

The ICJME has produced multiple editions of the Uniform Requirements for Manuscripts Submitted to Biomedical Journals. Over the years, issues have arisen that go beyond manuscript preparation, resulting in the development of a number of Separate Statements on editorial policy. The entire Uniform Requirements document was revised in 1997; sections were updated in May 1999 and May 2000. In May 2001, the ICMJE revised the sections related to potential conflict of interest. In 2003, the committee revised and reorganized the entire document and incorporated the Separate Statements into the text. The committee prepared this revision in 2004.

The total content of the Uniform Requirements for Manuscripts Submitted to Biomedical Journals may be reproduced for educational, not-for-profit purposes without regard for copyright; the committee encourages distribution of the material.

Journals that agree to use the Uniform Requirements are encouraged to state in their instructions to authors that their requirements are in accordance with the Uniform Requirements and to cite this version.

I.B. Potential Users of the Uniform Requirements
The ICMJE created the Uniform Requirements primarily to help authors and editors in their mutual task of creating and distributing accurate, clear, easily accessible reports of biomedical studies. The initial sections address the ethical principles related to the process of evaluating, improving, and publishing manuscripts in biomedical journals and the relationships between editors and authors, peer reviewers, and the media. The latter sections address the more technical aspects of preparing and submitting manuscripts. The ICMJE believes the entire document is relevant to the concerns of both authors and editors.

The Uniform Requirements can provide many other stakeholders—peer reviewers, publishers, the media, patients and their families, and general readers—with useful insights into the biomedical authoring and editing process.

I.C. How to Use the Uniform Requirements
The Uniform Requirements state the ethical principles in the conduct and reporting of research and provide recommendations relating to specific elements of editing and writing. These recommendations are based largely on the shared experience of a moderate number of editors and authors, collected over many years, rather than on the results of methodical, planned investigation that aspires to be "evidence-based." Wherever possible, recommendations are accompanied by a rationale that justifies them; as such, the document serves an educational purpose.

Authors will find it helpful to follow the recommendations in this document whenever possible because, as described in the explanations, doing so improves the quality and clarity of reporting in manuscripts submitted to any journal, as well as the ease of editing. At the same time, every journal has editorial requirements uniquely suited to its purposes. Authors therefore need to become familiar with the specific instructions to authors published by the journal they have chosen for their manuscript—for example, the topics suitable for that journal, and the types of papers that may be submitted (for example, original articles, reviews, or case reports)—and should follow those instructions. The Mulford Library at the Medical College of Ohio maintains a useful compendium of instructions to authors at www.mco.edu/lib/instr/libinsta.html.
. . .

IV. Manuscript Preparation and Submission
IV.A. Preparing a Manuscript for Submission to a Biomedical Journal
Editors and reviewers spend many hours reading manuscripts, and therefore appreciate receiving with manuscripts that are easy to read and edit. Much of the information in journals' instructions to authors is designed to accomplish that goal in ways that meet each journal's particular editorial needs. The guidance that follows provides a general background and rationale for preparing manuscripts for any journal.

BOX C-1 EXCERPT FROM UNIFORM REQUIREMENTS FOR MANUSCRIPTS SUBMITTED TO BIOMEDICAL JOURNALS: WRITING AND EDITING FOR BIOMEDICAL PUBLICATION—CONT'D

IV.A.1. GENERAL PRINCIPLES AND REPORTING GUIDELINES

IV.A.1.a. General Principles for Manuscript Preparation

The text of observational and experimental articles is usually (but not necessarily) divided into sections with the headings Introduction, Methods, Results, and Discussion. This so-called "IMRAD" structure is not simply an arbitrary publication format, but rather a direct reflection of the process of scientific discovery. Long articles may need subheadings within some sections (especially the Results and Discussion sections) to clarify their content. Other types of articles, such as case reports, reviews, and editorials, are likely to need other formats.

Publication in electronic formats has created opportunities for adding details or whole sections in the electronic version only, layering information, cross-linking or extracting portions of articles, and the like. Authors need to work closely with editors in developing or using such new publication formats and should submit material for potential supplementary electronic formats for peer review.

. Double spacing of all portions of the manuscript—including the title page, abstract, text, acknowledgments, references, individual tables, and legends—and generous margins make it possible for editors and reviewers to edit the text line by line, and add comments and queries, directly on the paper copy. If manuscripts are submitted electronically, the files should be double spaced, because the manuscript may need to be printed out for reviewing and editing.

During the editorial process reviewers and editors frequently need to refer to specific portions of the manuscript, which is difficult unless the pages are numbered. Authors should therefore number all of the pages of the manuscript consecutively, beginning with the title page.

IV.A.1.b. Reporting Guidelines for Specific Study Designs

Research reports frequently omit important information. The general requirements listed in the next section relate to reporting essential elements for all study designs. Authors are encouraged in addition to consult reporting guidelines relevant to their specific research design. For reports of randomized controlled trials authors should refer to the CONSORT statement (www.consort-statement.org). This guideline provides a set of recommendations comprising a list of items to report and a patient flow diagram. Reporting guidelines have also been developed for a number of other study designs that some journals may ask authors to follow. Some of these reporting guidelines can also be found at www.consort-statement.org. Authors should consult the information for authors of the journal they have chosen.

IV.A.2. TITLE PAGE

The title page should carry the following information:

1. The title of the article. Concise titles are easier to read than long, convoluted ones. Titles that are too short may, however, lack important information, such as study design (which is particularly important in identifying randomized controlled trials). Authors should include all information in the title that will make electronic retrieval of the article both sensitive and specific.
2. Authors' names and institutional affiliations. Some journals publish each author's highest academic degree(s), while others do not.
3. The name of the department(s) and institution(s) to which the work should be attributed.
4. Disclaimers, if any.
5. Corresponding authors. The name, mailing address, telephone and fax numbers, and e-mail address of the author responsible for correspondence about the manuscript (the "corresponding author;" this author may or may not be the "guarantor" for the integrity of the study as a whole, if someone is identified in that role. The corresponding author should indicate clearly whether his or her e-mail address is to be published.
6. The name and address of the author to whom requests for reprints should be addressed or a statement that reprints will not be available from the authors.
7. Source(s) of support in the form of grants, equipment, drugs, or all of these.
8. A running head. Some journals request a short running head or foot line, usually of no more than 40 characters (count letters and spaces) at the foot of the title page. Running heads are published in most journals, but are also sometimes used within the editorial office for filing and locating manuscripts.
9. Word counts. A word count for the text only (excluding abstract, acknowledgments, figure legends, and references) allows editors and reviewers to assess whether the information contained in the paper warrants the amount of space devoted to it, and whether the submitted manuscript fits within the journal's word limits. A separate word count for the Abstract is also useful for the same reason.
10. The number of figures and tables. It is difficult for editorial staff and reviewers to tell if the figures and tables that should have accompanied a manuscript were actually included unless the numbers of figures and tables that belong to the manuscript are noted on the title page.

Continued

| BOX C-I | EXCERPT FROM UNIFORM REQUIREMENTS FOR MANUSCRIPTS SUBMITTED TO BIOMEDICAL JOURNALS: WRITING AND EDITING FOR BIOMEDICAL PUBLICATION — CONT'D |

IV.A.3. CONFLICT OF INTEREST NOTIFICATION PAGE

To prevent the information on potential conflict of interest for authors from being overlooked or misplaced, it is necessary for that information to be part of the manuscript. It should therefore also be included on a separate page or pages immediately following the title page. However, individual journals may differ in where they ask authors to provide this information and some journals do not send information on conflicts of interest to reviewers. (*See Section II.D. Conflicts of Interest*)

IV.A.4. ABSTRACT AND KEY WORDS

An abstract (requirements for length and structured format vary by journal) should follow the title page. The abstract should provide the context or background for the study and should state the study's purposes, basic procedures (selection of study subjects or laboratory animals, observational and analytical methods), main findings (giving specific effect sizes and their statistical significance, if possible), and principal conclusions. It should emphasize new and important aspects of the study or observations.

Because abstracts are the only substantive portion of the article indexed in many electronic databases, and the only portion many readers read, authors need to be careful that abstracts reflect the content of the article accurately. Unfortunately, many abstracts disagree with the text of the article (6). The format required for structured abstracts differs from journal to journal, and some journals use more than one structure; authors should make it a point prepare their abstracts in the format specified by the journal they have chosen.

Some journals request that, following the abstract, authors provide, and identify as such, 3 to 10 key words or short phrases that capture the main topics of the article. These will assist indexers in cross-indexing the article and may be published with the abstract. Terms from the Medical Subject Headings (MeSH) list of Index Medicus should be used; if suitable MeSH terms are not yet available for recently introduced terms, present terms may be used.

IV.A.5. INTRODUCTION

Provide a context or background for the study (i.e., the nature of the problem and its significance). State the specific purpose or research objective of, or hypothesis tested by, the study or observation; the research objective is often more sharply focused when stated as a question. Both the main and secondary objectives should be made clear, and any pre-specified subgroup analyses should be described. Give only strictly pertinent references and do not include data or conclusions from the work being reported.

IV.A.6. METHODS

The Methods section should include only information that was available at the time the plan or protocol for the study was written; all information obtained during the conduct of the study belongs in the Results section.

IV.A.6.a. Selection and Description of Participants

Describe your selection of the observational or experimental participants (patients or laboratory animals, including controls) clearly, including eligibility and exclusion criteria and a description of the source population. Because the relevance of such variables as age and sex to the object of research is not always clear, authors should explain their use when they are included in a study report; for example, authors should explain why only subjects of certain ages were included or why women were excluded. The guiding principle should be clarity about how and why a study was done in a particular way. When authors use variables such as race or ethnicity, they should define how they measured the variables and justify their relevance.

IV.A.6.b. Technical information

Identify the methods, apparatus (give the manufacturer's name and address in parentheses), and procedures in sufficient detail to allow other workers to reproduce the results. Give references to established methods, including statistical methods (see below); provide references and brief descriptions for methods that have been published but are not well known; describe new or substantially modified methods, give reasons for using them, and evaluate their limitations. Identify precisely all drugs and chemicals used, including generic name(s), dose(s), and route(s) of administration.

Authors submitting review manuscripts should include a section describing the methods used for locating, selecting, extracting, and synthesizing data. These methods should also be summarized in the abstract.

Box C-1   EXCERPT FROM UNIFORM REQUIREMENTS FOR MANUSCRIPTS SUBMITTED TO BIOMEDICAL JOURNALS: WRITING AND EDITING FOR BIOMEDICAL PUBLICATION — CONT'D

IV.A.6.c. Statistics

Describe statistical methods with enough detail to enable a knowledgeable reader with access to the original data to verify the reported results. When possible, quantify findings and present them with appropriate indicators of measurement error or uncertainty (such as confidence intervals). Avoid relying solely on statistical hypothesis testing, such as the use of P values, which fails to convey important information about effect size. References for the design of the study and statistical methods should be to standard works when possible (with pages stated). Define statistical terms, abbreviations, and most symbols. Specify the computer software used.

IV.A.7. RESULTS

Present your results in logical sequence in the text, tables, and illustrations, giving the main or most important findings first. Do not repeat in the text all the data in the tables or illustrations; emphasize or summarize only important observations. Extra or supplementary materials and technical detail can be placed in an appendix where it will be accessible but will not interrupt the flow of the text; alternatively, it can be published only in the electronic version of the journal.

When data are summarized in the Results section, give numeric results not only as derivatives (for example, percentages) but also as the absolute numbers from which the derivatives were calculated, and specify the statistical methods used to analyze them. Restrict tables and figures to those needed to explain the argument of the paper and to assess its support. Use graphs as an alternative to tables with many entries; do not duplicate data in graphs and tables. Avoid non-technical uses of technical terms in statistics, such as "random" (which implies a randomizing device), "normal," "significant," "correlations," and "sample."

Where scientifically appropriate, analyses of the data by variables such as age and sex should be included.

IV.A.8. DISCUSSION

Emphasize the new and important aspects of the study and the conclusions that follow from them. Do not repeat in detail data or other material given in the Introduction or the Results section. For experimental studies it is useful to begin the discussion by summarizing briefly the main findings, then explore possible mechanisms or explanations for these findings, compare and contrast the results with other relevant studies, state the limitations of the study, and explore the implications of the findings for future research and for clinical practice.

Link the conclusions with the goals of the study but avoid unqualified statements and conclusions not adequately supported by the data. In particular, authors should avoid making statements on economic benefits and costs unless their manuscript includes the appropriate economic data and analyses. Avoid claiming priority and alluding to work that has not been completed. State new hypotheses when warranted, but clearly label them as such.

IV.A.9. REFERENCES

IV.A.9.a. General Considerations Related to References

Although references to review articles can be an efficient way of guiding readers to a body of literature, review articles do not always reflect original work accurately. Readers should therefore be provided with direct references to original research sources whenever possible. On the other hand, extensive lists of references to original work on a topic can use excessive space on the printed page. Small numbers of references to key original papers will often serve as well as more exhaustive lists, particularly since references can now be added to the electronic version of published papers, and since electronic literature searching allows readers to retrieve published literature efficiently.

Avoid using abstracts as references. References to papers accepted but not yet published should be designated as "in press" or "forthcoming"; authors should obtain written permission to cite such papers as well as verification that they have been accepted for publication. Information from manuscripts submitted but not accepted should be cited in the text as "unpublished observations" with written permission from the source.

Avoid citing a "personal communication" unless it provides essential information not available from a public source, in which case the name of the person and date of communication should be cited in parentheses in the text. For scientific articles, authors should obtain written permission and confirmation of accuracy from the source of a personal communication.

Some journals check the accuracy of all reference citations, but not all journals do so, and citation errors sometimes appear in the published version of articles. To minimize such errors, authors should therefore verify references against the original documents.

Continued

BOX C-1 EXCERPT FROM UNIFORM REQUIREMENTS FOR MANUSCRIPTS SUBMITTED TO BIOMEDICAL JOURNALS: WRITING AND EDITING FOR BIOMEDICAL PUBLICATION — CONT'D

IV.A.9.b. Reference Style and Format

The Uniform Requirements style is based largely on an ANSI standard style adapted by the National Library of Medicine (NLM) for its databases. (7) For samples of reference citation formats, authors should consult http://www.nlm.nih.gov/bsd/uniform_requirements.html.

References should be numbered consecutively in the order in which they are first mentioned in the text. Identify references in text, tables, and legends by Arabic numerals in parentheses. References cited only in tables or figure legends should be numbered in accordance with the sequence established by the first identification in the text of the particular table or figure. The titles of journals should be abbreviated according to the style used in *Index Medicus. Consult the List of Journals Indexed for MEDICINE,* published annually as a separate publication by the National Library of Medicine. The list can also be obtained through the Library's web site.

(http://www.nlm.nih.gov/tsd/serials/lji.html).

Journals vary on whether they ask authors to cite electronic references within parentheses in the text or in numbered references following the text. Authors should consult with the journal that they plan to submit their work to.

IV.A.10. TABLES

Tables capture information concisely, and display it efficiently; they also provide information at any desired level of detail and precision. Including data in tables rather than text frequently makes it possible to reduce the length of the text.

Type or print each table with double spacing on a separate sheet of paper. Number tables consecutively in the order of their first citation in the text and supply a brief title for each. Do not use internal horizontal or vertical lines. Give each column a short or abbreviated heading. Authors should place explanatory matter in footnotes, not in the heading. Explain in footnotes all nonstandard abbreviations. For footnotes use the following symbols, in sequence:

$$*, †, ‡, §, ||, **, ††, ‡‡$$

Identify statistical measures of variations, such as standard deviation and standard error of the mean.

Be sure that each table is cited in the text.

If you use data from another published or unpublished source, obtain permission and acknowledge them fully.

Additional tables containing backup data too extensive to publish in print may be appropriate for publication in the electronic version of the journal, deposited with an archival service, or made available to readers directly by the authors. In that event an appropriate statement will be added to the text. Submit such tables for consideration with the paper so that they will be available to the peer reviewers.

IV.A.11. ILLUSTRATIONS (FIGURES)

Figures should be either professionally drawn and photographed, or submitted as photographic quality digital prints. In addition to requiring a version of the figures suitable for printing, some journals now ask authors for electronic files of figures in a format (e.g., JPEG or GIF) that will produce high quality images in the web version of the journal; authors should review the images of such files on a computer screen before submitting them, to be sure they meet their own quality standard.

For x-ray films, scans, and other diagnostic images, as well as pictures of pathology specimens or photomicrographs, send sharp, glossy, black-and-white or color photographic prints, usually 127×173 mm (5×7 inches). Although some journals redraw figures, many do not. Letters, numbers, and symbols on Figures should therefore be clear and even throughout, and of sufficient size that when reduced for publication each item will still be legible. Figures should be made as self-explanatory as possible, since many will be used directly in slide presentations. Titles and detailed explanations belong in the legends, however, not on the illustrations themselves.

Photomicrographs should have internal scale markers. Symbols, arrows, or letters used in photomicrographs should contrast with the background.

If photographs of people are used, either the subjects must not be identifiable or their pictures must be accompanied by written permission to use the photograph (*See Section III.D.4.a*). Whenever possible permission for publication should be obtained.

Figures should be numbered consecutively according to the order in which they have been first cited in the text. If a figure has been published, acknowledge the original source and submit written permission from the copyright holder to reproduce the material. Permission is required irrespective of authorship or publisher except for documents in the public domain.

For illustrations in color, ascertain whether the journal requires color negatives, positive transparencies, or color prints. Accompanying drawings marked to indicate the region to be reproduced might be useful to the editor. Some journals publish illustrations in color only if the author pays for the extra cost.

Authors should consult the journal about requirements for figures submitted in electronic formats.

| Box C-1 | EXCERPT FROM UNIFORM REQUIREMENTS FOR MANUSCRIPTS SUBMITTED TO BIOMEDICAL JOURNALS: WRITING AND EDITING FOR BIOMEDICAL PUBLICATION — CONT'D |

IV.A.12. LEGENDS FOR ILLUSTRATIONS (FIGURES)

Type or print out legends for illustrations using double spacing, starting on a separate page, with Arabic numerals corresponding to the illustrations. When symbols, arrows, numbers, or letters are used to identify parts of the illustrations, identify and explain each one clearly in the legend. Explain the internal scale and identify the method of staining in photomicrographs.

IV.A.13. UNITS OF MEASUREMENT

Measurements of length, height, weight, and volume should be reported in metric units (meter, kilogram, or liter) or their decimal multiples.

Temperatures should be in degrees Celsius. Blood pressures should be in millimeters of mercury, unless other units are specifically required by the journal.

Journals vary in the units they use for reporting hematological, clinical chemistry, and other measurements. Authors must consult the information for authors for the particular journal and should report laboratory information in both the local and International System of Units (SI). Editors may request that the authors before publication add alternative or non-SI units, since SI units are not universally used. Drug concentrations may be reported in either SI or mass units, but the alternative should be provided in parentheses where appropriate.

IV.A.14. ABBREVIATIONS AND SYMBOLS

Use only standard abbreviations; the use of non-standard abbreviations can be extremely confusing to readers. Avoid abbreviations in the title. The full term for which an abbreviation stands should precede its first use in the text unless it is a standard unit of measurement.

IV.B. Sending the Manuscript to the Journal

An increasing number of journals now accept electronic submission of manuscripts, whether on disk, as attachments to electronic mail, or by downloading directly onto the journal website. Electronic submission saves time as well as postage costs, and allows the manuscript to be handled in electronic form throughout the editorial process (for example, when it is sent out for review). When submitting a manuscript electronically, authors should consult with the instructions for authors of the journal they have chosen for their manuscript.

If a paper version of the manuscript is submitted, send the required number of copies of the manuscript and figures; they are all needed for peer review and editing, and editorial office staff cannot be expected to make the required copies.

Manuscripts must be accompanied by a cover letter, which should include the following information.

- A full statement to the editor about all submissions and previous reports that might be regarded as redundant publication of the same or very similar work. Any such work should be referred to specifically, and referenced in the new paper. Copies of such material should be included with the submitted paper, to help the editor decide how to handle the matter.
- A statement of financial or other relationships that might lead to a conflict of interest, if that information is not included in the manuscript itself or in an authors' form
- A statement that the manuscript has been read and approved by all the authors, that the requirements for authorship as stated earlier in this document have been met, and that each author believes that the manuscript represents honest work, if that information is not provided in another form (see below); and
- The name, address, and telephone number of the corresponding author, who is responsible for communicating with the other authors about revisions and final approval of the proofs, if that information is not included on the manuscript itself.

The letter should give any additional information that may be helpful to the editor, such as the type or format of article in the particular journal that the manuscript represents. If the manuscript has been submitted previously to another journal, it is helpful to include the previous editor's and reviewers' comments with the submitted manuscript, along with the authors' responses to those comments. Editors encourage authors to submit these previous communications and doing so may expedite the review process.

Many journals now provide a pre-submission checklist that assures that all the components of the submission have been included. Some journals now also require that authors complete checklists for reports of certain study types (e.g., the CONSORT checklist for reports of randomized controlled trials). Authors should look to see if the journal uses such checklists, and send them with the manuscript if they are requested.

Copies of any permission to reproduce published material, to use illustrations or report information about identifiable people, or to name people for their contributions must accompany the manuscript.

Continued

BOX C-1 **EXCERPT FROM UNIFORM REQUIREMENTS FOR MANUSCRIPTS SUBMITTED TO BIOMEDICAL JOURNALS: WRITING AND EDITING FOR BIOMEDICAL PUBLICATION — CONT'D**

V. References

A. References Cited in this Document

1. Davidoff F for the CSE Task Force on Authorship. *Who's the Author? Problems with Biomedical Authorship, and Some Possible Solutions.* Science Editor. July-August 2000: Volume 23 - Number 4: 111-119.

2. Yank V, Rennie D. *Disclosure of researcher contributions: a study of original research articles in The Lancet.* Ann Intern Med. 1999 Apr 20;130(8):661–70.

3. Flanagin A, Fontanarosa PB, DeAngelis CD. *Authorship for research groups.* JAMA. 2002;288:3166-68.

4. Peer Review in Health Sciences. F Godlee, T Jefferson. London: BMJ Books, 1999.

5. World Medical Association Declaration of Helsinki: *ethical principles for medical research involving human subjects.* JAMA. 2000 Dec 20;284(23):3043–5.

6. Pitkin RM, Branagan MA, Burmeister LF. *Accuracy of data in abstracts of published research articles.* JAMA. 1999 Mar 24–31;281(12):1110–1.

7. Patrias K. *National Library of Medicine recommended formats for bibliographic citation.* Bethesda (MD): The Library; 1991.

B. Other Sources of Information Related to Biomedical Journals

World Association of Medical Editors (WAME) www.WAME.org

Council of Science Editors (CSE) www.councilscience editors.org

European Association of Science Editors (EASE) www.ease .org.uk

Cochrane Collaboration www.cochrane.org

The Mulford Library, Medical College of Ohio www.mco.edu/lib/instr/libinsta.html

From International Committee of Medical Journal Editors (ICMJE). (2003). *Uniform requirements for manuscripts submitted to biomedical journals: Writing and editing for biomedical publication.* Philadelphia, PA: American College of Physicians. pp. 1–5, 24–36. Retrieved August 16, 2004, from hyyp://www.icmje.org/index.html.

Standards for the Reporting and Publishing of Scientific Information; D. References to Legal Materials; and E. Sample Cover Letter.

In addition to the *Publication Manual* itself, the APA maintains on its Web site a link to frequently asked questions (FAQs) regarding certain features of this stylistic source. It is accessible at www.apaastyle.org/faqs.html. Although this particular electronic Web source spans only six pages, it does provide a brief illustration of certain prevalent bibliographic citation formats as well as referrals to additional resources for more in-depth coverage of the *Publication Manual*. Box C-2 displays these FAQs and the responses provided.

Box C-2   FREQUENTLY ASKED QUESTIONS ABOUT APA STYLE

APA Style | Frequently Asked Questions

http://www.apastyle.org/faqs.html   Q▾ Google

APA ONLINE
›HOME ›SITE MAP ›CONTACT

APA Style.org

SEARCH

› WEBSITE HELP

› APA STYLE HOME

› ABOUT APA STYLE

› PUBLICATION MANUAL

› APA STYLE TIPS

› ELECTRONIC
  REFERENCES

› FAQs

› WHAT'S NEW

› ETHICS OF PUBLICATION

› APA PRODUCTS
  Books
  Children's Books
  Journals
  Merchandise
  Monitor on Psychology
  Videos

› ELECTRONIC PRODUCTS
  APA Gold
  APA-Style Helper
  Continuing Education
  Graduate Study Online
  Prevention & Treatment
  Journal
  PsycARTICLES
  PsycBOOKS
  PsycCAREERS
  PsycEXTRA
  PsycINFO
  PsycPORT: News
  PsycVIDEO

▣ Frequently Asked Questions

APA's Publication Manual provides complete style guidelines and should be consulted first in all matters concerning APA style. Apastyle.org offers these FAQs to help clarify frequent areas of confusion.

Apastyle.org is an auxiliary companion to the Publication Manual, but is not intended as a replacement for it. To help style users, Apastyle.org provides — in addition to these FAQs — online guidelines for commonly asked questions concerning electronic references and a list of changes in the 5th edition. If your question involves more complex expressions of writing, visit our style tips area.

FAQS

› What is APA style? Can you send it to me? My paper is due, and it must be in APA style, especially references.

› Why is APA style needed?

› Why is there a specific APA style?

› Can you help with my research for my psychology paper? I'm looking for articles on a particular topic.

› The instructions in the Publication Manual for citing documents available on the Internet require inclusion of a date of publication or retrieval, yet Examples 73, 74, and 76 do not include "retrieved from" dates. Why is this?

› Does APA offer a workbook on APA style?

› In referencing periodicals, what's the difference between using "p." or "pp." for page numbers?

› I publish frequently in APA journals, and I've noticed that subjects is often changed in copyediting, most often to participants. Why?

› How do I format a bibliography in APA style?

› How do I cite an entire Web site (but not a specific document on that site)?

› How do I reference a Web page that lists no author?

› How do I cite Web site material that has no author, no year, and no page numbers?

› What format should I follow to cite an interview?

› How do I cite a source that I found in another source?

› In typing class I learned that two spaces always follow a period, but your Publication Manual says one space should follow all punctuation. Why is this?

Q: What is APA style? Can you send it to me? My paper is due, and it must be in APA style, especially references.

A: The reference format for APA style is described in the 5th edition of the Publication Manual of the American Psychological Association, which is a large reference book that contains hundreds of guidelines on how to format references, statistics, tables, punctuation, and grammar. It also contains writing tips and instructions about how to format manuscripts. You can find a full description and ordering information here. You may also find a copy of the Publication Manual in your school library or even a local bookstore.

› APA Style Helper 3
  Now Available!
  The electronic companion to APA's popular style guide has been improved and updated for the new, fifth edition.
  › More info

▦ E-References Guide
Get APA's complete style guide for citing electronic resources. Download online for $11.95.
› Order now.

Continued

BOX C-2   FREQUENTLY ASKED QUESTIONS ABOUT APA STYLE — CONT'D

Here are some basic reference forms to get you started:

Journal article:

Fine, M. A., & Kurdek, L. A. (1993). Reflections on determining authorship credit and authorship order on faculty-student collaborations. *American Psychologist, 48,* 1141-1147.

Book:

Nicol, A. A. M., & Pexman, P. M. (1999). *Presenting your findings: A practical guide for creating tables.* Washington, DC: American Psychological Association.

Book chapter:

O'Neil, J. M., & Egan, J. (1992). Men's and women's gender role journeys: Metaphor for healing, transition, and transformation. In B. R. Wainrib (Ed.), *Gender issues across the life cycle* (pp. 107-123). New York: Springer.

back to questions

Q: Why is APA style needed?

A: An author writing for a publication must follow the rules established by the publisher to avoid inconsistencies among journal articles or book chapters.

For example, without rules of style, three different manuscripts might use *sub-test, subtest,* and *Subtest* in one issue of a journal or book. Although the meaning of the word is the same (in this case, *subtest* is APA style), such variations in style may distract or confuse the reader.

The need for a consistent style becomes more apparent when complex material is presented, such as tables or statistics.

back to questions

Q: Why is there a specific APA style?

A: APA style focuses on the needs of presenting psychological information. APA style omits general rules explained in widely available style books and examples of usage with little relevance to the behavioral and social sciences.

Among the most helpful general guides to editorial style are *Words into Type* (Skillin & Gay, 1974) and the *Chicago Manual of Style* (University of Chicago Press, 1993).

Style manuals agree more often than they disagree. Where they disagree, the *Publication Manual,* because it is based on the special requirements of psychology, takes precedence for APA publications.

back to questions

Q: Can you help with my research for my psychology paper? I'm looking for articles on a particular topic.

A: We are not able to send you specific information related to your topic, but APA might have information in one of its databases that will help you to find literature that's already been written on your topic. These databases, which contain summaries of the literature and full-text APA articles, can serve as useful tools in completing your assignments.

APA's bibliographic databases and printed indexes provide summaries of journal articles, book chapters, books, and other scholarly documents in psychology and related disciplines. The bibliographic literature references are accessible via a number of resources, including the PsycINFO online database, the ClinPSYC CD-ROM databases, and the printed index *Psychological Abstracts.*

Box C-2   FREQUENTLY ASKED QUESTIONS ABOUT APA STYLE—CONT'D

Many university libraries and other research institutions subscribe or provide access to one or more of these resources. If you are unable to gain access through such an institution, however, another option is to establish an account through a commercial online service and do your own searching. Information is available on our PsycINFO Web site about your various access options, including access to online services via the Internet.

APA also provides "pay-per-view" access to these databases. You can get 24-hour access to APA's PsycINFO database (PsycINFO Direct) and retrieve individual APA journal articles (PsycARTICLES Direct). There is a fee for using these products.

We also recommend that you read APA's online pamphlet, "Library Research in Psychology: Finding It Easily." This pamphlet will help steer you toward additional resources.

back to questions

Q: How do I cite an entire Web site (but not a specific document on that site)?

A: When citing an entire Web site, it is sufficient to give the address of the site in just the text. For example, Kidspsych is a wonderful interactive web site for children (http://www.kidspsych.org).

back to questions

Q: The instructions in the *Publication Manual* for citing documents available on the Internet require inclusion of a date of publication or retrieval, yet Examples 73, 74, and 76 do not include "retrieved from" dates. Why is this?

A: This is an oversight. Each of these examples should include a retrieval date after the word *retrieved* and before the word *from*. Corrected examples appear in *APA Style Guide for Electronic Resources* as well as in the second and later printings of the manual.

APA Style Guide for Electronic Resources is a downloadable PDF that is available for $11.95 from our web site.
› Download *APA Style Guide for Electronic Resources* now

back to questions

Q: Does APA offer a workbook on APA style?

A: Yes. *Mastering APA Style* is a workbook for learning APA style.

back to questions

Q: In referencing periodicals, what's the difference between using "p." or "pp." for page numbers?

A: If a periodical includes a volume number, italicize it and then change to regular type and give the page range without "pp." If the periodical does not use volume numbers, include "pp." before the page numbers so the reader will understand that the numbers refer to pagination. Use "p." if the source is a page or less long.

back to questions

Q: I publish frequently in APA journals, and I've noticed that *subjects* is often changed in copyediting, most often to *participants*. Why?

A: A couple of guidelines in chapter 2's Guidelines to Reduce Bias in Language are at work here. One is to acknowledge human participation. The other is to be specific. *Subjects* is a fairly nondescriptive, passive term. Identifying human subjects as *participants, respondents, children, patients, clients,* and so forth increases specificity. (*Subjects* is perfectly appropriate when the person cannot him- or herself provide informed consent.)

back to questions

Continued

Box C-2   FREQUENTLY ASKED QUESTIONS ABOUT APA STYLE — CONT'D

Q: How do I format a bibliography in APA style?

A: APA style calls for a list of References instead of a bibliography. The requirements of a reference list are that all references cited in the text of a paper must be listed alphabetically by first author's last name in the list of References and that all references listed must be cited within the text. A bibliography, on the other hand, typically includes resources in addition to those cited in the text and may include annotated descriptions of the items listed. In general, the list of References is double-spaced and listed alphabetically by first author's last name. For each reference, the first line is typed flush with the left margin, and any additional lines are indented as a group a few spaces to the right of the left margin (this is called a *hanging indent*, see here for an example).

back to questions

Q: How do I reference a Web page that lists no author?

A: When there is no author for a Web page, the title moves to the first position of the reference entry:

> New child vaccine gets funding boost. (2001). Retrieved March 21, 2001,
>   from http://news.ninemsn.com.au/health/story_13178.asp

The text citation would then just cite a few words of the title to point the reader to the right area of your reference list: ...are most at risk of contracting the disease ("New Child," 2001).

back to questions

Q: How do I cite Web site material that has no author, no year, and no page numbers?

A: Because the material does not include page numbers, you can include any of the following in the text to cite the quotation (from p. 120 of the *Publication Manual*):

1. A paragraph number, if provided; alternatively, you could count paragraphs down from the beginning of the document.
2. An overarching heading plus a paragraph number within that section.
3. Nothing. Just put quotation marks around the words you're using, which the reader can use as a search string.

Because there is no date and no author, your text citation would include the first couple of words from the title and "n.d." for no date (e.g., para. 5, "Style List," n.d.). The entry in the reference list might look something like this:

> Style list for references. (n.d.). Retrieved January 1, 2001,
>   from http://www.apa.org

back to questions

Q: What format should I follow to cite an interview?

A: An interview is not considered recoverable data, so no reference to this is provided in the References. You may, however, cite the interview within the text as a personal communication. For example,

(J. Smith, personal communication, August 15, 2001)

back to questions

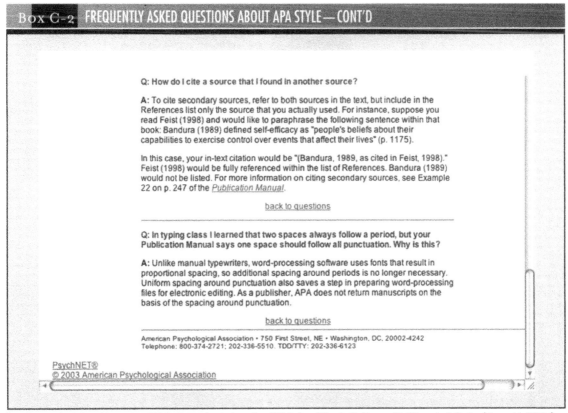

Box C-2   FREQUENTLY ASKED QUESTIONS ABOUT APA STYLE—CONT'D

Q: How do I cite a source that I found in another source?

A: To cite secondary sources, refer to both sources in the text, but include in the References list only the source that you actually used. For instance, suppose you read Feist (1998) and would like to paraphrase the following sentence within that book: Bandura (1989) defined self-efficacy as "people's beliefs about their capabilities to exercise control over events that affect their lives" (p. 1175).

In this case, your in-text citation would be "(Bandura, 1989, as cited in Feist, 1998)." Feist (1998) would be fully referenced within the list of References. Bandura (1989) would not be listed. For more information on citing secondary sources, see Example 22 on p. 247 of the *Publication Manual*.

back to questions

Q: In typing class I learned that two spaces always follow a period, but your Publication Manual says one space should follow all punctuation. Why is this?

A: Unlike manual typewriters, word-processing software uses fonts that result in proportional spacing, so additional spacing around periods is no longer necessary. Uniform spacing around punctuation also saves a step in preparing word-processing files for electronic editing. As a publisher, APA does not return manuscripts on the basis of the spacing around punctuation.

back to questions

American Psychological Association • 750 First Street, NE • Washington, DC, 20002-4242
Telephone: 800-374-2721; 202-336-5510. TDD/TTY: 202-336-6123

PsychNET®
© 2003 American Psychological Association

From American Psychological Association. (2004). *Frequently asked questions (FAQs) about APA style.* Washington, DC: APA. pp. 1–6. Retrieved August 16, 2004, from http://www.apastyle.org/faqs.html.

REFERENCES

American Psychological Association (APA). (2001). *Publication manual of the American Psychological Association* (5th ed.). Washington, DC: American Psychological Association.

American Psychological Association. (2004). *Frequently asked questions (FAQs) about APA style.* Washington, DC: APA. Retrieved August 16, 2004, from www.apastyle.org/faqs.html.

Browner, W. S. (1999). *Publishing and presenting clinical research.* Baltimore, MD: Lippincott Williams & Wilkins.

Byrne, D. W. (1998). *Publishing your medical research paper: What they don't teach in medical school.* Philadelphia: Lippincott Williams & Wilkins.

International Committee of Medical Journal Editors (ICMJE). (2003). *Uniform requirements for manuscripts submitted to biomedical journals: Writing and editing for biomedical publication.* Philadelphia: American College of Physicians. Retrieved August 16, 2004, from www.icmje.org/index.html.

ADDITIONAL RECOMMENDED RESOURCES

American Medical Association. (1998). *American Medical Association manual of style: A guide for authors and editors* (9th ed.). Philadelphia: Lippincott Williams & Wilkins.

Belgrave, L. L., Zablotsky, D., & Guadagno, M. A. (2002). How do we talk to each other? Writing qualitative research for quantitative readers. *Qualitative Health Research, 12*(10), 1427–1439.

Gelfand, H., & Walker, C. J. (Eds.). (2002). *Mastering APA style: Student's workbook and training guide.* Washington, DC: American Psychological Association.

Health Care Communication Group. (2001). *Writing, speaking, & communication skills for health professionals.* New Haven, CT: Yale University Press.

Nicol, A. A. M., & Pexman, P. M. (2003). *Displaying your findings: A practical guide for creating figures, posters, and presentations.* Washington, DC: American Psychological Association.

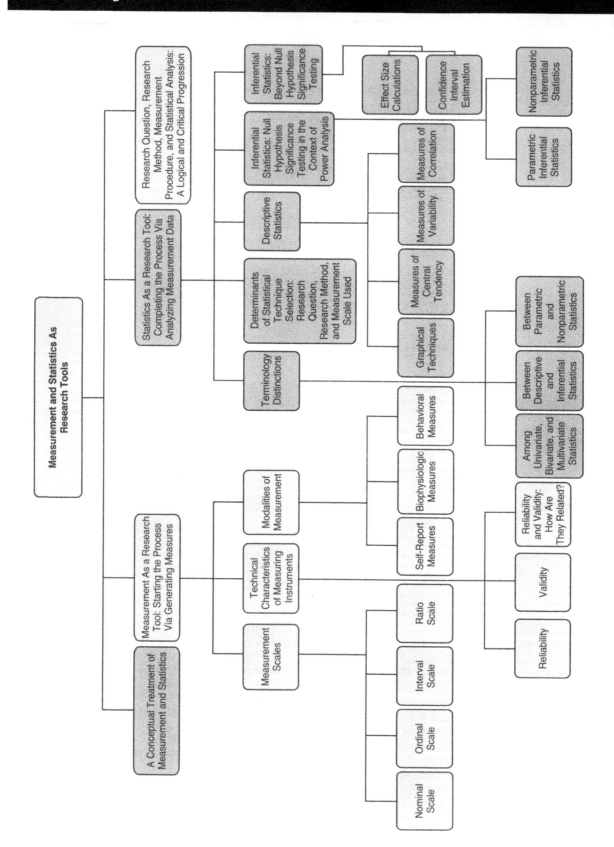

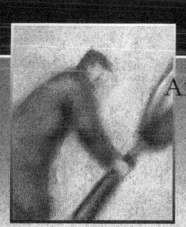

OUTLINE

OBJECTIVES

Upon completion of this appendix, the reader will have the information necessary to perform the following tasks:

1 Distinguish between measurement and statistics at a conceptual level.

2 Characterize and recognize examples of each of the following four measurement scales: nominal, ordinal, interval, and ratio.

3 Define *reliability* as a technical characteristic of a measuring instrument.

4 Distinguish among, and recognize examples of, the following types of reliability: test-retest reliability, equivalent or parallel forms reliability, reliability of internal consistency (or homogeneity), inter-rater reliability, and intra-rater reliability.

5 Regarding reliability of internal consistency, discuss the meaning of the following: split-half reliability, Spearman-Brown prophesy formula, Kuder-Richardson formula 20, and Cronbach's alpha.

6 Explain the purpose served by Cohen's kappa relative to inter-rater reliability.

7 Distinguish among, and recognize examples of, the following types of validity: face validity, content validity, criterion-related validity as manifested via predictive validity and concurrent validity, and construct validity.

8 Discuss the relationship between reliability and validity.

9 Characterize and recognize examples of each of the following three modalities of measurement: self-report measures, biophysiologic measures, and behavioral measures.

10 Distinguish among, and recognize examples of, the following statistics-related terms: *univariate, bivariate, multivariate, descriptive, inferential, parametric,* and *nonparametric statistics.*

KEY TERMS

Archival research
Association-oriented statistical techniques
Behavioral measures
Behavioral observation
Biophysiologic measures
Bivariate statistics
Cohen's kappa
Concurrent validity
Confidence interval estimation
Construct validity
Content analysis
Content validity
Criterion-related validity
Cronbach's alpha
Descriptive statistics
Determinants of statistical technique
   selection
Difference-oriented statistical techniques

Effect size calculations
Equivalent or parallel forms
   reliability
Face validity
Graphical techniques
In vitro measurements
In vivo measurements
Inferential statistics
Inter-rater reliability
Interval measurement scale
Intra-rater reliability
Kuder-Richardson formula 20
Measurement
Measurement scales
Measures of central tendency
Measures of correlation
Measures of variability
Modality of measurement

Multivariate statistics
Nominal measurement scale
Nonparametric statistics
Normal distribution curve
Null hypothesis significance testing (NHST)
Ordinal measurement scale
Parametric statistics
Predictive validity
Ratio measurement scale
Reliability
Reliability of internal consistency
   (or homogeneity)
Self-report measures
Spearman-Brown prophesy formula
Statistics
Test-retest reliability
Univariate statistics
Validity

11 Explain how the selection of an appropriate statistical technique is determined by the following: the research question, research method, and measurement scale used.

12 Characterize and recognize examples of each of the following four categories of descriptive statistical techniques: graphical techniques, measures of central tendency, measures of variability, and measures of correlation.

13 Define, illustrate, and characterize the normal distribution curve.

14 Explain the relationship between (a) inferential statistics and (b) null hypothesis significance testing in the context of power analysis.

15 Characterize and recognize examples of each of the following two divisions of inferential statistics: parametric inferential statistics and nonparametric inferential statistics.

16 Characterize and recognize examples of each of the following two subdivisions under parametric and nonparametric inferential statistics: association-oriented and difference-oriented statistical techniques.

17 Discuss the roles played by effect size calculations and confidence interval estimations relative to augmenting or supplementing null hypothesis significance testing.

18 Explain the logical and critical progression across the following aspects of the research process: research question, research method, measurement procedure, and statistical analysis.

A CONCEPTUAL TREATMENT OF MEASUREMENT AND STATISTICS

We initially discussed measurement and statistics as research tools in Chapter 3. You may recall that **measurement** is the term typically used to designate that procedure whereby numerical and/or verbal data are collected to characterize, in as valid and reliable a manner as possible, a factor or variable of interest to a researcher. As an example, any effort to test an outcome of interest (e.g., range of motion [ROM]) represents an instance of measurement. Once the measurement data are collected, the area of applied mathematics known as **statistics** is used to analyze and better understand what the data are demonstrating.

This appendix provides more detail than covered elsewhere in the book regarding both measurement and statistics as tools that are indispensable to the researcher. In so doing, our treatment of the topics covered will be *conceptual* in nature rather than computational. A computational treatment is beyond the scope and intent of this book. Ample resources are recommended in this appendix for those readers who have an interest in pursuing the measurement and statistical topics beyond the conceptual coverage provided here.

MEASUREMENT AS A RESEARCH TOOL: STARTING THE PROCESS VIA GENERATING MEASURES

Generating data on variables of interest in a research study is a critical starting point in the process of investigating a research question. The following discussion of measurement as a research tool spans these three principal areas: *measurement scales* labeled nominal, ordinal, interval, and ratio; *technical characteristics* of measuring instruments known as reliability and validity; and *modalities of measurement* including self-report, biophysiologic, and behavioral measures.

MEASUREMENT SCALES: NOMINAL, ORDINAL, INTERVAL, AND RATIO

There are four **measurement scales** on which data may be collected: the nominal, ordinal, interval, and ratio scales. The **nominal measurement scale** uses numbers simply to name or identify variations on a variable. For example, using the numbers 1 and 2 to distinguish between males and females in a study represents a nominal scale of measurement. Nothing at all is implied beyond the simple task of naming or identifying; rank order is not even part of the interpretation. The **ordinal measurement scale** serves not only to name or identify, but also to rank order. As an illustration, severity of tension headache may be recorded by a client as moderate (a 1), severe (a 2), or debilitating/critical (a 3). These measures certainly identify headache severity and serve to rank order the degree of pain experienced; however, this scale does not necessarily imply that the quantity or quality of the variable measured between a 1 and a 2 is equivalent to that measured between a 2 and a 3. In other words, we cannot assume equal intervals between any two pairs of consecutive points on the scale.

To make that assumption, we would have to use an **interval measurement scale**. There the numbers on the scale serve to name, rank order, and permit the assumption of equal intervals between any two pairs of consecutive points on the scale. This scale, however, does not involve a true or absolute zero point. Examples here would include measures of intelligence (IQ), the Celsius temperature sale, or numerical achievement test performance scored from 0 to 100. In the case of a Celsius temperature reading of 0° C, this is simply the designated freezing point of water rather than the absence of heat.

If we were to move to the Kelvin scale, however, then a Kelvin temperature reading of 0 K would imply the absence of heat. A measurement scale, therefore, that allows us to name, rank order, assume equal intervals, and acknowledge a true or absolute zero point is called a **ratio measurement scale**. Other illustrations of the ratio scale include weight, height, blood pressure, and heartbeats.

TECHNICAL CHARACTERISTICS OF MEASURING INSTRUMENTS

The two principal technical characteristics of any measuring instrument are its reliability and validity.

Reliability

The **reliability** of an instrument refers to the consistency with which the measurements occur. This technical characteristic involves four realms in which the reliability or consistency of measurement may be considered. These include *test-retest* reliability, *equivalent or parallel forms* reliability, reliability of *internal consistency or homogeneity*, and *inter-/intra-*reliability relative to a rater or subject.

Test-Retest Reliability. **Test-retest reliability** involves the degree to which a given instrument measures a certain variable consistently for the same group of individuals across two different points in time. For example, the rank ordering of clients' self-esteem at point A in time might be correlated with their rank ordering on the same instrument at point B in time (say, one month later). Because self-esteem is a relatively stable human characteristic, we would expect the two rank orderings to remain basically the same across the two measurement episodes. This can be quantified by way of a simple correlational study, as discussed in Chapter 6. A resulting positive correlation would suggest a direct relationship between the two sets of self-esteem measures, thereby indicating a certain degree of stability in the test-retest process.

Equivalent or Parallel Forms Reliability. Occasionally in educational settings, an instrument will be needed to measure, for example, the achievement of students who are perhaps completing a segment of a course in a staggered fashion. Administering the same achievement test to different students as they complete the course segment at different points in time would obviously not work well. Consequently, it becomes necessary for the educator to prepare two or more versions, or forms, of the same test, known as **equivalent or parallel forms reliability**. In the case of, say, two forms of the same test, the content coverage and performance objectives are identical, but the actual test items on each of the two forms of the test are different. Presumably, the educator has two equivalent or parallel forms of the test. This can be verified by administering form A to a group of students at point A in time and administering form B to the same group at point B in time. If indeed the two sets of scores correlate positively, then we can infer that the two forms of the same test are indeed equivalent or parallel given the consistency of student performance across the two different forms.

Reliability of Internal Consistency (or Homogeneity).

In addition to consistency of measurement across two points in time and across two presumably equivalent forms of the same test, there is another type of reliability that "looks internally." It is referred to as **reliability of internal consistency (or homogeneity)**. In the instance of internal consistency reliability, we examine the stability or consistency of measurement *within* the test itself. This is accomplished by "splitting" the test in half, and then proceeding to examine the correlation between the two resulting sets of scores. For example, we might correlate the performance of examinees on the odd-numbered items with their performance on the even-numbered items. Here, too, a positive correlation suggesting a direct relationship between the two sets of scores would indicate a certain consistency of measurement within the test itself.

When this type of *split-half reliability* is calculated, the resulting correlation coefficient (*r*) is actually a conservative estimate (meaning slightly lower in magnitude) of the true or actual reliability coefficient. This is because the correlation calculations are based on what seems to be an instrument only half the actual size of the test's true length. And because the number of items on an instrument directly influences the size of the correlation coefficient, the resulting correlation coefficient is smaller in magnitude than would be the case if the calculations were based on the test's actual length. To compensate for this underestimation seen in the split-half reliability coefficient, we could use what is known as the **Spearman-Brown prophesy formula** (known as the *Spearman-Brown R*). This calculation allows the original split-half reliability coefficient to be adjusted in an upward direction to indicate what is in all likelihood a more accurate estimate of the

instrument's authentic reliability reflective of its true length.

The example given here of splitting a test in half by viewing the odd- and even-numbered items as two sets of data to be correlated is just one of many ways in which an instrument can be divided into two parts. In response to this fact, the **Kuder-Richardson formula 20** estimates the average of all the possible split-half correlations that might be derived from all of the possible ways of splitting an instrument in half (cf. Kuder & Richardson, 1937; and Gravetter & Forzano, 2003). This average of all possible split-half correlations is designated as *K-R 20* for short and may assume values extending from 0 to 1.0. The limitation to this technique, however, is that it applies only to a test that involves a binary decision response to each item (for example, true/false, valid/invalid, yes/no, fact/opinion, agree/disagree, etc.).

To compensate for this binary decision-based limitation of the *K-R 20*, Cronbach (1951) modified the *K-R 20* formula so as to accommodate instruments on which the items might have more than two possible responses. This resulted in the so-called **Cronbach's alpha**, which likewise measures the split-half reliability of an instrument by estimating the average correlation that would result from all possible ways of splitting a test in half. Cronbach's alpha also extends from 0 to 1.0, with a higher value being interpreted as indicating a higher degree of internal consistency or reliability.

Inter-Rater Reliability, Cohen's Kappa, and Intra-Rater Reliability.

In certain measurement situations involving clinical assessments or behavioral observations, it might be necessary for two or more observers/raters to assign scores regarding a subject's responses. When this type of measurement scenario relates to observing behavior at a given point in time, we then can speak in terms of the degree of consistency, or agreement, between/among the two or more observers/raters. This constitutes what is known as an issue of **inter-rater reliability**. It takes the form of percentage of agreement, say, between two observers/raters regarding the behavior observed at the same point in time. And because there is always the possibility that this percentage of agreement may reflect a certain degree of chance agreement, we always run the risk that the value of the percent agreement is somewhat inflated. To compensate for this possibility, **Cohen's kappa** can be calculated to index a measure of agreement that corrects for chance (cf. Cohen, 1961).

It is possible for a situation to exist wherein only one observer/rater records on two or more occasions a target behavior of interest. **Intra-rater reliability** here refers to the consistency with which the observer/rater assigns score ratings to the observed behavior across the two or more occasions. For example, research on the nature of client-therapist verbal interactions immediately following a massage session may be videotaped for subsequent analysis. When the videotape is viewed on two later occasions, it is possible that variations *within* the rater will account for inconsistencies in what is recorded/noted about the client-therapist interaction. This type of inconsistency must be minimized as much as possible if indeed the measurement effort is to be regarded as having an appropriate degree of intra-rater reliability.

Validity

The **validity** of an instrument refers to the extent to which the instrument measures what it claims or purports to be measuring. Because different instruments exist to fulfill different purposes, it stands to reason that there are various types of validity. This section, then, addresses the following types of validity: *face validity, content validity, criterion-related validity* in the form of *predictive validity* and *concurrent validity,* and *construct validity.*

Face Validity. **Face validity** is a subjective assessment that appeals to the apparent validity of an instrument for its stated purpose. It relates to the extent to which the instrument looks or appears to be pertinent to the measurement task at hand. An observational checklist of possible variations in client posture "on the face of its appearance" may be judged to possess appropriate validity for the purpose intended.

Content Validity. A typical occasion for interest in **content validity** is that of an achievement test of subject matter mastery by students. An anatomy examination, for example, would be judged to have appropriate content validity if a panel of subject matter experts assessed the test items to be appropriate and representative samples of the course content addressed by the exam. This type of validity also relates to the types of items that constitute a questionnaire designated for a particular purpose.

Criterion-Related Validity. As the expression implies, **criterion-related validity** has as its reference point an external criterion by which the validity of the instrument in question is assessed. In this context, criterion-related validity is manifested by both predictive validity and concurrent validity. **Predictive validity** is the degree to which an instrument actually predicts a certain outcome for which it is designed. A popular example here is the Student Achievement Test (SAT), which purports to predict student success in college. The correlation, then, between SAT scores and subsequent grade point average in college is an indication of the predictive validity of the SAT. The external criterion used here is college grade point average. In the health sciences, for instance, an instrument that generates initial evaluation scores and thus enables a researcher or practitioner to predict the period of time until recovery from an injury would be characterized as having predictive validity. Regarding **concurrent validity**, the external criterion against which a new instrument of interest is being validated would be an already well established instrument for the designated purpose. In this case, the concurrent validity of the newly designed instrument would be established if indeed its measurements correlated in a positive manner with measurements on the established instrument.

Construct Validity. An instrument is said to possess **construct validity** if it can be demonstrated that it indeed measures the particular abstract concept, or construct, it purports to measure. An instrument that claims to measure the construct of pain would need to demonstrate a correlation with other indicators of the experience of pain. As an illustration, a newly designed questionnaire purporting to measure chronic pain might be expected to demonstrate associations with three other characteristic indices of the pain experience such as restrictions in work style, leisure activity reductions, and disturbed quality of sleep patterns. Each of these four indicators of the chronic pain construct would presumably manifest an association or correlation with the other three, thereby establishing the construct validity of the newly designed instrument.

Reliability and Validity: How Are They Related?

Reliability is a prerequisite for validity in that a measurement procedure cannot be valid unless it is reliable. Inconsistent or unreliable measurements of a variable, therefore, suggest that the actual measures generated have no real meaning relative to the variable of interest.

Validity, however, is not a prerequisite for reliability. We could conceivably measure someone's height and claim that we are measuring pain.

Although the measurement procedure is indeed invalid, it may proceed reliably by virtue of a series of consistent measurements being recorded. Accordingly, consistency of measurement is no guarantee of a valid instrument.

MODALITIES OF MEASUREMENT

Sometimes variables measured in a research study are constructs. Examples of constructs might include such variables as pain, depression, self-esteem, fatigue, anxiety, intelligence, stress, and mood. A construct is a hypothetical and abstract concept that cannot be observed directly, yet it can be manifested or displayed in different ways that allow observation and measurement. Researchers, therefore, need to determine which of several possible external displays of a construct best reveals its underlying dimension. Following that determination, the investigator must then decide which of several types or modalities of measurement is appropriate for revealing the construct. In this section we consider three possibilities: *self-report measures*, *biophysiologic measures*, and *behavioral measures*. Using stress as the construct of interest, it should become apparent in the following discussion that a researcher might use any one or more of these three modalities to measure this variable.

Self-Report Measures: Open-Ended, Restricted, and Rating Scale Question Types

The *self-report* **modality of measurement** relies on the individual responding to questions that may be asked regarding the construct under investigation. In **self-report measures**, the precipitating questions may take the form of being *open-ended*, thereby allowing the respondent to answer in one's own words. Another option is a series of *restricted questions* whereby the individual is given a limited number of response alternatives or possibilities. A third option here in the self-report modality is that of *rating scale questions* such that the individual responds to a predetermined scale displaying several numerical values that quantify the construct of interest. A prevalent example of this latter option is the so-called Liker-type scale on which an individual responds to a 5-point continuum extending from "strongly disagree" at one pole to "strongly agree" at the other end. Returning to our illustration of measuring stress, participants in a study may be asked to report on their own perceived stress level by responding to open-ended, restricted, or rating scale questions.

Biophysiologic Measures: In Vivo and In Vitro

As noted by Polit and Beck (2004), **biophysiologic measures** fall into one of two principal categories: (a) **in vivo measurements** that occur directly in or on a living organism and include as examples blood pressure and body temperature measures and (b) **in vitro measurements** occurring outside the organism's body as is the case with blood chemistry analyses. With either option, the researcher is examining manifestations of an underlying construct by appealing to biophysiologic indicators that may span cardiovascular, pulmonary, blood, urine, saliva, chemistry, and immunodiagnostic studies. In the example of stress suggested earlier, one might measure such indicators as galvanic skin response (GSR), cortisol level, and heart rate to determine the degree of stress present in the subject.

Behavioral Measures: Observations and Content/Archival Analyses

The third of three possible modalities of measurement is that of **behavioral measures** that lend themselves to constructs whose nature can be displayed overtly. When such is the case, an appeal to *behavioral observations, content analyses,* and *archival research* is a rather direct route.

The process of **behavioral observation** entails direct observation along with the requisite record of the behavior(s) examined. This approach to measurement calls for the research to decide on both the *method for generating numerical values* for the behavior observed as well as the *method for sampling* the behavior itself. Regarding the former, Gravetter and Forzano (2003) suggested observing behavior relative to its frequency of occurrence, its duration, or its occurrence within designated time intervals. Regarding the latter issue of sampling method, they further suggest time sampling (i.e., alternating observation and recording activities across a series of time intervals during which the behavior may occur), event sampling (i.e., shifting the actual event or behavior observed from one time interval to the next), and individual sampling (i.e., shifting the individual observed from one time interval to the next).

Content analysis here is a form of behavioral measurement "using the techniques of behavioral observation to measure the occurrence of specific events in literature, movies, television, programs, or similar media that present replicas of behaviors" (Gravetter & Forzano, 2003, p. 106). Closely related to content analysis is **archival research** whereby historical documents (or archives) are examined in search of past behaviors or events.

STATISTICS AS A RESEARCH TOOL: COMPLETING THE PROCESS BY ANALYZING MEASUREMENT DATA

Once a data set is established via measurement procedures, we then have to analyze it to gain insight regarding its meanings. Primarily–though not exclusively–in quantitative research this task brings into play the area of applied mathematics known as statistics. As we noted earlier, in certain realms of both qualitative and integrative research we likewise must appeal to some form of statistical analysis.

Our treatment of statistics as a research tool, once again, will be conceptual in nature for the reasons given at the outset of this appendix. In so doing we will address the following five general areas: (a) terminology distinctions involving univariate, bivariate, multivariate, descriptive, inferential, parametric, and nonparametric statistics; (b) research method and measurement scale used as determinants of statistical technique selection; (c) categories of descriptive statistics; (d) inferential statistics for hypothesis testing purposes; and (e) inferential statistics for establishing effect sizes and interval estimations.

TERMINOLOGY DISTINCTIONS
Among Univariate Statistics, Bivariate Statistics, and Multivariate Statistics

The three realms of statistics identified here actually refer to the number of variables analyzed in each case. As the term implies, **univariate statistics** include all those techniques that focus on quantifying *one* particular variable of interest. Such is the case, for example, when we calculate the arithmetic average, or mean, for a set of scores reflecting the stress level for a group of clients receiving therapeutic massage in a study. Again, the focus here is on our analysis of only one variable by way of only one statistical technique.

Bivariate statistics encompass all those statistical methods that allow us to analyze the relationship between *two* variables of interest. The Pearson correlation coefficient (r) introduced in earlier chapters, for example, enables us to analyze statistically the relationship between two dependent variables (DVs). A possible application of this bivariate technique might be that of correlating measures of client progress regarding trunk flexion ROM

(i.e., DV_1) and measures of therapist verbal acknowledgment/approval (i.e., DV_2) to ascertain if the two DVs are positively correlated (i.e., directly related) or negatively correlated (i.e., inversely related).

Multivariate statistics include those techniques that allow us to analyze the relationship among *three or more* variables of interest. In an extension of the illustration cited previously, the use of *multiple linear regression* as a statistical technique would allow us to analyze the relationship among the following three variables: extent of client progress on trunk flexion ROM (the criterion variable here), measures of therapist verbal acknowledgment/approval (one of two predictor variables), and measures of client compliance with a between-session stretching regimen assigned by the therapist (the second of two predictor variables).

Between Descriptive Statistics and Inferential Statistics

Descriptive statistics is the name given to one of the two major families of statistical techniques that are popularized in both professional and nonprofessional circles. As the name implies, descriptive statistics include those methods that allow us to characterize, portray, or literally describe a data set in succinct and economical ways. A graphical display of data, for example, is a descriptive technique for characterizing the contents of a data set in a succinct fashion.

Inferential statistics is the name for the second of the two major statistical technique families. These include those statistical analysis options that allow us (a) to test hypotheses regarding a study's sample and/or (b) to calculate effect sizes and interval estimations as supplements to hypothesis testing. One of two major focal points in inferential statistics is that of testing a study's null hypothesis for the purpose of eventually inferring decisions back to the corresponding research and alternative hypotheses. A second major focal point here is that of gaining insight regarding the characteristics of a sample (known as statistics) in order to make inferences regarding the corresponding characteristics in the population from which the sample was derived (and those population characteristics are known as parameters). Augmenting or supplementing the use of inferential statistics for hypothesis testing purpose are inferential techniques that allow us to calculate what is known as effect sizes and interval estimations (both of which were introduced earlier in this text and are addressed again later in this appendix).

Between Parametric Statistics and Nonparametric Statistics

The inferential family of statistics is further subdivided into parametric and nonparametric statistical techniques. The techniques involved in using **parametric statistics** make certain assumptions about the distribution of a study's variables in the population from which the sample came. These assumptions pertain to the normal distribution of a study's DV in the population as well as equal variances in the two or more segments of the population from which, for example, the two or more comparison groups in a study were derived. Parametric statistics also necessitate either an interval or ratio scale on which the DV has been measured.

Nonparametric statistics, by contrast, do not make any assumptions of normality or equal variance regarding the distribution of a study's variables in the population from which the sample was derived. Consequently, they are sometimes referred to as distribution-free statistics. Furthermore, nonparametric statistics are appropriate when the variable being analyzed has been measured on either a nominal or ordinal scale.

DETERMINANTS OF STATISTICAL TECHNIQUE SELECTION: RESEARCH QUESTION, RESEARCH METHOD, AND MEASUREMENT SCALE USED

Three major considerations determine the statistical technique that should be selected for any data analysis purpose: (a) the nature of the research question investigated, (b) the research method used to investigate the research question, and (c) the measurement scale on which the data have been collected. A continuum exists, then, that starts with the research question, proceeds to the research method used as well as the measurement scale on which the data are generated, and finally ends with what should be a clear indication of the proper statistical technique to invoke.

Our earlier clarifications regarding difference-oriented, association-oriented, and descriptive-oriented research strategies are relevant as illustrations at this point. If our research question is descriptive oriented in nature, then presumably we are using a descriptive-oriented research method to investigate it. In so doing, we would invoke one or more appropriate descriptive statistical techniques to analyze the study's resulting data. And within the context of the descriptive statistics available, the measurement scale used would also help to inform our decision as to which statistical technique is most appropriate.

This theme of three **determinants of statistical technique selection** will become even more apparent as we continue our conceptual coverage into the subdivisions of both descriptive and inferential statistics that follows.

DESCRIPTIVE STATISTICS

Expanding on our characterization of descriptive statistics, this family of statistical techniques includes the following categories: *graphical techniques, measures of central tendency, measures of variability*, and *measures of correlation* when hypothesis testing is not the intent.

The **graphical techniques** include among the most common such displays as histograms, bar graphs, pie charts, and stem and leaf plots. The **measures of central tendency** identify values relative to a data set that are, in a sense, most representative of the "tending" or "tendency" of the group of scores as a whole. Included here are the mean, median, and mode. The mean is simply the arithmetic average; the median is the midpoint above and below which 50% of the scores fall; and the mode is the most frequently appearing score in the data set. Regarding the **measures of variability**, each of these is a value that represents from a given perspective the extent of "spread," "variation," or "diversification" in a set of scores. The most commonly recognized measures of variability are the range, variance, and standard deviation. The range is the distance between the highest and lowest scores in a data set whereas the variance might be thought of as somewhat of an "average" extent to which the individual scores vary or deviate from the mean. The standard deviation, in turn, is simply the square root of the variance. Regarding **measures of correlation**, these techniques are typically not thought of as belonging to the descriptive statistics family. When not used for the purpose of hypothesis testing, however, they are considered descriptive in nature. Perhaps the best example here is the Pearson correlation coefficient that we have already seen elsewhere in this book.

Regarding the measures of central tendency and variability, the **normal distribution curve** is a standard context within which measures such as the mean and the standard deviation are frequently introduced. Vogt (1999) characterized the *normal distribution* as

> *a theoretical continuous probability distribution in which the horizontal axis represents all possible values of a variable and the vertical axis represents the probability of those values occurring. The scores on the variable . . .*

are clustered around the mean in a symmetrical, unimodal pattern known as the bell-shaped curve or normal curve. In a normal distribution, the mean, median, and mode are all the same. There are many different normal distributions, one for every possible combination of mean and standard deviation. (p. 194)

Figure D-1 displays the normal curve with the following features illustrated: symmetrical; bell-shaped; mean, median, and mode coinciding; standard deviation units above (positive values) and below (negative values) the mean; and proportions of area under the curve "captured" within ±1 standard deviation, ±2 standard deviations, and ±3

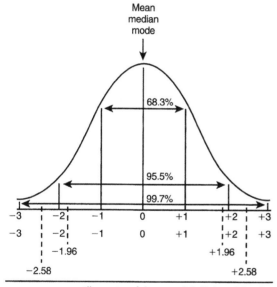

FIGURE D-1 ■ Illustration of the normal, bell-shaped distribution curve. (From Burns, N., & Grove, S. K. [2003]. *Understanding nursing research* [3rd ed.]. Philadelphia: W.B. Saunders. p. 318.)

standard deviations of the mean—namely, 68.3%, 95.5%, and 99.7%, respectively.

INFERENTIAL STATISTICS: NULL HYPOTHESIS SIGNIFICANCE TESTING (NHST) IN THE CONTEXT OF POWER ANALYSIS

Here, too, we are building on earlier discussions of this inferential family of statistical techniques. The majority of our references to inferential statistics thus far have been in terms of techniques used for hypothesis testing purposes. These discussions of hypothesis testing have been couched in terms of the requisite *statistical power analysis* that consistently should be performed. Chapter 3 provided a characterization of power analysis as another probability context within which a null hypothesis is tested. As a reminder, it refers to the probability or mathematical odds that the statistical analysis of the data will result in a rejection of the null hypothesis when in reality the null is false and should, therefore, be rejected.

There are several other strategic considerations regarding hypothesis testing in the context of a power analysis being in place. Earlier in this appendix we made the distinction between parametric and nonparametric statistics, the two major divisions of the inferential family. There is an even further distinction that we can now make within the parametric and nonparametric divisions that has each subdivided into **association-oriented statistical techniques** and **difference-oriented statistical techniques**. Box D-1 provides an overview of the divisions and subdivisions existing in the inferential family of statistics used for hypothesis testing purposes. It also names a few of the more prevalent statistical methods positioned in each category.

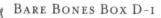

BARE BONES BOX D-1

Overview of the Divisions and Subdivisions Constituting Inferential Statistics for Null Hypothesis Significance Testing Purposes

- Inferential Statistics: Hypothesis Testing Purposes
  - Parametric
    - Association-Oriented (e.g., Pearson correlation, partial correlation, and simple and multiple linear regression)
    - Difference-Oriented (e.g., t-test and analysis of variance [ANOVA])
  - Nonparametric
    - Association-Oriented (e.g., Spearman rank-order correlation)
    - Difference-Oriented (e.g., chi square, Mann-Whitney U, and Kruskal-Wallis one-way ANOVA)

INFERENTIAL STATISTICS: BEYOND NULL HYPOTHESIS SIGNIFICANCE TESTING

Since the mid-1990s there has been escalating debate regarding the traditional reliance on **null hypothesis significance testing (NHST)** (cf. Cohen, 1994; Estes, 1997; Hunter, 1997; Hunter & Schmidt, 1990; Loftus, 1996; Wilkinson & the Task Force on Statistical Inference, 1999). A major part of this discussion has focused on statistical techniques such as *effect size calculations* and *confidence interval estimation* as either supplements or alternatives to the traditional use of null hypothesis significance testing. Chapter 3 provided a brief consideration of these two additional approaches.

Effect Size Calculations

Effect size calculations can be demonstrated in several different ways. Perhaps the most basic is calculating the degree/extent of influence or "effect" of the independent variable in a study on the DV. This can be quantified in one of two possible ways. One way is in terms of calculating, for example, an *eta-squared* value that shows the proportion of variance on the DV that can be explained or accounted for by the IV. A second approach uses, for instance, *Cohen's d statistic* (as discussed in Chapter 9) in that it quantifies the size of the difference between the means for two comparison groups as indicated in standard deviation units. Still another approach to effect size calculations as seen in the case of a correlational study involves squaring the correlation coefficient *r* value. This results in a *coefficient of determination* (r^2) that indicates the proportion of variance on one DV that is explained by the other DV.

Confidence Interval Estimation

In addition to effect size calculations, another option is **confidence interval estimation**. This type of statistic allows us to calculate a range of numerical values that has a certain probability (95% or 99%) of including or "capturing" the true population parameter being investigated in a study. As an illustration, a 95% confidence interval would specify both the lower and upper limits of a range of values that we are 95% confident actually contains the true population parameter being studied. Note that we are not actually identifying the precise value of the population parameter. Instead, we are simply estimating a numerical range of values that we are confident—at a certain probability level—does indeed contain the true population parameter value. Hence, we use the expression *confidence interval estimation*.

RESEARCH QUESTION, RESEARCH METHOD, MEASUREMENT PROCEDURE, AND STATISTICAL ANALYSIS: A LOGICAL AND CRITICAL PROGRESSION

One desired outcome of this appendix is the realization of the *interdependency* existing among such features of the research process as the initiating *research question*, the *research method* used to investigate the question, the *measurement procedures* chosen to document the variables of interest, and the *statistical techniques* invoked to analyze the resulting data.

This progression is quite logical and suggests a critical feature of what makes scientific research systematic. The interdependency among these aspects of scientific inquiry allows for a reasoned, justified, compatible, and effective approach to exploring critical professional issues expressed in the form of empirical and operational research questions.

Beyond the resources already cited in the brief overview provided in this appendix are several others that speak to both the conceptual and computational features of the measurement and statistical topics covered. These include the following: Batavia (2001); Braitman (1991); Burns and Grove (2003); Domholdt (2000); Greenfield, Kuhn, and Wojtys (1996); Healey (2005); Polgar and Thomas (2000); Sim and Arnell (1993); and Zechmeister and Posavac (2003).

REFERENCES

Batavia, M. (2001). *Clinical research for health professionals: A user-friendly guide.* Boston: Butterworth/Heinemann.

Braitman, L. E. (1991). Confidence intervals assess both clinical significance and statistical significance. *Annals of Internal Medicine, 114*(6), 515–517.

Burns, N., & Grove, S. K. (2003). *Understanding nursing research* (3rd ed.). Philadelphia: W.B. Saunders.

Cohen, J. (1961). A coefficient of agreement for nominal scales. *Educational and Psychological Measurement, 20,* 37–46.

Cohen, J. (1994). The earth is round (*p* < .05). *American Psychologist, 49,* 997–1003.

Cronbach, L. J. (1951). Coefficient alpha and the internal structure of tests. *Psychometrika, 16,* 297–334.

Domholdt, E. (2000). *Physical therapy research: Principles and applications* (2nd ed.). Philadelphia: W. B. Saunders.

Estes, W. K. (1997). On the communication of information by displays of standard errors and confidence intervals. *Psychonomic Bulletin & Review, 4,* 330–341.

Gravetter, F. J., & Forzano, L. B. (2003). *Research methods for the behavioral sciences.* Belmont, CA: Thomson Wadsworth.

Greenfield, M. L. V. H., Kuhn, J. E., & Wojtys, E. M. (1996). A statistics primer: p values–probability and clinical significance. *The American Journal of Sports Medicine, 24*(6), 863–865.

Healey, J. F. (2005). *Statistics: A tool for social research* (7th ed.). Belmont, CA: Thomson Wadsworth.

Hunter, J. E. (1997). Needed: A ban on significance tests. *Psychological Science, 8,* 3–7.

Hunter, J. E., & Schmidt, F. L. (1990). *Methods of meta-analysis: Correcting error and bias in research.* Newbury Park, CA: Sage.

Kuder, G. F., & Richardson, M. W. (1937). The theory of estimation of test reliability. *Psychometrika, 2,* 151–160.

Loftus, G. R. (1996). Psychology will be a much better science when we change the way we analyze data. *Current Directions in Psychological Science, 5,* 161–171.

Polgar, S., & Thomas, S. A. (2000). *Introduction to research in the health sciences* (4th ed.). New York: Churchill Livingstone.

Polit, D. F., & Beck, C. T. (2004). *Nursing research: Principles and methods* (7th ed.). Philadelphia: Lippincott Williams & Wilkins.

Sim, J., & Arnell, P. (1993). Measurement validity in physical therapy research. *Physical Therapy, 73*(2), 102–115.

Vogt, W. P. (1999). *Dictionary of statistics & methodology* (2nd ed.). Thousand Oaks, CA: Sage.

Wilkinson, L., & the Task Force on Statistical Inference. (1999). Statistical methods in psychology journals. *American Psychologist, 54,* 594–604.

Zechmeister, E. B., & Posavac, E. J. (2003). *Data analysis and interpretation in the behavioral sciences.* Belmont, CA: Thomson Wadsworth.

ADDITIONAL RECOMMENDED RESOURCES

Bailar, J. C., & Mosteller, F. (1992). *Medical uses of statistics* (2nd ed.). Boston: NEJM Books.

Baumgardner, K. P. (1997). A review of key research design and statistical analysis issues. *Oral Surgery, 84*(5), 550–556.

Bland, M., & Peacock, J. (2000). *Statistical questions in evidence-based medicine.* New York: Oxford University Press.

Fischbach, F. (2000). *A manual of laboratory & diagnostic tests* (6th ed.). Philadelphia: Lippincott Williams & Wilkins.

Goodman, S. N., & Berlin, J. A. (1994). The use of predicted confidence intervals when planning experiments and the misuse of power when interpreting results. *Annals of Internal Medicine, 121,* 200–206.

Jaccard, J., & Becker, M. A. (2002). *Statistics for the behavioral sciences* (4th ed.). Belmont, CA: Thomson Wadsworth.

Munro, B. H. (1997). *Statistical methods for health care research* (3rd ed.). Philadelphia: Lippincott Williams & Wilkins.

Nolan, M. T., & Mock, V. (2000). *Measuring patient outcomes.* Thousand Oaks, CA: Sage.

Riegelman, R. K. (2000). *Studying a study and testing a test: How to read the medical evidence* (4th ed.). Philadelphia: Lippincott Williams & Wilkins.

GLOSSARY

A-B Design One of several possible research designs included under the single-case experimental research method. It involves documenting over a period of time—say, several days or weeks, for example—the signs/symptoms/behavior presented by a client who (a) is initially in need of treatment not yet provided and (b) is then provided with the treatment. The initial phase, called the *baseline phase* and designated by the letter "A," is that period of time during which no treatment is introduced and the targeted signs/symptoms/behaviors are measured. This is followed by the *treatment phase*, designated by the letter "B," that spans a period of time during which a treatment is introduced and measures are continued on the targeted outcome(s).

A-B-A Design A slight extension of the A-B design in that it involves an additional third phase wherein the treatment is removed and, consequently, the subject is returned to the baseline phase. The intent is to demonstrate the outcome or consequence of a return to the subject's initial status of not receiving treatment.

A-B-A-B (or Reversal) Design A slight extension of the A-B-A design in that it involves an additional fourth phase wherein the treatment is reintroduced, thereby creating an intermittent reversal from baseline to treatment that is repeated.

Allied and Complementary Medicine (AMED) A database maintained by the Health Care Information Service of the British Library. It addresses resources available in complementary medicine, palliative care, and numerous professions allied with medicine.

Alpha Level (α) The alpha level also known as the probability of a Type I error. When testing a null hypothesis, a decision to reject the null is always accompanied by an admission that there is a certain probability or likelihood that one may be making an error in doing so, thereby committing the so-called Type I error. That probability level is called the alpha level, and it is typically established before the actual statistical analysis is completed. In the behavioral sciences, an alpha level of .05 is customary; in many of the basic and health science areas of research, though, a lower and more demanding alpha level is set (e.g., at .01).

Alternative Hypothesis (H_A or H_1) An alternative hypothesis (a) is a well-justified prediction of a study's anticipated outcome in the context of the study's population; (b) is consistent with the prediction of the research hypothesis, although referring to the study's population; and (c) typically contradicts the prediction of the null hypothesis and, hence, is literally an alternative to the null.

Anonymity This provision in a research study ensures that the researcher has no way of associating a research subject's identity with any information received from that individual.

APA (2001) Publication Manual This manual represents the stylistic format and requirements for scientific communication in many health science and behavioral science areas. It is published by the American Psychological Association (APA) and was most recently updated in 2001 (5th ed.).

Archival Indicators See Behavioral Measures.

Association-Oriented Research Strategy One of three research strategies included under the quantitative research category. As its name implies, this research strategy is oriented to investigating a relationship between/among variables with an initial focus on the possible existence of an association between/among them. This association can take the form of two possibilities: (a) a co-relationship, or correlation, between two dependent variables; and (b) an already established correlation between two dependent variables such that one dependent variable can be predicted from the other dependent variable.

Assurance of Compliance (with 45 CFR 46) A statement of an institution's policy and procedures for protecting human subjects that assures compliance with 45 CFR 46. Given that 45 CFR 46 is an overarching framework for the protection of human research subjects, its actual implementation is overseen by the DHHS's Office for Human Research Protections (OHRP). Any institution engaged in human subjects research that is conducted or supported by any agency of the DHHS must have an OHRP-approved *assurance of compliance* (or simply *assurance*).

Behavioral Measures A modality of measurement that lends itself to constructs whose nature can be displayed overtly. When such is the case, an appeal can be made to behavioral observations, content analyses, and archival indicators. Behavioral observations entail direct observation, along with the requisite record, of the behavior(s) observed. Content analyses involve a form of behavioral observation that focuses on specific events occurring in various media context such as literature, film, television, and comparable replicas of behavior. Archival research focuses on indicators of past behaviors and/or events via a reliance on historical documents.

Belmont Report (1979) In 1979 the National Commission for the Protection of Human Subjects of Biomedical and Behavioral Research issued the *Belmont Report,* which speaks to several ethical principles and guidelines covering three major areas: (a) the boundaries between practice and research; (b) basic ethical principles pertaining to respect for persons, beneficence, and justice; and (c) applications of these principles in terms of informed consent, the assessment of risk and benefits, and the selection of subjects.

Beneficence One of three basic ethical principles addressed in the Belmont Report (1979), *beneficence* refers to an obligation to ensure the well-being of individuals by (a) doing no harm and (b) maximizing potential benefits while minimizing possible harm.

Best-Evidence Synthesis Research Method One of six research methods included under the synthesis-oriented research strategy. It is operationally defined as a research method characterized by several research procedures/features: (a) it builds on the principal advantages of—yet represents an alternative to—the traditional narrative review, critical systematic review, and meta-analytic review methods; (b) it combines attention to both the traditional review's individual studies and methodological and substantive issues and conventional meta-analysis's quantification of effect sizes and systematic study selection procedures; (c) it corrects for a major drawback in conventional meta-analysis wherein the all-inclusive and exhaustive collection of primary studies may include studies not representing the best available evidence in a given research domain; (d) it is *selectively exhaustive* in its identification and collection of primary studies that are eventually meta-analyzed; (e) it appeals to a legal analogy whereby the same evidence that would be essential in one case might be disregarded in another because in the second case there is better evidence available; (f) it is predicated, therefore, on the principle of best evidence and the corresponding a priori criteria used for identifying episodes of best evidence; (g) a priori criteria for best evidence determinations can be proposed for individual research subfields via examining earlier narrative, critical systematic, and meta-analytic reviews; and (h) it focuses, therefore, on the *best evidence* available in a research domain, that is, studies highest in internal and external validity, using well-specified and defended a priori inclusion/exclusion criteria, and using effect size indices as an adjunct to a full discussion of the literature being reviewed.

Between-Subjects Independent Variable (or Design) A between-subjects independent variable, sometimes also known as a between-subjects design, refers to a manner in which participants become affiliated with the two or more comparative groups in a study such that each level of the independent variable involves a separate and distinct group of individuals affiliated with it.

Biophysiologic Measures As the name suggests, this modality of measurement allows a researcher to examine manifestations of an underlying construct by appealing to biological/physiological indicators that may span cardiovascular, pulmonary, blood, urine, saliva, and immunodiagnostic studies. Such measures fall into two possible categories: (a) in vivo measurements that occur directly in or on a living organism and include as examples blood pressure and body temperature measures and (b) in vitro measurements occurring outside the organism's body as is the case with blood chemistry analyses.

Bivariate Statistics Those statistical techniques that allow one to analyze the relationship between *two* variables of interest; hence, *bi-variate* means *two variables*. For example, the Pearson correlation coefficient (r) indicates the degree of relationship between two dependent variables of interest.

Blended-Methods Approach See Mixed-Methods Approach.

Blinding (or Masking) The research procedure whereby one or more parties in a study (i.e., participant, investigator, and/or evaluator) are unaware of the level of the independent variable to which participants belong. Also see Single-Blind Procedure, Double-Blind Procedure, and Evaluator- (or Analysis) Blind Procedure.

Boolean Operators Refers to words such as AND, OR, and NOT that are used when two or more key words are employed in the electronic searching of databases. They make a given search strategy either more exclusive or inclusive, depending on the Boolean operator(s) used.

Boundaries Between Practice and Research As articulated in the Belmont Report (1979), *practice* refers to biomedical or behavioral interventions providing diagnosis, preventive treatment, or therapy to a patient or client with a reasonable expectation of enhancing the individual's well-being. In contrast, *research* is an activity implemented to investigate a hypothesis, allow conclusions to be drawn, and consequently advance generalizable knowledge typically conveyed in theories, principles, and statements of relationships uncovered. Admittedly, research and practice may conceivably be addressed in tandem, as is the case when research aims to evaluate a given therapy's safety and efficacy.

CAM on PubMed Another feature of PubMed specific to complementary and alternative medicine that was developed by the National Library of Medicine (NLM) in tandem with the National Center on Complementary and Alternative Medicine (NCCAM). Its intent is to facilitate the search and retrieval of needed articles on CAM from the approximately 220,000 citations that constitute CAM on PubMed.

Case Report Research Method One of four research methods included under the descriptive-oriented research strategy. It is operationally defined as a research method characterized by several principal research procedures/features: (a) the focal point is primarily on a detailed description of the clinical practice itself that defines the treatment plan for a client, (b) this clinical practice treatment plan is described in the context of both the client's profile and the supporting justification for the intervention selected, and (c) in the preceding context, this method then describes the sequence of clinical visits as well as the ongoing and final results of the treatment's effectiveness. Compare with Single-Case Experimental Research Method, Single-Case Quantitative Analysis Research Method, and Case Study Research Method.

Case Study Research Method One of four research methods included under the contextual/interpretive-oriented research strategy. It is operationally defined as a research method characterized by several principal research procedures/themes: (a) the identification of a case entity as a single individual, organization, issue, activity, event, or program of interest that is bounded by certain time and space delimitations; (b) an intensive description and analysis of the case entity reflecting its context and multiple data sources; and (c) the availability of three case study options, namely, an *intrinsic* case study to acquire more insight on the uniqueness of a particular case, an *instrumental* case study to refine or alter a theoretical explanation of an issue or event, and a *collective* case study of several case entities to gain insight on the phenomenon represented across the several cases. Compare with Single-Case Experimental Research Method, Single-Case Quantitative Analysis Research Method, and Case Report Research Method.

Centralized Information Service for Complementary Medicine (CISCOM) An electronic database maintained by the Research Council for Complementary Medicine, United Kingdom. It contains randomized trials and bibliographic citations and abstracts pertaining to major complementary therapies.

ClinicalTrials.gov A source that provides disease treatment information, inclusive of CAM-oriented therapies, modalities, and substances.

Cochrane Collaboration Initiated in 1993 by the National Health Service (NHS) in the United Kingdom and organized around 15 Cochrane Centers established throughout the world. The Cochrane Library is an electronic database produced by the Cochrane Collaboration to document and disseminate high-quality evidence for enhanced decision making by those providing and receiving health care as well as those engaged in health care research, education, and administration. Database components of the Cochrane Library include (a) The Cochrane Database of Systematic Reviews, (b) the Cochrane Controlled Trial Register in bibliographic form, (c) the Database of Abstracts of Reviews of Effectiveness, and (d) the Cochrane Review Methodology Database in bibliographic form regarding the science of research synthesis.

Code of Federal Regulations, Title 45, Part 46; or (45 CFR 46) Also known as the *Common Rule*, 45 CFR 46 codifies the federal government's role in protecting human research subjects. Originally it applied only to research conducted or supported by the Department of Health and Human Services (DHHS); however, in 1991 the regulations were revised and made applicable to all federally supported research. This legislation represents a framework, rather than a set of rigidly applied rules, for ensuring the rights and welfare of human research subjects. Its most recent revision occurred in 2001.

Coefficient of Determination (r^2) A measure of effect size that indexes the proportion of variations on one dependent variable that can be explained by the variations on a second dependent variable.

Cohen's d Statistic See Effect Size.

Combined-Methods Approach See Mixed-Methods Approach.

Common Rule See Code of Federal Regulations, Title 45, Part 46; or 45 CFR 46.

Competency "*Competency* . . . is a two-dimensional construct [cf. White, 1959]. The first dimension is . . . mastery. In other words, *mastery* can be thought of as the intellectual component of competency. A competent learner has acquired a variety of learning products. However, competency also consists of the attainment of self-confidence or the sense of being able to cope. This attainment of *self-confidence* is the emotional or affective component of competency" (emphases added) (Block & Anderson, 1977, p. 165).

Concurrent Validity One of two possible forms of criterion-related validity. Regarding concurrent validity, the external criterion against which a new instrument of interest is being validated would be an already well established instrument or activity for the designated purpose. If indeed the measurements on the newly designed instrument correlated in a positive manner with measurements on the established instrument or activity, then concurrent validity could be inferred.

Confidence Interval (CI) Although various types of confidence intervals may be reported in the results section of a research report, in its most basic form a confidence interval refers to a range of numerical values that has a certain probability of capturing the true population parameter under investigation in a study.

Confidentiality This provision in a research study means that although the researcher potentially or actually can associate a research subject's identity with information received from that individual, assurances are given that such associations of one's identity and information will be kept strictly secret, private, and undisclosed.

Confounding Variable Any factor in a research study related to the study's participants or the characteristics of the study's setting/circumstance that (a) is initially present as a potentially problematic extraneous variable; (b) is not adequately planned for or accommodated by the researcher; and, hence, (c) has the effect of confusing or obfuscating—quite literally, confounding—the eventual outcome and interpretation of the study.

Construct Validity An instrument is said to possess construct validity if it can be demonstrated that it indeed measures the particular abstract concept, or construct, it purports to measure. For instance, an instrument that claims to measure the construct of pain would need to demonstrate a positive correlation with other indicators of the experience of pain.

Constructivism Defined as "a relativist ontology (there are multiple realities), a subjective epistemology (knower and subject create understandings), and a naturalistic (in the natural world) set of methodological procedures" (Denzin & Lincoln, 1994, p. 13, as cited by Miller et al., 2003). Constructivism is the philosophical basis or perspective underlying qualitative research and represents a less extreme view of reality, truth, and values than its historical successor, postmodernism.

Content Analyses See Behavioral Measures.

Content Validity A typical occasion for interest in content validity is that of an achievement test of subject matter mastery by students. This type of validity refers to the degree of correspondence that exists between (a) an instrument's test items and (b) the learning/performance objectives and associated content coverage taught to the students and for which they are held accountable via the test.

Contextual/Interpretive-Oriented Research Strategy This is the singular research strategy that operationalizes the qualitative research category. As its name implies, this generic research strategy is oriented to investigations that emphasize three principal themes: (a) researcher immersion in the setting or context of the study's participants; (b) interpretation of a study's dynamics and findings as rooted in the participants' ascribed meanings and understandings; and (c) the preceding themes of immersion and interpretation as occurring in three related yet different contexts, namely, the study's unique set of participants, the nature of the interaction and discourses that occur between/ among the participants, and the sociocultural context in which the phenomena being studied occur.

Control Group (CG) Used as a basis of comparison to one or more treatment (or experimental) groups, a control group is a comparable group of participants that is not exposed to the experimental treatment or intervention.

Control Variable A control variable is any factor in a research study related to the study's participants or the characteristics of the study's setting/circumstance that (a) is initially present as a potentially problematic extraneous variable; (b) is planned for or accommodated by the researcher to ensure that its influence does not confound or confuse the eventual outcome and interpretation of the study; and, hence, (c) typically allows the assumption of group equivalence at the outset of a study when the research focus is on comparing two or more groups regarding a dependent variable.

Correlational Research Method One of two research methods included under the association-oriented research strategy. It is operationally defined as a research method characterized by the following three research procedures/features: (a) the existence of a sample of participants that may or may not have been formed by random selection; (b) the measurement of each participant in the sample on two or more dependent variables; and (c) the application of correlational statistical techniques to analyze the data set generated by the measures of the dependent variables.

Criterion-Related Validity As the expression implies, criterion-related validity is a generic type of validity that has as its reference point an external criterion by which the validity of the instrument in question is assessed. In this context, then, criterion-related validity is manifested by two subcategories of validity: (a) predictive validity and (b) concurrent validity. Also see Predictive Validity and Concurrent Validity.

Criterion Variable (CV) That variable in the predictive research method that is predicted quantitatively by means of another variable of interest (called the predictor variable) using the statistical technique of linear regression.

Critical Systematic Review Research Method One of six research methods included under the synthesis-oriented research strategy. It is operationally defined as a research method characterized by several principal research procedures/features: (a) it is conducted with a view toward applying scientific strategies in an unbiased way to collect, critique, and synthesize all relevant primary studies that address a specific clinical question; (b) its research question is narrow, falls in the clinical realm, and is defined explicitly regarding the areas of population and setting, condition of interest, exposure to a treatment, and/or one or more specific outcomes; (c) potential researcher bias is controlled via the use of explicit inclusion/exclusion criteria for study selection; (d) it conducts an *exhaustive* search of all relevant primary studies using the explicit inclusion/exclusion criteria; (e) the primary studies' designs, characteristics, data analyses, and results are critiqued and interpreted; (f) the resulting critique and interpretation of the primary studies lead to an objective synthesis of pertinent literature useful for informing clinical practice and suggesting needed research; (g) the absence of meta-analysis precludes the systematic aggregating and integrating of empirical data across the several primary studies for the purpose of better estimating the effects of treatments; and (h) it facilitates decision making and problem solving by clinicians more readily than is typical with only results from a single study, yet does not substitute for appropriate clinical reasoning.

Cronbach's Alpha An index of the split-half reliability of an instrument arrived at by estimating the average correlation that would result from all possible ways of splitting an instrument in half.

Cross-Sectional Design One of two possible designs considered to be developmental or time sequence designs. In this design, the researcher identifies representative samples of individuals at the specific age or time interval levels of interest and then measures them on the dependent variable at only one point in time.

Cumulative Index of Nursing and Allied Health Literature (CINAHL) As its name implies, this is a database established in 1956 to accommodate the professional literature needs of nonmedical health professionals in the nursing and allied health areas.

Debriefing The planned postinvestigation explanation of a study's purpose that is given to the research participants. This feature is particularly important in studies that involve any form of deception.

Deception This possible feature of a research study involves the researcher either intentionally withholding information about the study from participants (an act of *omission,* or passive deception) or intentionally misleading the participants regarding the true nature of a study (an act of *commission,* or active deception). Naturally, a risks/benefits assessment is critical in this regard and certainly relates to the ethical principle of beneficence.

Declaration of Helsinki (1964/2000) In 1964 the World Medical Association (WMA) adopted the *Declaration of Helsinki* that articulates certain ethical principles and guidelines for biomedical research involving human subjects. This was done in response to the need for guidelines more comprehensive than the Nuremberg Code provided. This declaration has been amended several times by the WMA since 1964, with the most recent occurring in 2000.

Dependent Variable Also known as a DV, the dependent variable is that factor of interest in a research study that (a) is an outcome measure of concern to the researcher either on its own stand-alone merit or in relation to an independent variable or some other dependent variable and (b) has as possible synonyms such expressions as response variable, output variable, outcome variable, consequent variable, or perhaps effect variable.

Descriptive-Oriented Research Strategy One of three research strategies included under the quantitative research category. As its name implies, this research strategy is oriented to investigating one or more dependent variables with a view toward characterizing, portraying, profiling, or—quite literally—describing the one or more dependent variables of interest. There is no attempt, however, to investigate relationships between/among the dependent variables when two or more are considered. Furthermore, because there is no independent variable involved, the issue of examining a relationship between an independent variable and a dependent variable is nonexistent.

Descriptive Statistics The family of quantitative analysis techniques that allows one to characterize, portray, or literally describe a data set in succinct and economical ways.

Developmental or Time Sequence Designs One of several research designs included under the nonexperimental comparative groups research method. In these designs, the researcher investigates human development changes or the sequencing of behaviors/conditions over time. The nonmanipulated independent variable here is either age or time interval specific.

Difference-Oriented Research Strategy One of three research strategies included under the quantitative research category. As its name implies, this research strategy is oriented to investigating

whether or not a difference exists between/among the levels of an independent variable relative to a dependent variable. (As a reminder, the levels of an independent variable refer to the two or more comparison groups that represent varying manifestations of the independent variable.)

Dismantling or Component Analysis Design One of several possible research designs included under the single-case experimental research method. Representing somewhat of an elaboration of the multiple treatment design, this design allows a researcher to use a series of treatment phases in contrast with a baseline phase in order to investigate a complex type of intervention. This is accomplished by the researcher adding or subtracting sequentially those individual components that together actually constitute the complex treatment.

Double-Blind Procedure A research procedure whereby neither the investigator nor the participant is aware of the participant's group membership (or affiliated level of the independent variable).

Effect Size Although various types of effect sizes may be reported in the results section of a research report, one basic form of an effect size refers to the degree or extent of influence or effect of the independent variable on the dependent variable in a study. Accordingly, it may be quantified as (a) the proportion of variation on the dependent variable measures that can be explained or accounted for by the independent variable (i.e., *eta-squared*) and/or (b) the size of the difference between the means of two comparison groups as indicated in standard deviation units (i.e., *Cohen's d statistic*). In the case of a correlational study involving two dependent variables, a second basic form of an effect size measure is the *coefficient of determination* (r^2), which indicates the proportion of variance on one dependent variable that is explained by the other dependent variable.

Effectiveness A determination that a therapeutic intervention is feasible and has measurable beneficial effects applicable to a broad population of clients/patients in real-world settings. Effectiveness studies typically do not have the degree of research design control present in efficacy studies; however, they tend to emphasize external validity and the generalizability of treatments for which some evidence of efficacy has already been demonstrated. Compare with Efficacy.

Efficacy The benefits of a therapeutic intervention demonstrated by way of a comparison between one or more experimental treatments and one or more control or comparison treatments performed in the context of a highly controlled clinical trial. Efficacy studies must be designed so as to encourage replication. This typically implies at least four critical components: (a) a well-defined group of study clients/patients whose condition has been objectively identified via rigorous inclusion/exclusion criteria; (b) the presence of an appropriate control condition for comparison to the experimental condition; (c) the random assignment of participants to the comparison conditions; and (d) close attention to documenting and ensuring compliance with treatment protocol specifications. Compare with Effectiveness.

Equivalent or Parallel Forms Reliability This type of reliability involves the degree to which two forms/versions of the same instrument measure a certain variable consistently for the same group of individuals, with each form/version of the instrument being administered at a different point in time than the other.

Eta-Squared See Effect Size.

Ethics One of two subdivisions of that branch of philosophy known as axiology. Whereas axiology speaks to the issue of values in general, ethics is its subdivision that addresses values in the context of human behavior. (The second subdivision of axiology is that of aesthetics and concerns itself with values in the context of the appreciation of beauty.)

Ethnographic Research Method One of four research methods included under the contextual/interpretive-oriented research strategy. It is operationally defined as a research method characterized by several principal research procedures/features: (a) the focal point is on understanding and interpreting human behavior as embedded in a given cultural context; (b) behavior is studied from within the culture of interest (i.e., the *emic* approach) or from outside the culture with cross-cultural interests (i.e., the *etic* approach); (c) reliance primarily is on participant observation and in-depth interviews for data collection purposes; and (d) participant observation implies the role of the researcher as an instrument, that is, the researcher observes in the context of becoming a participant in the culture.

Evaluation The process of making a value judgment or an assessment of merit concerning one or more variables of interest that have been measured and analyzed. For example, grading is an instance of evaluation. (Consider the following verbal analogy: Measurement is to testing as evaluation is to grading.)

Evaluator- (or Analysis-) Blind Procedure A research procedure whereby the research team member responsible for the statistical analysis of the study's data is unaware of which treatment (if any) the various study participants received.

***Ex Post Facto* (After the Fact) Designs** This set of research designs is one of several included under the nonexperimental comparative groups research method. In these designs, the participants selected have (a) already been exposed to a particular treatment/condition or (b) already exhibit a particular trait, characteristic, or outcome.

Exclusion Criteria As the expression implies, these are criteria or standards used as a basis for determining which potential participants being considered for a study will indeed be excluded from the study.

Experimental (or Treatment) Group Used as a basis of comparison to a control group or yet another variation of the experimental/treatment group, an experimental or treatment group refers to a comparable group of participants to whom the study's treatment or intervention is applied.

External Validity The extent to which the conclusions reached in a study can be generalized with confidence from the sample back to the accessible population from which the sample was derived.

Extraneous Variable An extraneous variable is any factor in a research study related to the study's participants or the characteristics of the study's setting/circumstance that (a) is not the principal or primary focus of the investigation; (b) is considered — quite literally — extraneous to the study's major emphasis; (c) has the potential to confound or confuse the eventual outcome and interpretation of the study; and, hence, (d) should be accommodated or planned for in the design and implementation of the study.

Face Validity A subjective assessment that appeals to the apparent validity of an instrument for its stated purpose. It relates to the extent to which the instrument looks or appears to be pertinent to the measurement task at hand.

Grounded Theory Research Method One of four research methods included under the contextual/interpretive-oriented research strategy. It is operationally defined as a research method characterized by several principal research procedures/features: (a) most applicable to areas characterized by a paucity of previous research or to establish research areas necessitating new viewpoints; (b) the focal point is on a conceptual or theoretical model that explains an experience or phenomenon in a particular setting that is both relevant to, and problematic for, the study's participants; (c) the researcher attempts to uncover the process useful to the participants in resolving the problem; (d) the foundational construct is social interactionism, which explores how people define reality and how their beliefs impact their behavior; and (e) research activities progress interactively from data generation/analysis to construct identification to theoretical formulation, with the emergent theory rooted or grounded in the original data.

Holistic Therapy Reflects (a) the interrelatedness of body, mind, and spirit in the healing process and (b) the diversity of disciplines, professions, and traditions in the pursuit of well-being for the whole person. This eclectic view of the individual also encompasses the social, cultural, and environmental milieu in which the person functions. Health care, accordingly, is responsive not only to conventional interventions but also to those traditions and systems of beliefs and practices that maximize the individual's options for the control of illness and the attainment of wellness.

Hypothesis A statement that (a) is founded or justified by way of some conceptual, theoretical, experiential, and/or research basis and (b) predicts a research outcome regarding a study's sample and/or population.

Inclusion Criteria As the expression implies, these are criteria or standards used as a basis for determining which potential participants being considered for a study will indeed be included in the study.

Independent Variable Also know as an IV, the independent variable is that factor of interest in a research study that (a) is investigated for a possible relationship to a dependent variable; (b) may be manipulated or governed by the researcher; (c) may be nonmanipulable in nature and, hence, a reflection of study participants' characteristics, conditions, or features; and (d) has as possible synonyms such expressions as stimulus variable, input variable, treatment variable, or perhaps causal variable.

Inferential Statistics The family of quantitative analysis techniques that allows one not only to test hypotheses in a study, but also to calculate effect sizes and confidence interval estimations as supplements to hypothesis testing.

Informed Consent One of three applications of the basic ethical principles addressed in the Belmont Report (1979), *informed consent* by research subjects is the moral requirement derived primarily from the ethical principle of *respect for persons.* Though somewhat controversial, consensus does exist in that informed consent must encompass three critical elements as the researcher attempts to ensure that prospective subjects have all of the required information necessary to make a rational decision regarding their participation in a study. These three elements involve (a) the extent and nature of study-related information provided to potential research subjects, (b) the comprehensibility of the study-related information, and (c) the voluntary nature of the consent if and when it is forthcoming.

Institutional Review Board (IRB) Regarding the protection of human and animal subjects in the research process, any institution or agency engaged in such research must designate a review board for the purpose of ensuring both the scientific and ethical integrity of the investigative effort. The Department of Health and Human Services (DHHS), for example, mandates such a review process via an IRB by any agency or institution receiving government funding for human subjects research. This essentially includes all colleges, universities, hospitals, and clinics wherein the research endeavor involves human subjects.

Integrative Research Category One of three possible research categories characterized as follows: (a) philosophically driven by somewhat of a hybrid view of reality and truth that recognizes the equally valuable possibilities that exist in both the objective analyses and the subjective interpretations of whatever experiences are investigated; (b) rooted in both numerical and verbal data, but with a concerted effort to synthesize research that has already been generated in the quantitative and/or qualitative realms; and (c) representative of research that highlights two

basic themes, namely, "the whole may indeed be greater than simply the sum of its parts" and "patterns of meaning may unfold in an area of research if a synthesizing approach is taken."

Internal Validity The extent to which the dependent variable measures in a study can be traced back exclusively to the influence of the independent variable.

Inter-Rater Reliability The degree of consistency, or agreement, between/among two or more observers/raters when assessing a subject's responses at a given point in time.

Interval Scale One of four measurement scales, the interval scale uses numbers to name, rank order, and permit the assumption of equal intervals between any two pairs of consecutive points on the scale. This scale, however, does not involve a true or absolute zero point. Examples here include measures of intelligence (IQ), the Celsius temperature scale, or numerical achievement test performance scored from 0 to 100.

Intervening Variable Any factor in a research study that is theorized, speculated about, or proposed as a possible explanation of why the researcher obtained the results that were uncovered in the investigation. In a sense, this variable is that factor that explains "why we got what we got" in a study and, accordingly, is also known as an explanatory variable. In the context of a difference-oriented research strategy, this variable is that factor presumed (a) to have *intervened* between the onset of the independent variable and the eventual measurement of the dependent variable and, hence, (b) to explain the uncovered relationship between the independent variable and the dependent variable.

Intra-Rater Reliability The degree of consistency with which one observer/rater assigns score ratings to the observed target behavior across two or more occasions.

Justice One of three basic ethical principles addressed in the Belmont Report (1979), justice here is understood in the context of "fairness in distribution" or "what is deserved" regarding the possible benefits of research as well as the assumption of its burdens.

Longitudinal Design One of two possible designs considered to be developmental or time sequence designs. In this design, the researcher selects a single group of participants and then measures them on the dependent variable of interest at each of several points across time corresponding to the age levels or time intervals defining the independent variable.

Masking See Blinding (or Masking).

Massage Research Agenda Workgroup (MRAW) An interdisciplinary group of health science professionals convened for a three-day conference in March 1999 by the Massage Therapy Foundation. Its outcomes document identifies five specific recommendations regarding the advancement of research in the massage therapy profession: (a) build a massage research infrastructure; (b) fund research on the safety and efficacy of massage therapy; (c) fund studies of physiological (or other) mechanisms by which massage therapy achieves its effects; (d) fund studies stemming from a wellness paradigm; and (e) fund studies of the profession of therapeutic massage.

Massage Therapy A generic term that denotes both (a) the promotion of health and well-being by way of soft tissue manipulation and movement of the body and (b) a health care profession engaged in by massage practitioners. Specialties within the massage therapy profession are defined by virtue of those client populations served, health conditions treated, and intervention techniques used.

Massage Therapy Research Database (MTRD) This database maintained by the Massage Therapy Foundation represents the only consolidated, comprehensive listing of bibliographic citations to the scientific research literature on therapeutic massage and bodywork. It currently contains more than 4000 entries and serves as a reference source to help professionals and the public at large locate articles and other relevant documents.

Measurement A research procedure whereby numerical and/or verbal data are collected so as to portray, in as valid and reliable a manner as possible, a factor or variable of interest to an investigator. For instance, testing is a measurement procedure.

MEDLINE This electronic successor to the print-based *Index Medicus* includes entries from 1966 to the present and is perhaps the most recognized and widely used of the biohealth databases.

Meta-Analytic Systematic Review Research Method One of six research methods included under the synthesis-oriented research strategy. It is operationally defined as a research method characterized by several principal research procedures/features: (a) it is an "analysis of analyses" in that it is the quantitative analysis of a large collection of results from earlier primary studies for the purpose of integrating the findings; (b) it views as "subjects" the results from various primary studies that have been systematically selected for scrutiny by way of explicitly declared inclusion/exclusion criteria; (c) already existing analyses across the assembled primary studies are analyzed; (d) characteristics of the assembled primary studies are classified and coded, and these represent the independent variables; (e) outcome measures from the assembled primary studies are converted to a common scale or metric mainly via effect size calculations, and the converted common metric is the dependent variable; (f) advantages include but are not limited to the following: explicitly documented study protocol; inclusiveness of primary studies assembled; systematic investigation of patterns across primary studies via the classifying, coding, and aggregating procedures used; greater statistical power than primary studies; and thorough and objective description of current status in a research domain; and (g) disadvantages include

but are not limited to the following: rarity of exemplary primary studies being described in detail; biases inherent in one or more primary studies potentially undetected and, hence, present in meta-analysis; mechanistic procedures evident at times due to heightened concern over researcher bias; and potential loss of focus on better comprehending the research domain under study.

Methodological Triangulation See Mixed-Methods Approach.

Mixed-Methods Approach A research approach that uses two or more research methods from both the quantitative and qualitative research categories. It is also sometimes referred to as the blended methods approach, combined methods approach, or methodological triangulation.

Multiple Coefficient of Determination (R^2) Represents the proportion of variability on the criterion variable that can be explained by the combined set of two or more predictor variables.

Multiple Correlation Coefficient (R) Represents the correlation between a combined set of two or more predictor variables and the one predicted criterion variable.

Multiple-Predictor Design One of two possible research designs included under the predictive research method. This design is an extension of the single-predictor design in that here two or more predictor variables are used to predict one criterion variable. The inferential statistical technique used to carry out this design is called multiple linear regression (*multiple* because two or more predictor variables are used).

Multiple Treatment Design One of several possible research designs included under the single-case experimental research method. Representing somewhat of an extension of the basic A-B design, this design contrasts a baseline phase with two or more treatment phases involving two or more different types of interventions designated, for instance, as "B," "C," and so on.

Multivariate Statistics Those statistical techniques that allow one to analyze the relationship among *three or more* variables of interest; hence, *multi-variate* means *three or more variables*. For example, multiple linear regression permits a researcher to use two predictor variables to predict quantitatively a criterion variable, thereby informing the relationship among the three variables of interest.

Naturalistic/Structured Observational Research Method One of four research methods included under the descriptive-oriented research strategy. It is operationally defined as a research method characterized by several principal research procedures/features: (a) the focus is on an individual subject or a group of subjects whose behavior in a typical setting or circumstance is of interest; (b) it investigates one or more dependent variables in the form of the behavior of individuals as enacted in their typical environment or setting; (c) the researcher ensures a detached and neutral observation of the subject(s) so as to safeguard a highly objective description of the target behaviors (dependent variables); (d) it typically is used for exploratory purposes with the intent of generating a database for decision making and/or hypotheses for future study; (e) it may also be used for confirmatory purposes when actual hypothesis testing is done; and (f) potential difficulties regarding observer bias, subject reactivity, and ethical dilemmas must be anticipated and accommodated via established means.

No Treatment (or "Do Nothing") Control Group Used as a basis of comparison to one or more treatment (or experimental) groups, this type of control group refers to a comparable group of participants for whom no treatment or involvement is planned.

Nominal Scale One of four measurement scales, the nominal scale uses numbers simply to name or identify variations on a variable. For example, using the numbers "1" and "2" to distinguish between males and females in a study represents the nominal scale of measurement.

Nonequivalent, Control-Group, Interrupted Time Series Design One of several possible research designs included under the quasi-experimental research method. It is almost identical to the nonequivalent, control-group, pretest-posttest design, except for the presence here of multiple pretest and multiple posttest measures over time.

Nonequivalent, Control-Group, Pretest-Posttest Design One of several possible research designs included under the quasi-experimental research method. It entails the presence of intact groups in lieu of the random assignment of subjects, pretesting before the independent variable is introduced, a control group in comparison to the experimental/treatment group, and posttesting after the independent variable has been introduced.

Nonexperimental Comparative Groups Research Method One of four research methods included under the difference-oriented research strategy. It is operationally defined as a research method characterized by the following two research procedures/features: (a) the use of a nonmanipulated independent variable and (b) the designation of comparative groups based on a trait, characteristic, or previous treatment/ condition exposure of the participants that already exists rather than a new treatment to which the participants are now being subjected. Regarding this latter feature, the group membership of the participants is a matter of already being "in place" or "intact" as members, or perhaps being randomly selected from two or more strata in the accessible population.

Nonparametric Statistics One of two subdivisions of inferential statistics, nonparametric techniques do not make any assumptions of normality or equal variance regarding the distribution of a study's variables in the population from which the sample was derived. Also, nonparametric techniques are appropriate when data are collected on a nominal or ordinal measurement scale.

Normal Distribution Curve A graphical display of a distribution of events that appears as a symmetrical bell-shaped curve wherein the values for the mean, median, and mode are identical. It is sometimes referred to as the "Gaussian distribution."

Null Hypothesis (H_0) Also known as the statistical hypothesis, the null hypothesis is that prediction of a study's outcome that (a) asserts the absence of a statistically significant relationship between/among the study's variables, (b) speaks to one or more characteristics or properties of the study's population, (c) is the focal point in a study's statistical analysis, and (d) provides the basis for inferring a decision back to the study's research hypothesis and alternative hypothesis.

Null Hypothesis Significance Testing (NHST) The statistical testing of a study's null hypothesis by way of inferential techniques, done in the context of an alpha level being cited and a power analysis being performed, has been the traditional reliance in the quantitative research realm. Recent calls have been made, though, for NHST to be augmented by *effect size calculations* as well as *confidence interval estimations*.

Nuremberg Code (1947) The Nuremberg Code, one outcome of the Nuremberg Military Tribunal of 1946 that tried 23 Nazi physicians for crimes against prisoners of war, is that codification identifying 10 conditions that must be met to justify research with human subjects. Of the 10 conditions cited, the two most critical are (a) the need for voluntary informed consent of the subjects and (b) a scientifically justifiable research design capable of potentially beneficial outcomes for the good of society.

Open Study A study wherein there is a complete absence of any form of blinding or masking.

Ordinal Scale One of four measurement scales, the ordinal scale serves not only to name or identify, but also to rank order. As an illustration, severity of tension headache may be recorded by a client as moderate (a 1), severe (a 2), or debilitating/critical (a 3). This scale does not necessarily imply that the quantity or quality of the variable measured between a 1 and a 2 is equivalent to that measured between a 2 and a 3.

P Value (p) Also known as the level of significance, the p value signifies the probability or likelihood of obtaining by chance the results of our statistical analysis if indeed the null hypothesis is actually valid.

Parameter A characteristic, property, feature, or attribute of a population.

Parametric Statistics One of two subdivisions of inferential statistics, parametric techniques make certain assumptions about the distribution of a study's variables in the population from which the sample came. These assumptions pertain to the normal distribution of a study's dependent variable in the population as well as equal variances, for instance, in the two or more segments of the population from which the two or more comparison groups in the study were derived. Parametric techniques also necessitate either an interval or ratio scale on which the dependent variable has been measured.

Partial Correlation ($r_{12.3}$) Signified by the expression $r_{12.3}$, partial correlation indexes the correlation between dependent variables 1 and 2, with the influence of dependent variable 3 held constant (or partialed out).

Partial Correlational Design One of three possible research designs included under the correlational research method. In this design, the researcher investigates the correlation between the two dependent variables of principal interest, that is, DV_1 and DV_2, but with an adjustment made so that the influence of a third dependent variable, DV_3, is cancelled or "partialed" out. This allows a more accurate reading on the correlation between the first two dependent variables in that the unwanted influence of the third dependent variable is mathematically eliminated.

Pearson r Signifies the correlation coefficient for two dependent variables and indexes both the strength and direction of the linear relationship between the two.

PEDro An electronic database that provides a broad range of reviews and rated trials in rehabilitation and physiotherapy.

Phenomenological Research Method One of four research methods included under the contextual/interpretive-oriented research strategy. It is operationally defined as a research method characterized by several principal research procedures/features: (a) the focal point is primarily on the lived experience of each participant in the study; (b) recognition of the ongoing interdependency or interaction between the person and the environment is paramount; (c) the study participant is the only reliable source of insight regarding the meaning of that person's lived experience; and (d) the researcher's strategic role is that of transforming verbal data derived from multiple sources.

Placebo-Attention Control Group Used as a basis of comparison to one or more treatment (or experimental) groups, this type of control group refers to a comparable group of participants who are not receiving the investigative treatment, but are instead exposed to a stimulus experience that is inert regarding any direct anticipated impact on the outcome being studied. Although inert, the stimulus experience is typically in the form of interpersonal contact and support that provides those participants with a sense of being attended to and involved.

Placebo-Sham Treatment Control Group Used as a basis of comparison to one or more treatment (or experimental) groups, this type of control group refers to a comparable group of participants who are not receiving the investigative treatment, but are instead exposed to a simulated treatment that feigns the intervention of a viable treatment. The *presumed* dynamic treatment provided to the control group is actually a pretended or impostor-type intervention with no actual dynamic or viable potential to influence the study's outcome measure(s).

Population In a research context, population refers to that group, set, universe, or macrocosm of study participants that is the focus of an investigation. When such a set of study participants is accessible to the extent that each member can potentially be selected for inclusion in the study, it is then known as an accessible population.

Positivism Known as the naïve realist position, this philosophical perspective maintains that there is a reality out there that can be studied objectively and understood (Denzin & Lincoln, as cited by Miller et al., 2003). Positivism is the historical predecessor to postpositivism, a less extreme view of reality, truth, and values that is the philosophical basis underlying quantitative research.

Postmodernism Known as the radical doubt position, postmodernism counters the naïve realist position of positivism by asserting that "there can never be a final, accurate representation of what is meant or said, only different textual representations of different experiences" (Denzin, 1996, p. 132, as cited by Miller et al., 2003). Postmodernism is the historical successor to constructivism, a less extreme view of reality, truth, and values that is the philosophical basis underlying qualitative research.

Postpositivism "Postpositivism rests on the assumption that reality can never be fully apprehended, only approximated. Postpositivists use multiple methods to capture as much of reality as possible; emphasize the discovery and verification of theories; and apply traditional evaluative criteria, such as validity" (Denzin & Lincoln, as cited by Miller et al., 2003, p. 220). Postpositivism is the philosophical basis or perspective underlying quantitative research and represents a less extreme view of reality, truth, and values than its historical predecessor, positivism.

Posttesting Posttesting is a research procedure whereby the study participants are measured on the study's dependent variable(s) for either of two possible purposes: (a) to rely exclusively on the contrast between/among the two or more levels of the independent variable relative to the posttest measure only or (b) to examine the contrast between pretest and posttest performances, relative to the dependent variable, within each level of the independent variable.

Predictive Research Method One of two research methods included under the association-oriented research strategy. It is operationally defined as a research method characterized by the following six research procedures/features: (a) the existence of a sample of participants that may or may not have been formed by random selection, (b) the availability of a correlational data set reflecting two or more original dependent variables, (c) the measurement of each participant in the sample on one or more of the original dependent variables, (d) the designation of one of the original dependent variables as a criterion variable, (e) the designation of one or more of the original dependent variables as one or more predictor variables, and (f) the application of correlation-based statistical techniques that reflect the earlier original data set of two or more dependent variables and that allow predictions.

Predictive Validity One of two possible forms of criterion-related validity. Predictive validity is the degree to which an instrument actually predicts a certain outcome for which it is designed. In the health sciences, for instance, an instrument that generates initial evaluation scores and thus enables a researcher or practitioner to predict accurately the period of time until recovery from an injury would be characterized as having predictive validity.

Predictor Variable (PV) As the name implies, a predictor variable is that variable in the predictive research method that predicts quantitatively another variable of interest (called the criterion variable) by means of a statistical technique known as linear regression.

Pretesting A research procedure whereby the study participants, prior to the introduction of the independent variable, are measured on one or more variables for either of two possible purposes: (a) to establish a baseline record of the participants' reactions regarding the dependent variable under consideration before any type of intervention is introduced or (b) to collect data that become the basis for subsequently identifying the two or more levels of the independent variable.

Proficiency "*Proficiency* refers to the efficiency with which the individual makes use of the acquired learning products. While *mastery* refers to the *effectiveness* of the learning process in producing the desired learning product, *proficiency* refers to the *efficiency* of the learning product once it has been acquired" (emphases added) (Block & Anderson, 1977, p. 165).

Prospective Cohort Design One of three possible designs considered to be *ex post facto* (or after the fact) designs. In this design the two or more comparative groups are formed in the *present* based on an *already existing exposure* to treatment/condition variations and then followed forward into the *future* with a view toward one or more outcomes being measured.

PsycINFO The computerized version of *Psychological Abstracts* maintained by the American Psychological Association (APA). It is an excellent resource for the mind-body aspect of CAM in that it obviously speaks directly to CAM interventions regarding mental disorders, stress management, and behavioral processes as well as neuroimmunology.

PubMed An information system inaugurated by the National Library of Medicine (NLM) in 1997 for the purpose of providing free Web access to MEDLINE. Although obviously inclusive of MEDLINE, PubMed contains additional entries that augment the MEDLINE records. Such additional records include in-process citations not yet assigned a medical subject heading (MeSH) as well as supplied-by-publisher records that likewise will eventually be given a MeSH.

Qualitative Meta-Summary Research Method One of six research methods included under the synthesis-oriented research strategy. As the name implies, it represents a systematic review method from the perspective of the qualitative research tradition, and is operationally defined as a research method characterized by several principal research procedures/features: (a) it accommodates the need for qualitative researchers to translate the integrative function of the research process into an approach consistent with the constructivist perspective and its corresponding research methods; (b) it focuses on qualitative reports whose findings are summarized rather than synthesized and, hence, these reports do not lend themselves to a meta-synthesis; (c) it is a form of systematic review or integration of qualitative research findings in a target domain that are themselves topical or thematic summaries or surveys of data; and (d) the summarized findings of these qualitative studies are reminiscent of survey features, typically assume the form of lists and frequency counts of topics and themes, and rely more on naming concepts than interpreting them. (cf. Finfgeld, 2003; and Sandelowski & Barroso, 2003.)

Qualitative Meta-Synthesis Research Method One of six research methods included under the synthesis-oriented research strategy. As the name implies, it represents a systematic review method from the perspective of the qualitative research tradition, and is operationally defined as a research method characterized by several principal research procedures/features: (a) it accommodates the need for qualitative researchers to translate the integrative function of the research process into an approach consistent with the constructivist perspective and its corresponding research methods; (b) it incorporates a broad, global, encompassing, umbrella term designating the synthesis of research findings (not simply data) across several qualitative studies so as to render a new interpretation; (c) focus is on integrating qualitative research findings in a target domain that are themselves interpretive syntheses of data, including phenomenologies, ethnographies, grounded theories, and other integrated and coherent descriptions of phenomena or events; (d) the synthesizing function is interpretive given the qualitative research focus as opposed to the more aggregative function found, e.g., in a quantitative meta-analysis; and (e) its major goal is to generate a new and integrative interpretation of findings that is more substantive than those resulting from individual investigations.

Qualitative Research Category One of three possible research categories characterized as follows: (a) philosophically driven by a view of reality and truth that emphasizes the subjective, contextual, and highly individualistic perceptions of all that is observed and experienced; (b) rooted primarily in verbal data that by its nature lends itself to alternative interpretations on the part of both the observed and the observer; and (c) representative of research that has historically been emphasized in disciplines such as anthropology and sociology, but with a somewhat recent emergence in psychology and various health science professions.

Qualitative Systematic Review Research Methods Two of the six research methods included under the synthesis-oriented research strategy. They represent systematic review methods from the perspective of the *qualitative* research tradition and are identified as follows: (a) the qualitative meta-synthesis research method and (b) the qualitative meta-summary research method. These two research methods address the qualitative systematic review function from two polar perspectives, namely, a global/general vantage point (i.e., the meta-synthesis) and a particular/specific view (i.e., the meta-summary). (Please see individual entries for each of these two methods elsewhere.)

Quantitative Research Category One of three possible research categories characterized as follows: (a) philosophically driven by a view of reality and truth that emphasizes the objective and unbiased approach to scientific investigation; (b) rooted primarily in numerical data that are statistically analyzed once the measurements have been demonstrated to be valid and reliable; and (c) representative of the vast majority of research that has historically dominated the basic, behavioral, and health sciences.

Quasi-Experimental Research Method This is one of four research methods included under the difference-oriented research strategy. It is operationally defined as a research method characterized by the following two research procedures/features: (a) the use of "intact" groups of participants (that is, two or more participant groups already formed or in place) for comparison purposes, rather than randomly assigning the study's participants to the comparison groups, and (b) the use of a manipulated independent variable as the study's treatment or intervention.

Random Assignment An aspect of the randomization process whereby each member of a sample has an equal and nonzero chance of being included in any one of two or more comparison groups of a study (also known as levels of the study's independent variable).

Random Selection An aspect of the randomization process whereby each and every member of an accessible population has an equal and nonzero chance of being included in a sample.

Randomized Clinical Trial Research Method See Randomized Controlled Trial (or True Experimental) Research Method for subtle distinction and clarification.

Randomized, Control-Group, Posttest-Only Design One of several possible research designs included under the true experimental (or randomized controlled trial) research method. It entails the random assignment of subjects, a control group in comparison to the experimental/treatment group, and a posttest.

Randomized, Control-Group, Pretest-Posttest Design One of several possible research designs included under the true experimental (or randomized controlled trial) research method.

It entails the random assignment of subjects, pretesting before the independent variable is introduced, a control group in comparison to the experimental/treatment group, and posttesting after the independent variable has been introduced.

Randomized Controlled Trial (or True Experimental) Research Method One of four research methods included under the difference-oriented research strategy. It is operationally defined as a research method necessitating two major research procedures/features: (a) the random assignment of participants to the two or more comparison groups (i.e., the levels of the independent variable) and (b) the use of a manipulated independent variable as the study's treatment or intervention. (Please note that the term *controlled* in the expression *randomized controlled trial* designates that the group being compared to the experimental group is a *no treatment or "do nothing" control group* or, possibly, a *waiting-list control group*. As suggested by Hagino (2003), the expression randomized *clinical* trial is preferred when the comparison to the experimental group involves a *comparison treatment control group* as is the case with a *standard treatment control group, placebo-attention control group,* or *placebo-sham treatment control group*.)

Ratio Scale One of four measurement scales, the ratio scale uses numbers to name, rank order, assume equal intervals, and acknowledge a true or absolute zero point. Examples here would include the Kelvin temperature scale, weight, height, blood pressure, and heartbeats.

Reliability (of Measurement) The reliability of a measuring instrument refers to the consistency of measurement that the instrument is demonstrating.

Reliability of Internal Consistency (or Homogeneity) In the instance of internal consistency reliability, one examines the stability or consistency of measurement *within* the instrument itself. This is accomplished by "splitting" the instrument in half for data analysis purposes and then proceeding to examine the consistency (via correlational measures) between the two resulting sets of scores. This procedure generates what is sometimes known as a "split-half" reliability.

Research At its most basic level, research is a process that explores one or more areas of interest (called factors or variables) by analyzing numerical and/or verbal data so as to advance our understanding. More specifically, research is an activity that allows one to accomplish one or more of the following tasks: (a) to characterize a variable of interest by an appeal to numerical and/or verbal data, (b) to investigate a possible relationship between two or more variables, and (c) to integrate or synthesize data from already published sources concerning one or more variables of interest.

Research Category The most global or general level at which the research process is considered. Three research categories exist: (a) the *quantitative* research category, (b) the *qualitative* research category, and (c) the *integrative* research category.

Research Competency The mastery of desired research-specific learning outcomes at acceptable levels of performance and the self-confidence usually associated with such mastery. Compare with Competency.

Research Design Regarding most, though not all, research methods, this is the first level of specificity or detail beyond the research method to which it belongs and attempts to operationalize. For example, the randomized, control-group, pretest-posttest research design (a) belongs to or is included under the true experimental or randomized controlled trial research method and (b) attempts to operationalize in a specific way that particular research method. Any given research design is driven by the investigator's inclusion/exclusion of certain study components such as random assignment, pretesting, posttesting, and the number and nature of comparison groups, to name but a few.

Research Hypothesis (H_R) A well-justified prediction of a study's anticipated outcome in the context of the study's sample that is typically stated at the outset of a study when the research question is being formulated against the backdrop of what the relevant professional literature has to say about the research problem area.

Research Literacy and Capacity "Research literacy is the ability to find, understand, and critically evaluate research evidence for application in professional practice. Research capacity is the ability to conduct research" (Dryden & Achilles, 2003, p. 1).

Research Method The first level of specificity or detail beyond the research strategy to which it belongs and attempts to operationalize. For example, the true experimental or randomized controlled trial research method (a) belongs to or is included under the difference-oriented research strategy and (b) attempts to operationalize in a specific way the difference-oriented research strategy. Any given research method is driven by the degree of control the investigator can exercise over the study's variables.

Research Procedure The first level of specificity or detail beyond the research design to which it belongs and attempts to operationalize. For example, the research procedure of manipulating an independent variable (a) belongs to or is included under the randomized, control-group, pretest-posttest research design and (b) attempts to operationalize in a specific way that particular research design. Any given research procedure is driven by the one or more activities that actually define and operationalize the procedure. For instance, the protocol used in a massage therapy intervention entails certain activities that define and operationalize the experimental level of an independent variable that is being manipulated in a study.

Research Strategy The first level of specificity or detail beyond the general research category to which it belongs and attempts to operationalize. For example, the difference-oriented research strategy (a) belongs to or is included under the quantitative research category and (b) attempts to operationalize in a specific

way the quantitative research category. Any given research strategy is driven by the research question that the strategy is investigating.

Respect for Persons One of three basic ethical principles addressed in the Belmont Report (1979), *respect for persons* requires, at the very least, a twofold obligation: (a) to accommodate the autonomy of individuals by acknowledging their opinions and choices and refraining from impeding their behavior unless their actions are harmful to others and (b) to safeguard those individuals who suffer diminished autonomy due to their being immature or incapacitated to an extent that seriously compromises their capacity for self-determination.

Retrospective Case-Control Design One of three possible designs considered to be *ex post facto* (or "after the fact"). In this design, the two comparative groups are formed in the *present* based on the *presence of an outcome* (i.e., the case) and the *absence of the same outcome* (i.e., the control), and then they are traced backward in time with a view toward *past exposure* to a treatment/condition.

Retrospective Cohort Design One of three possible designs considered to be *ex post facto* (or "after the fact") designs. In this design, the two or more comparative groups were formed in the *more distant past* based on a previous exposure to treatment/condition variations, and then they are followed forward to the *more recent past* with a view toward one or more outcomes having been measured.

Risks/Benefits Assessment One of three applications of the basic ethical principles addressed in the Belmont Report (1979), the *assessment of risks and benefits* is the moral requirement derived primarily from the ethical principle of *beneficence*. This assessment should be viewed not only as a responsibility but also as an opportunity for the researcher, a review committee, and a prospective research subject. For all three parties involved, it allows for the systematic gathering of comprehensive information about the research being proposed, with each party to the process having a unique set of concerns regarding the study's potential risks and benefits.

Sample In a research context, sample refers to that subgroup, subset, or microcosm of study participants identified/selected according to specific criteria for inclusion in an investigation.

Scatterplot A graphical technique frequently used with the correlational research method to display pictorially the nature of the relationship between two dependent variables that are plotted along the x- and y-axes.

Science Citation Index (SCI) A database that allows the bibliographic information for, say, a significant article of interest to be traced forward in time so as to identify those later or subsequent sources that cited the article in their reference lists. Someone using SCI, therefore, can identify and retrieve those later or subsequent sources that are presumably germane to the area of interest because they cited the original significant article.

Selection of Subjects   One of three applications of the basic ethical principles addressed in the Belmont Report (1979), the *selection of subjects* relates to the moral requirement derived primarily from the ethical principle of *justice*. Justice here is considered at two levels: (a) *individual justice* mandates the selection of subjects in an equitable manner such that preferential or biased factors do not come into play; and (b) *social justice* speaks to the issue of classes or groups of subjects, and the distinction that must be made regarding which classes ought or ought not participate in certain kinds of research based on ability to bear the burdens of research.

Self-Report Measure   The self-report modality of measurement relies on the individual responding to questions that may be asked regarding the construct under investigation. The precipitating questions may take the form of being open-ended questions, restricted questions, or rating scale questions.

Simple Correlational Design   One of three possible research designs included under the correlational research method. It allows a researcher to investigate the relationship between two dependent variables by exploring whether or not there is an association between the two variables (i.e., whether or not they co-relate, or are correlated, with each other).

Simple Interrupted Time Series Design   One of several possible research designs included under the quasi-experimental research method. It is almost identical to the nonequivalent, control-group, interrupted time series design, except for the absence here of a control group for comparison purposes.

Single-Blind Procedure   A research procedure whereby a study participant is unaware of his or her group membership (or affiliated level of the independent variable).

Single-Case Experimental Research Method   One of four research methods included under the difference-oriented research strategy. As its name implies, it is operationally defined as a research method characterized by the following four research procedures/features: (a) it focuses on one specific participant, rather than a group of participants; (b) the one specific participant is exposed to a given treatment or intervention representing a manipulated independent variable; (c) the treatment phase, during which the single participant is exposed to the manipulated independent variable, is typically alternated with the absence/withdrawal of the manipulated independent variable, thereby defining the baseline phase; and (d) the original treatment phase may also be alternated with a variation of the original treatment and/or an entirely different treatment, thereby defining alternative treatment phases. Compare with Single-Case Quantitative Analysis Research Method, Case Report Research Method, and Case Study Research Method.

Single-Case Quantitative Analysis Research Method   One of four research methods included under the descriptive-oriented research strategy. It is operationally defined as a research method characterized by the following five research procedures/features: (a) the focus is on a single participant rather than a group of participants; (b) there is no possible manipulation of an independent variable in that one is not present; (c) instead, there is passive observation/measurement of one or more dependent variables as reflected in the quantitative data collected; (d) it is considered a *confirmatory* single-case quantitative analysis if done for hypothesis testing purposes; and (e) it is considered an *exploratory* single-case quantitative analysis if done for hypothesis generating purposes. Compare with Single-Case Experimental Research Method, Case Report Research Method, and Case Study Research Method.

Single-Predictor Design   One of two possible research designs included under the predictive research method. This design builds on an earlier simple correlational study in which the Pearson *r* was calculated to index the correlation between two original dependent variables. Once these correlational data are in place, the single-predictor design allows the prediction of one of the original dependent variables (now known in this context as the criterion variable) based on a knowledge of the other original dependent variable (now known as the predictor variable). This design makes use of an inferential statistical technique called simple linear regression ("simple" because only one predictor variable is used).

Standard Treatment Control Group   Used as a basis of comparison to one or more treatment (or experimental) groups, this type of control group refers to a comparable group of participants receiving whatever health care treatment or intervention is recognized as standard or typical for their condition.

Statistic   A statistic is a characteristic, property, feature, or attribute of a sample.

Statistical Inference   The appropriate use of measurement and statistical testing are critical procedures that allow a researcher to make two important inferences: (a) The statistical analysis of data collected on a given dependent variable enables the researcher to test the null hypothesis. The decision made regarding the null hypothesis, namely, to reject or fail to reject the null, then permits an inferential decision back to both the alternative and research hypotheses. (b) If indeed a study has employed random selection of participants from an accessible population for the purpose of forming the sample, then the statistical analysis of the study's hypotheses allows an inference of what is learned about the sample back to the accessible population.

Statistical Power   Also known as power analysis, the statistical power that exists when the data on a given dependent variable are statistically analyzed refers to the probability or mathematical odds that the analysis will result in a rejection of the null hypothesis when in reality the null is indeed false and, hence, should be rejected.

Statistics A research tool involving one or more mathematical techniques used to analyze and better understand a data set generated by earlier measurement procedures; an area of applied mathematics that has as its two major subdivisions both descriptive and inferential quantitative analysis techniques.

Survey Research Method One of four research methods included under the descriptive-oriented research strategy. It is operationally defined as a research method characterized by several principal research procedures/features: (a) it relies on a direct appeal to a representative/unbiased sample of participants, drawn from a clearly defined population, from whom input is derived on one or more dependent variables; (b) the sampling, data gathering, and instrumentation techniques used emphasize appropriate validity and reliability; (c) it typically is used for exploratory purposes with the intent of generating a database for decision making and/or hypotheses for future study; and (d) it may also be used for confirmatory purposes when actual hypothesis testing is done.

Synthesis-Oriented Research Strategy The singular research strategy that operationalizes the integrative research category. As its name implies, this generic research strategy is oriented to investigations that emphasize three principal themes: (a) combining the accumulation of research studies available in a given area so as to allow the efforts of earlier researchers to have more of a collective impact than would be the case if only individual studies were considered; (b) this combining or accumulating of previous research in a given area into a more manageable and meaningful whole involves, quite literally, an act of integrating or synthesizing the earlier studies whether they occurred in the quantitative or qualitative tradition; and (c) this effort of combining, accumulating, integrating, or synthesizing earlier studies occurs with respect to several varied study features as the following: research problems investigated, populations studied, size of sample derived, methodologies used, degrees of control exerted, data collection instruments employed, data analyses completed, interpretations rendered, conclusions drawn, and needed areas of research recommended.

Test-Retest Reliability The degree to which a given instrument measures a certain variable consistently for the same group of individuals across two different points in time.

Time-Lagged, or Cross-Lagged, Correlational Design One of three possible research designs included under the correlational research method. In this design, the study's participants are measured on two dependent variables at each of two different points across time. Once this is done, the researcher can then calculate the Pearson *r* for the two dependent variables at both time point 1 and time point 2. More important, one can then examine

further the correlation coefficients for several pairs of dependent variables in different combinations at various points in time.

Traditional Narrative Review Research Method One of six research methods included under the synthesis-oriented research strategy. It is operationally defined as a research method characterized by several principal research procedures/features: (a) its intent is to characterize the current state of knowledge in a given research area by giving a broad-based perspective on the topic; (b) it provides a *selective*—though not necessarily exhaustive—coverage of previous independent studies on a given research problem; (c) it is most appropriate for portraying the history or development of a problem area, describing encouraging developments if available research is sparse or limited by faulty methodologies, and conceptually integrating two or more previously unrelated areas of research; (d) its focus may be on either original data-based studies wherein numerical and/or verbal data were analyzed or possibly studies primarily conceptual or theoretical in nature that inform a chosen research problem area; (e) it relies on a narrative summary of the procedures and results of various studies addressing a focused problem area; (f) it attempts to formulate conclusions across various studies so as to inform the theory surrounding the problem area; (g) it potentially provides insight on those mechanisms underlying the results of the individual studies reviewed; (h) it potentially forms theory-based categories of studies and compares their findings, thus resulting in conclusions not possible via any one earlier study; (i) it potentially summarizes the current state of research in a problem area and suggests needed avenues of future research; and (j) it is limited by the following: seldom exhaustive in coverage of studies in a research area, possible research bias in selection of studies to review, frequent absence of specific inclusion/exclusion criteria for study selection, typical absence of systematic weighting of different study features, inconsistency in identifying which studies constitute the bulk of research evidence, and questionable value in providing detailed quantitative insight on specific clinical issues.

Treatment (or Experimental) Group See Experimental (or Treatment) Group.

True Experimental (or Randomized Controlled Trial) Research Method See Randomized Controlled Trial (or True Experimental) Research Method.

Uniform Requirements for Manuscripts Submitted to Biomedical Journals Represents the stylistic format and requirements for scientific communication in many health science areas. It is produced and maintained by the International Committee of Medical Journal Editors (ICMJE) and was most recently updated in November 2003.

Univariate Statistics Refers to those statistical techniques that focus on quantifying *one* particular variable of interest; hence, *uni-variate* means *one variable.* For example, the mean or arithmetic average of a set of scores is a univariate statistic.

Validity (of Measurement) Refers to the degree or extent to which the instrument is actually measuring what it claims or purports to be measuring.

Variable That aspect or factor of interest in a research study that has the potential to vary, change, or be altered.

Waiting-List Control Group Used as a basis of comparison to one or more treatment (or experimental) groups, this type of control group refers to a comparable group of participants who are not initially receiving the investigative treatment or intervention during the actual conduct of the study, but are instead literally on a "waiting list" scheduled to receive the treatment once the study is completed.

Within-Subjects (or Repeated Measures) Independent Variable (or Design) A within-subjects (also known as repeated measures) independent variable (or design) refers to a manner in which participants become affiliated with the two or more levels of the independent variable in a study such that a specific group of participants actually experiences each and every level of the independent variable.

REFERENCES

Anderson, L. W., & Block, J. H. (1977). Mastery learning. In D. J. Treffinger, J. K. Dent, & R. E. Ripple (Eds.), *Handbook on teaching educational psychology* (pp. 163–185). New York: Academic Press.

Denzin, N. K., & Lincoln, Y. S. (Eds.). (1994). *Handbook of qualitative research.* Thousand Oaks, CA: SAGE Publications, as cited by Miller et al., 2003.

Dryden, T., & Achilles, R. (2003). *Massage therapy research curriculum kit.* Evanston, IL: AMTA Foundation.

Finfgeld, D. L., (2003). Metasynthesis: The state of the art—so far. *Qualitative Health Research, 13*(7), 893–904.

Sandelowski, M., & Barroso, J. (2003). Creating meta-summaries of qualitative findings. *Nursing Research, 52*(4), 226–233.

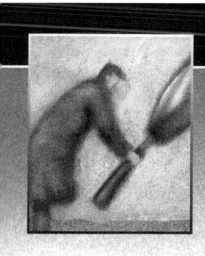

INDEX*

*A "b" following a page number indicates a box; a "t" indicates a table.

Printed and bound by CPI Group (UK) Ltd, Croydon, CR0 4YY

03/10/2024

01040364-0009